NEW TREATMENTS FOR OPIATE DEPENDENCE

THE GUILFORD SUBSTANCE ABUSE SERIES
Howard T. Blane and Thomas R. Kosten, *Editors*

NEW TREATMENTS FOR OPIATE DEPENDENCE

EDITED BY

Susan M. Stine, M.D., Ph.D.
Thomas R. Kosten, M.D.

THE GUILFORD PRESS
New York London

©1997 The Guilford Press
A Division of Guilford Publications, Inc.
72 Spring Street, New York, NY 10012

Printed in the United States of America

This book is printed on acid-free paper.

Last digit is print number: 9 8 7 6 5 4 3 2 1

Library of Congress Cataloging-in-Publication Data

New treatments for opiate dependence / edited by Susan M. Stine and
   Thomas R. Kosten.
      p.   cm.
   Includes bibliographical references and index.
   ISBN 1-57230-190-2
   1. Opioid habit—Chemotherapy.   2. Opioid habit—Treatment.
I. Stine, Susan M.   II. Kosten, Thomas R.
   [DNLM: 1. Narcotic Dependence—therapy. 2. Opium—adverse
effects.   WM 286 N532 1997]
RC568.O45N49   1997
616.86'3206—dc21
DNLM/DLC
for Library of Congress   97-3244
                                                              CIP

CONTRIBUTORS

S. Kelly Avants, Ph.D., Department of Psychiatry, Yale University School of Medicine, New Haven, CT

Beatrice R. Burns, M.S.N., A.P.R.N., Department of Psychiatry, VA Connecticut Healthcare System, Yale University School of Medicine, West Haven, CT

Grace Chang, M.D., M.P.H., Department of Psychiatry, Harvard Medical School; Division of Psychiatry, Brigham and Women's Hospital, Boston, MA

Peggy Compton, R.N., Ph.D., UCLA School of Nursing, Los Angeles, CA

Conor K. Farren, M.B., M.R.C.P.I., M.R.C.Psych., Department of Psychiatry, Yale University School of Medicine, New Haven, CT

Therese A. Kosten, Ph.D., Department of Psychiatry, Yale University School of Medicine, New Haven, CT

Thomas R. Kosten, M.D., Department of Psychiatry, VA Connecticut Healthcare System, Yale University School of Medicine, West Haven, CT

Walter Ling, M.D., Los Angeles Addiction Treatment Research Center, Los Angeles, CA

Arthur Margolin, Ph.D., Department of Psychiatry, Yale University School of Medicine, New Haven, CT

Eric J. Nestler, M.D., Ph.D., Department of Psychiatry, Yale University School of Medicine, New Haven, CT

Patrick G. O'Connor, M.D., M.P.H., Primary Care Center, Yale University School of Medicine, New Haven, CT

Robert Ohlin, Psy.D., Atlantic Health Services, New Haven, CT

Alison Oliveto, Ph.D., Department of Psychiatry, Yale University School of Medicine, New Haven, CT

Stephanie O'Malley, Ph.D., Department of Psychiatry, Yale University School of Medicine, New Haven, CT

Marc Rosen, M.D., Department of Psychiatry, VA Connecticut Healthcare System, Yale University School of Medicine, West Haven, CT

Bruce Rounsaville, M.D., Department of Psychiatry, Yale University School of Medicine, New Haven, CT

Peter A. Selwyn, M.D., M.P.H., Yale AIDS Care Program, Yale University School of Medicine, New Haven, CT

Susan M. Stine, M.D., Ph.D., Opiate Substitution Program, Department of Psychiatry, VA Connecticut Healthcare System, Yale University School of Medicine, West Haven, CT

PREFACE

This book has grown out of our work on a previous volume on cocaine, the *Clinician's Guide to Cocaine Addiction: Theory, Research, and Treatment.* In that volume, we responded to the then peaking cocaine epidemic, and for it we drew on active clinical and laboratory research collaborations at Yale. This volume, on opiate treatment, is both a continuation of the collaborative academic tradition at Yale that produced the cocaine book and also a much-needed response to the current epidemic in opiate use. This recent spread of opiate use, fortunately, has coincided with the availability of new treatments, a synchronicity which energized our efforts to produce an urgently needed update volume.

This book begins by providing a scientific basis, both behavioral and biological, for the subsequent clinical chapters. The clinical chapters consider the unique characteristics of opiate dependence, its stigma, and the ambivalence of health care practitioners and society in general toward treating it. (This is especially clear in those chapters that touch on the history of methadone maintenance programs and dosing issues.) Chronic ambivalence to treating opiate users was followed, because of the role of opiate use in the HIV epidemic, by vigorous attention to treatment, and this has caused a discontinuity in the way opiate treatments have been refined: after a long period of dormancy in the 1980s, following the development of methadone treatment in the 1960s and 1970s, there has been a sudden surge in new psychosocial and pharmacological treatments in the 1990s.

Although this book draws largely on work conducted at Yale, we have included a chapter from a noted outside expert in the pharmacotherapy field, Walter Ling, M.D., concerning one of the new medications available, LAAM. Nevertheless, much of the development of other new treatments, especially buprenorphine, has taken place at Yale, both at the APT foundation and at VA Connecticut—and it is still ongoing.

ACKNOWLEDGMENTS

The West Haven VA Medical Center was recently one site in the large-scale, multisite study funded by the NIDA Medication Development Center and the VA Cooperative Studies Program Center (CSP 93/999A+AE), which has just been completed. VA Connecticut is now involved in a second NIDA study (CSP 93/1008A), with Susan M. Stine, M.D., Ph.D., as the principal investigator for the West Haven site. Dr. Stine also acknowledges support from a NIDA two-site study, Matching Methadone Patients to Psychosocial Treatments (DA 08754).

Thomas R. Kosten, M.D., gratefully acknowledges support from the NIDA Medication Development Center (P50-DA09250) and the CRC (P50-DA04060), as well as a scientist career grant. We would like to thank NIDA directors Alan Leshner, Ph.D., and Robert Schuster, Ph.D., for their vision in supporting these research centers and research career development programs.

SUSAN M. STINE, M.D., PH.D.
THOMAS R. KOSTEN, M.D.

CONTENTS

Chapter 1

INTRODUCTION AND OVERVIEW

Thomas R. Kosten, M.D.
Susan M. Stine, M.D., Ph.D.

During the last 5 years, a substantial new epidemic of heroin abuse has been developing in the United States and spreading to middle-class users who were formerly more likely to abuse only cocaine. In December 1994, *Pulse Check,* a publication by the Office of National Drug Control Policy (ONDCP), reported some key trends in heroin use: more teenagers and young adults and more middle- and upper-middle-class people are using purer heroin, and the proportion of people inhaling or smoking heroin as well as the number of people seeking treatment continue to increase. Heroin use and availability is also higher in the Northeast and Midwest and relatively lower in most of the South and the West. From the 35–40 million cocaine users who were produced in the United States over the last 10–15 years, a residual of about 3–4 million cocaine-dependent individuals are increasingly turning to heroin either alone or in combination with cocaine. New users who "spread the contagion" in this epidemic add to the problem. *The National Drug Control Strategy* reports that the strongest sign of an epidemic is the entry of a large number of new users (new initiates), and this new influx of heroin users defines such an epidemic. New users are particularly problematic because they have had less exposure and fewer health and legal adverse consequences and are therefore more likely to recruit other new users. The scope of this new epidemic is evident in recent articles from major newspapers that have reported overdoses by middle-class Americans. Emergency rooms are also filled with large numbers of heroin overdoses as the purity of the drug has improved.

This transition from a cocaine to a heroin epidemic is a result of several factors. First among these is an increasing recognition of the medical toxicity and psychological problems of sustained cocaine abuse. As was first recognized after the last cocaine epidemic at the turn of the century, the sustained stimulation from drugs such as cocaine cannot be maintained, whereas the sedation from drugs such as heroin leads to a sustainable long-term dependence. Second, there has been a change in the supply side of heroin. New sources of heroin have become available from Mexico and South America with a much greater purity and lower cost than was available 5 years ago. Many of the cartels that were formerly importing cocaine into the United States have been reported to turn increasingly to heroin distribution. Third, heroin usage has become more acceptable because the increase in its purity has made smoking and snorting, not just intravenous use, possible. With low-quality heroin, intravenous use is necessary in order to develop a high or rush; but as the purity increases to about 15–20%, then the other routes of administration by snorting and smoking become not only possible but preferable as ways to reduce the risk of acquiring HIV (a group of retroviruses) infection and AIDS (acquired immunodeficiency syndrome).

This expanding market for heroin has been increasing treatment challenges in the substance abuse field, but such expanded use comes at a time when a variety of new treatments have become available. These new treatments include ways to optimize the delivery of methadone maintenance (the mainstay of opiate pharmacotherapies during the last 20 years) and ways to introduce alternatives to methadone, such as levo-alpha-acetylmethadol (LAAM) and buprenorphine. These alternative treatment interventions have evolved out of a more clearly understood neurobiology of opioid dependence and a greatly improved understanding of the behavioral psychology of addiction and dependence. Chapters 2 and 3 of this book review the behavioral and neurobiological foundations that have led to these clinical advances and are followed by chapters on new developments in methadone maintenance treatment and then by a series of chapters on alternative pharmacotherapies to methadone.

FOUNDATIONS FOR NEW TREATMENTS

The behavioral psychology of addiction and of dependence on opiates has been carefully studied in a variety of animal models. As reviewed by Therese A. Kosten (Chapter 2), these animal models include self-administration, place conditioning, drug discrimination, and acute withdrawal from opiates. This withdrawal can be spontaneous or precipitated by antagonists such as naloxone. Animal models of acute withdrawal have been used to screen new detoxification agents that might relieve the signs and symptoms of opiate detoxification. The self-administration, drug discrimination, and place conditioning models have been particularly useful for understanding what properties of opiates lead to their continued abuse. These models also act as screens for new synthetic opiates, to determine the abuse liability of a new compound, such as buprenorphine.

The chronic pharmacological effects of opiates in producing tolerance and dependence can only be understood in the context of learning principles that govern conditioned stimuli. Conditioning has a profound effect on the relapse back to opiate dependence in humans. Conditioned cues in the environment are frequently associated with relapse to opiate dependence long after acute detoxification has been completed. The application of learning principles to treatment approaches is critical. Relapse prevention strategies need to combine pharmacological agents, such as methadone and naltrexone, with learning and conditioning approaches. Overall, the optimal treatment for opioid-dependent patients will always involve a combination of pharmacological and behavioral treatments that have their foundations in the neurobiology and behavioral psychology of opioid dependence.

Recent work links the behavioral effects of opiates with underlying neurobiological pathways in specific brain regions, and individual vulnerability is being increasingly understood in genetic terms, as specific strains of animals with high and low tendencies for drug self-administration are examined. These fundamental studies are also demonstrating similarities between the neurobiological effects of learning itself and the brain changes induced by different types of abused drugs. These similarities are central to our understanding of the common learning pathways in the brain that may lead to drug abuse vulnerability and to individual differences in this vulnerability. From these genetic behavioral studies, new strategies for prevention and treatment intervention should develop.

As Eric J. Nestler (Chapter 3) shows, animal studies have also led to important advances: an appreciation of the role of specific brain neurotransmitters in opioid withdrawal and in the maintenance of dependence has led to a deeper understanding of current pharmacotherapy as well as the development of new pharmacotherapies. While dopamine brain systems are critical for the reinforcement associated with a wide range of abused drugs, including both cocaine and opioids, acute withdrawal from opioid dependence appears much more determined by activity in noradrenergic areas, such as the locus coeruleus. These acute withdrawal phenomena in the brain are related to chronic changes that occur in brain cells after long-term opiate exposure. The chronic changes with opiate dependence involve the cyclic AMP (adenosine monophosphate) second messenger systems beyond the opiate receptor and even structural changes in brain proteins such as microtubules. Basic molecular machinery, such as the DNA in cell nuclei, are activated during the development of opiate dependence. This DNA activation is needed to manufacture new proteins as well as to change existing brain proteins. All of these neurobiological changes indicate how profoundly the brain is altered by opiates and also suggest how a wide variety of pharmacological interventions might target these alterations.

At least three signal transduction pathways are involved in opiate withdrawal: an intrinsic noradrenergic system, an extrinsic excitatory amino acid system, and the dopaminergic reinforcement system. The intrinsic noradrenergic system uses cyclic AMP as a postreceptor signaling pathway. Profound adaptations occur in this intrinsic signal-transduction pathway during opiate tolerance, dependence, and eventual withdrawal symptoms. This cyclic AMP-dependent signal transduction system is closely related to phosphorylation of several proteins critical for nerve cell firing. An "extrinsic pathway" is important in opiate withdrawal and involves activation of cells that are dependent on excitatory amino acids, such as glutamate. Finally, the mesolimbic dopamine system is altered during opioid dependence. This dopamine system affects the reinforcing properties of opiates and the tolerance to this reinforcement over time. These basic molecular neurobiology studies have suggested specific target neurons for reversing the chronic action of opiates in order to treat abstinence syndromes and to reduce craving for these drugs. These studies are also linked to the behavioral studies in identifying genetic factors that predispose individuals to opiate dependence.

OPTIMIZING CURRENT TREATMENTS

Refining the Use of Pharmacotherapy

Part II of this book focuses on improvements in the traditional treatment modalities of methadone maintenance and on the pharmacological alternative to methadone, detoxification, and naltrexone maintenance. The first strategy for optimizing treatment consists of the considerable improvement in the use of the pharmacotherapeutic agents themselves (Section A). Methadone maintenance has been carefully studied over the last 20 years as an intervention for heroin addicts. As reviewed by Susan M. Stine (Chapter 4), methadone maintenance has demonstrated excellent success in reducing opiate use, in increasing such prosocial activities as employment, in reducing illegal activities, and in promoting psychological well-being. The assessment of a large number of programs has suggested that optimal methadone dosing is in the 65–80 mg/day range, which is somewhat higher than the mean dose generally used within the United States. Thus, patients in methadone may be routinely underdosed. A variety of specific medical issues have become clearly relevant to the individualized management of methadone dosage in patients, including the interaction of methadone with other treatment medications. These medications include antitubercular medications that may induce methadone metabolism, thereby leading to withdrawal symptoms. Other medications, such as cimetidene and several other compounds, can prolong the action of methadone and can be therapeutically useful for the 5–10% of rapid metabolizers of methadone. These patients benefit from having their methadone metabolism slowed down, thereby making daily dosing comfortable and practical. A special case of this rapid metabolism is the treatment of pregnant women who frequently need more than daily dosing in order to maintain adequate drug levels of methadone. Another critical medical area has been the interaction of AZT (azidothymidine) with methadone; methadone appears to increase blood levels of AZT, thereby potentially increasing AZT toxicity in the methadone-maintained AIDS patient. Another issue of interest in methadone dosing has been the potential reduction in abuse of cocaine in some patients as methadone dosages are increased.

The next two chapters focus on traditional pharmacotherapy alternatives to methadone maintenance. The major pharmacotherapy alternative to methadone, namely, naltrexone, has been available for a number of years. Long considered a pharmacologically ideal medication for opioid dependence, naltrexone has been relatively little used by clinicians and poorly accepted by patients. In the transition from opioid dependence to naltrexone maintenance during detoxification significant advances have been made that have the potential to increase the utilization of naltrexone. These advances reduce the time required for this transitional procedure, from over 2 weeks to as little as 3 days.

The history of and new developments in the treatment of opiate detoxification are described by Marc Rosen in Chapter 5. The pharmacological treatment of opiate withdrawal was advanced significantly at the Addiction Research Center during the 1960s by researchers who gave a clear description of the opiate withdrawal syndrome and by the development of opiate antagonists for precipitating withdrawal. From the work of those researchers, there have evolved effective methods of detoxification, including opioid substitution, stabilization, and tapering by using methadone. Methadone enabled once-daily dosing rather than the four- to five-times-per-day dosing that was necessary for stabilization or detoxification with such short-acting opiates as morphine. More recently, buprenorphine (discussed more completely in Part III of this volume) has been utilized in detoxification. This medication is a partial opioid and has a relatively mild withdrawal syndrome that only lasts about 5 days if untreated. However, several approaches to detoxification with nonopioid agents can be used to relieve these withdrawal symptoms. Some of the most successful work has focused on clonidine. In a randomized clinical trial comparing clonidine to methadone tapering among outpatients, success rates were equivalent at 40%, although inpatient studies have demonstrated up to 90% success with clonidine. More rapid detoxification has been accomplished by using the opioid antagonist naloxone or naltrexone in combination with clonidine or benzodiazepines. An important question for future research is the role of protracted withdrawal in precipitating relapse for several months after detoxification is complete. Because of this potential for protracted withdrawal, a major role for detoxification is to prepare patients for maintenance pharmacotherapy with the antagonist naltrexone.

Recent developments in naltrexone maintenance are discussed by Conor K. Farren, Stephanie O'Malley, and Bruce Rounsaville in Chapter 6. Naltrexone is an orally active narcotic antagonist with a relatively long half-life that enables it to be given as little as two to three times per week. Because naltrexone will precipitate withdrawal in opiate-dependent individuals, detoxification is a critical first step for induction into naltrexone therapy. Naltrexone does best in highly motivated patients, such as health care professionals who can be well monitored for compliance with the medication and who therefore cannot engage in illicit opiate use. Naltrexone can also be successful in work release programs tied to the criminal justice system. Overall, treatment with naltrexone needs to last at least a year in order to insure suitable psychosocial rehabilitation, since treatment is not simply the stopping of illicit opiate use. In order to optimize the delivery of naltrexone, psychosocial interventions can include family therapy or contingency payment. Furthermore, pharmacological adjuncts during the initial weeks of naltrexone treatment can minimize protracted withdrawal symptoms. While naltrexone has certain advantages over methadone, including naltrexone's nonaddicting properties and its complete blockade of opiate effects in comparison to methadone, naltrexone treatment has had less acceptability than methadone maintenance. The above developments in detoxification have reduced the duration as well as the intensity of withdrawal symptoms by the use of nonopioid and nondependence-producing medications that make the medication more acceptable. Since naltrexone treatment shortens the length of time required for detoxification, such treatment may prove to be a valuable clinical option in this age of economic limitation and managed care. Naltrexone also has become of recent interest as a medication for treating alcohol dependence and therefore may be particularly useful for the alcoholic opiate addict. Since 25% or more of heroin addicts can have significant alcohol problems, a very important target population may be alcoholic opiate addicts.

The comorbid abuse of opiates and cocaine has become a critical problem requiring special attention in most programs, and different pharmacotherapies have been tested with some encouraging results. Abuse of cocaine in methadone-maintained patients has become an especially acute problem because there is a high prevalence of it in patients beginning treatment, and it continues in up to 50% of patients who are undergoing methadone treatment. Many of the significant benefits of methadone maintenance treatment, including rapid socialization with a dramatic decrease in intravenous heroin use, is undermined by continued intravenous and freebase cocaine use. Furthermore, opiate-dependent patients with comorbid cocaine abuse tend to have high rates of psychopathology and are frequently HIV infected. In our methadone programs, we found a strong association between cocaine abuse and HIV infection. Continuing cocaine abuse accounted for 75% of the HIV-positive treatment failures, but for only 30% of the non-HIV-positive treatment failures. A wide range of treatments has been applied to these patients, including intensive psychosocial interventions (as outlined above) and conjunctive pharmacotherapies (such as the tricyclic antidepressant desipramine or the serotonergic antidepressant fluoxetine). Success has been limited with these adjunctive pharmacotherapies, even though some of these pharmacotherapies have demonstrated much greater success in a nonmethadone population with comorbid depression and cocaine abuse. Alcohol abuse also has historically been problematic in methadone programs and continues to be a treatment challenge. The use of Antabuse in such cases has been shown to be effective. The clinical management of these comorbid drug problems is discussed by Beatrice Burns in Chapter 7 with particular focus on alcohol and cocaine.

Psychosocial Treatment and Treatment Matching for Special Populations

Two other critical issues are the duration of treatment and the provision of psychosocial interventions for methadone patients. Several studies have found that longer-term treatment in methadone maintenance, particularly treatment beyond 2 years, is associated with a much better outcome and allows patients to develop a lifestyle that no longer includes illicit drug use. Thus, strategies clearly are needed to improve patient retention in methadone maintenance, since many programs have an average retention time of 1 year or less. An important factor in improving retention in methadone treatment is the availability of ancillary services in addition to the simple provision of methadone. These services focus on the development of a drug-free lifestyle, as well as on psychiatric consultation and primary medical care. Medical care has become particularly important as the rate of HIV infection has gone above 20–30% in many methadone programs, and the methadone program provides the most consistent site for obtaining medical attention.

Another strategy for optimizing current treatment is the recent progress in psychosocial treatment and the development of ancillary services for special populations. Intensive psychosocial interventions, including daily treatment, also can improve treatment outcome and are reviewed by S. Kelly Avants, Robert Ohlin, and Arthur Margolin in Chapter 8. In response to the overwhelming demand for methadone maintenance in many cities and the inadequate resources available to provide this treatment for all patients, a low-intensity type of methadone program was approved by the U.S. Food and Drug Administration. These interim methadone clinics simply dispense methadone, and patients are provided with only minimal AIDS counseling and referral services. In spite of this minimal intervention, as many as 20% of patients may have a substantial reduction of illicit opiate use and may reduce their AIDS risk behaviors. However, 80% of patients need more intensive case management and counseling. Beyond dispensing and minimal counseling, a variety of behavioral interventions have been applied to methadone-maintained patients, including such negative contingencies as lowering the methadone dose and ultimate detoxification. More sophisticated cue exposure therapies based on a conditioning model of dependence also have been used. Individual psychotherapy and group psychotherapies have been included, because of the relatively high rates of psychopathology, particularly depression and anxiety disorders. These interventions may compose an intensive day treatment that can address physical and emotional health, substance abuse, community development, and the development of alternative reinforcements and basic daily living skills. The community reinforcement approach, which includes occupational training, reciprocal marriage counseling, social skills training, relapse prevention counseling, and a contingency management system, can be provided in a 6-month framework for both the substance abuser and a significant other who is not a substance abuser. This type of intensive intervention has been particularly useful in the early treatment of methadone-maintained patients in order to improve treatment retention and reduce illicit heroin and cocaine abuse.

Current research is attempting to determine if these more intensive interventions are cost effective for the additional reduction in illicit drug use that may accrue. An important economic consideration is that the cost of residential treatment is from $12,000 to $30,000 per year, whereas these additional outpatient methadone services cost less than half that price. Furthermore, the cost of illegal activities committed by a single heroin addict can range from $50,000 to $200,000 per year, and incarceration costs from $25,000 to $80,000 per year. Finally, the cost of caring for a single AIDS patient can range from $50,000 to $200,000 in the final 2 years of his or her life. Thus, intensive psychosocial interventions, particularly in the early stages of methadone maintenance treatment, are being investigated to determine whether they are effective in improving retention and whether they are ultimately more cost effective than no treatment at all or than such alternative interventions as incarceration or residential treatment.

Among the more creative approaches that have been applied to the problem of cocaine abuse among methadone patients has been acupuncture, or the insertion of needles in specific points of the body, which has been practiced for many centuries, although its mechanism is essentially unknown. It has been applied extensively with approximately 200 clinics nationwide, including over 20 methadone clinics that have offered auricular acupuncture as treatment for cocaine abuse. Several randomized clinical trials assessing acupuncture as a treatment for cocaine abuse have shown some promise when compared to alternative drug treatment modalities, and acupuncture has been shown to be consistently better than needle-insertion control. In general, a suitable needle-insertion control group has yet to be identified. The methodological issues in designing these studies are similar to the issues raised by studies of psychotherapy rather than to the issues raised by studies of pharmacological interventions. A relaxation control condition is needed for these comparisons, because relaxation is an important component of the 45-minute procedure that is given three to five times per week. Arthur Margolin and S. Kelly Avants in Chapter 9 describe an ongoing acupuncture study, including its control condition, and its attempt to match patients to treatment in order to identify for whom acupuncture is effective. Critical components of that match include HIV status, severity of drug dependence, and depression. Overall, acupuncture, as with other psychosocial interventions, needs to be offered in a context that can provide for the multiple psychosocial problems, vocational, interpersonal, and medical, that these cocaine-abusing opiate addicts frequently have.

In optimizing methadone maintenance treatment, important advances have been made in the special treatment issues of opiate-dependent women. Developments in this area are summarized by Grace Chang in Chapter 10. Psychosocial treatment directed toward women must recognize a variety of baseline needs that are gender specific: there are higher rates of unemployment, depression, and anxiety disorders and more severe medical problems in women than in men. Because traumatic events also appear to be more common among women, the treatment of posttraumatic stress disorders needs to be a critical component of these services. Additionally, HIV-positive women in methadone maintenance are noted for their sexual risks and for their inability to insist that their partners use condoms. An all-female staff and child care services are well received by female opiate abusers and clearly show a program's increased sensitivity to women's particular needs.

The pregnant opiate user is an excellent candidate for methadone maintenance but requires multiple services and careful management. Management of methadone dosage can be complex because of the increased metabolism of methadone and the desire to minimize opiate dosages in order to reduce the possibility of withdrawal in the newborn. Abuse of other drugs, particularly benzodiazepines, is not uncommon during pregnancy; and benzodiazepine detoxification can be complex and protracted. Positive contingencies for reducing illicit drug use can improve neonatal outcome and can increase the use of prenatal care by these women, but more study is clearly needed. Outreach efforts should be directed towardsthese pregnant women, and methadone programs with waiting lists will often preferentially admit pregnant women ahead of other candidates on a waiting list for methadone maintenance. Thus, opiate-abusing women appear to have a range of more severe problems than male abusers do and may need some special services that include a focus on pregnancy, child care, and HIV-risk behaviors.

Further developing the issues of medical comorbidity and HIV infection, Patrick G. O'Connor and Peter A. Selwyn provide a comprehensive update for the clinician in Chapter 11. Since the 1980s, much research has been directed at understanding and fighting HIV infections. As a result of these studies and clinical experiences, the Centers for Disease Control and Prevention (CDC) revised the AIDS case definition in 1993 to use the importance of CD4-positive T-lymphocyte counts. Most recently, the importance of viral load has emerged and is becoming paramount in classifying the severity of HIV infection. This chapter considers HIV risk factors associated with opioid dependence, medical management of HIV infection, treatment of opportunistic infections, and other medical problems associated with opioid dependence (hepatitis B, C [and A and D]), other HIV-like retroviruses, bacterial infections, fever, tuberculosis, sexually transmitted diseases, heroin-induced nephropathy, and cancer. Particular attention is then given to treatment and risk reduction in this population.

NEW ADVANCES IN PHARMACOTHERAPY

A major newly available medication is LAAM, a long-acting form of methadone that can be given three times per week. In Chapter 12, this medication is reviewed by Walter Ling and Peggy Compton, who have for many years been involved in its development. Although this long-acting derivative of methadone has been clinically available since 1993 and has over 20 years of data on its safety and efficacy, it has long been an "orphan drug," and its marketing has only recently been facilitated. The clinical pharmacology of LAAM includes slow absorption after oral administration, with peak blood levels 4–8 hours after administration. It builds up very slowly over several weeks; and because of this slow onset and build up, initial retention on LAAM during the first month of treatment has been lower than retention on methadone. After the initial induction period, safety and efficacy of LAAM are generally similar to methadone in 6- to 12-month trials with comparable treatment retention, clinic attendance, reductions in illicit opiate use, and reduction in illegal activities. Additionally, this long-acting form of methadone can address problems of diversion of take-home methadone dosages, and it has less potential for overdose. Patient selection for LAAM is no different from the selection of suitable patients for methadone maintenance, but special advantages may be had by patients who have problems with transportation or with the scheduling of medication or who have a past history of methadone failure or fear of methadone maintenance. Induction into LAAM treatment and the dosage regimen can be somewhat more complex than induction into methadone treatment, but the typical LAAM dosage of 60–100 mg is needed only three times per week, thus diminishing the need for take-home doses. Eventual detoxification from LAAM, as well as procedures for missed medication, has not been as fully studied as detoxification with methadone. Side effects are rare, and overdose is relatively difficult with LAAM compared to other opiates. Because of the three-times-per-week dosing schedule, less staff and less nursing hours are required for the same number of patients, and special groups of patients, such as pregnant women, may benefit from LAAM treatment. Overall, LAAM treatment has become a solid alternative to methadone treatment and may be particularly useful for the more stabilized and healthy opiate addict who does not need daily clinic attendance.

The most recent alternative to methadone is buprenorphine. This partial opioid agonist, discussed in Chapter 13 by Alison Oliveto and Thomas R. Kosten, needs no more than once-daily dosing, and it may be possible to administer it on an every-other-day basis. It has a relatively lower abuse liability than other opioids do and has shown good treatment potential for both detoxification and maintenance. The chapter on buprenorphine examines its pharmacology and summarizes the clinical studies that have examined its efficacy in reducing opiate abuse in humans. These human studies have suggested some abuse liability for buprenorphine, but its abuse liability appears to be lower than that of full opioid agonists such as methadone. Tolerance and dependence also develop with buprenorphine, but the withdrawal syndrome following discontinuation of buprenorphine is milder than with full opioid agonists and only lasts about 1 week. In large-scale outpatient treatment studies, buprenorphine at a daily dosage of 8–16 mg has shown efficacy equivalent to that of methadone in reducing illicit opioid use, although some studies found better retention on methadone than on buprenorphine. An interesting effect of buprenorphine, as shown in some initial studies, is the possible reduction in cocaine use in a dose-dependent manner, with less cocaine use as the dosage of buprenorphine is increased. However, the efficacy of buprenorphine for opioid and cocaine dependence needs further examination since most studies have shown no superiority to methadone for these cocaine abusers. Approval by the U.S. Food and Drug Administration of buprenorphine for opioid dependence is expected in 1998. An approved formulation will probably combine buprenorphine with naloxone in order to minimize the former's diversion to illicit intravenous abuse.

The major challenge now facing clinicians who work with opiate addicts is to appropriately match patients to the variety of treatment alternatives. In an era of diminishing resources for medical care, it is important that cost-effectiveness be considered and that the most effective treatment alternative be considered. In some cases, this alternative may be methadone maintenance with a minimal use of psychosocial services, or perhaps LAAM treatment in a three-times-weekly context with minimal services. As many as 20% of opioid abusers will respond to this low-intervention modality. However, the bulk of abusers need more intensive outpatient treatment in the context of methadone maintenance or possibly can benefit from alternative agents to methadone, such as buprenorphine, or from opiate detoxification followed by naltrexone maintenance. Many of the specific treatment-matching issues are discussed throughout this volume. But this issue is at the leading edge of this rapidly changing field, and the outlook for the future is considered by Thomas R. Kosten in Chapter 14.

Part I

FOUNDATIONS FOR THE NEW INTERVENTIONS

Chapter 2

BEHAVIORAL MODELS
OF OPIATE ABUSE IN ANIMALS

Therese A. Kosten, Ph.D.

Opiate abuse continues to be a major problem in the United States today, and treatment successes remain limited. The problems associated with injection drug abuse have intensified recently because of the increased risk of HIV and other blood-borne infections through needle sharing. Thus, it is necessary to continue to understand the etiology and phenomenology of opiate abuse in order to develop more effective treatment strategies. One treatment strategy is pharmacotherapy, that is, the use of medications to treat either opiate withdrawal symptoms or to help maintain opiate abstinence. Potential pharmacotherapies for opiate abuse are often investigated initially through the use of animal models. Animal models have many advantages, including the ability to manipulate and control the drug exposure parameters; and such models provide the capacity to examine etiology, something not ethically possible to study in human subjects. Concepts derived from animal research can then be tested in human laboratory and clinical studies to help direct new pharmacotherapy treatment approaches. In addition to the use of animal research in the pharmacotherapy of drug abuse, research with animals on the behavioral effects of psychoactive drugs and the role of conditioning factors has helped to guide certain psychotherapy approaches to drug abuse.

The purpose of this chapter is to examine the use of animal models to understand opiate abuse. First, we will discuss the rationale for and role of animal models in substance abuse. Second, we will illustrate the behavioral techniques used to assess opiate exposure effects. Third, we will review the acute behavioral and physiological effects of opiate exposure in animal studies that are relevant to characteristics of human opiate abuse and its treatment. Fourth, we will present the consequences of chronic opiate exposure that are involved in these characteristics. Finally, we will describe the ways in which data obtained from animal models of opiate abuse are applicable to current and potential treatment strategies for opiate abuse.

HOW ANIMAL MODELS CAN APPLY TO OPIATE ABUSE

Advantages and Limitations

Animals are used extensively in behavioral research, and the benefits of this approach have been discussed in detail (Gallup & Suarez, 1985; Miller, 1985). One advantage of using animal models is that it allows control over a variety of factors, such as genetic background, environmental influences, and types and lengths of prior experiences, such as drug exposure. Such factors are difficult to control in studies of psychoactive drug effects on human subjects. An advantage of the ability to control these various factors is that it allows for more efficient and more statistically powerful experimental designs because there is less variability among subjects. For example, one research area of interest is the study of factors that predispose an individual to develop drug abuse. To examine these factors in humans is the most directly relevant way, yet it requires large-scale prospective epidemiological studies or smaller-scale retrospective studies that would provide inferior data compared to prospective data. In contrast, animal models can be designed to examine such factors by controlling genetic background, manipulating environmental influences, or making comparisons between differing amounts and types of drug exposure. Information gained from such studies would give direction to human epidemiological studies; such direction should allow smaller-scale studies to provide adequate information about the human addiction processes. Another advantage of animal models is that one can use many experimental manipulations directed at understanding the neuropharmacological processes of psychoactive drug effects. With the exception of a few procedures, such as neuroimaging techniques and examination of neurotransmitter metabolite levels in cerebral spinal fluid obtained via spinal taps, both of which are costly and have limitations, neuropharmacological processes cannot be examined in human subjects.

Compared to other areas of medicine, the use of animal models in psychiatry is complicated because the etiology and mechanisms of behavioral disorders in humans are either not known or have multiple possible causes. Indeed, psychiatric disorders are specifically defined by their signs and symptoms (e.g., the American Psychiatric Association's [1994] DSM-IV) to avoid references to etiology. However, unlike other psychiatric disorders, such as depression or anxiety, animal models of substance abuse are less ambiguous because part of the etiology of the disorder is due to the effects of psychoactive drug exposure. Yet, although all animal models of substance abuse will involve drug exposure, this aspect is not uniform. Parameters of dose, timing, length, and route of exposure will vary across studies and can often be associated with different results. Moreover, psychoactive drug exposure is only one aspect of substance abuse and is likely only a small part of the etiology of these disorders. Indeed, drug abuse reflects the complex interaction of social, behavioral, genetic, and physiological factors since many individuals can be exposed to psychoactive drugs but do not move on to abuse them. Even among those who become drug abusers, there are likely various types and degrees of these factors that were involved in the development of the drug abuse disorder. Clearly, no one animal model of substance abuse can be designed to be an ideal parallel to human substance abuse disorders. Thus, it is best to assess a variety of animal models that vary in the ways in which they were designed to resemble human drug abuse disorders.

Types of Animal Models

Animal models have been categorized into four types based on their purpose in comprehending a human disorder, according to Henn and McKinney (1987). First, animal models can be designed to reflect behavioral similarity to the human disorder. Models of this type in substance abuse include those designed to test the abuse liability of new substances. The degree to which the new substance resembles a known abused substance, for example, in its effect on behavior, can be used to appraise its potential for abuse in humans. Second, animal models can be aimed at testing an etiology. For example, genetic factors that are likely involved in the predisposition to substance abuse can be assessed in animal models by the use of inbred strains. Or the question of whether prenatal or early postnatal drug exposure enhances the propensity to abuse drugs in adulthood can be more easily assessed in animal models where genetic and environmental conditions are controlled. Third, animal models can be used to test mechanisms. For example, understanding the neurobiological mechanisms of substance abuse is of great interest. These mechanisms can be investigated in animals through the use of established neurobiological techniques, with the most useful data being obtained through the simultaneous investigation of drug-using behaviors. Finally, animal models can be directed at testing potential pharmacological treatments. Once there are data from neurobiological studies that suggest pharmacological mechanisms, agents can be tested by using established behavioral paradigms in animal models of substance abuse. Often, a study that uses pharmacological manipulations can address either the mechanisms of the disorder (third type of model) or a possible treatment (fourth type of model), but not both, because agents that can be potential treatments do not necessarily have specific actions and can only be given systemically. Thus, data obtained from this kind of study are limited in their ability to inform about neuropharmacological mechanisms.

BEHAVIORAL TECHNIQUES USED
TO ASSESS EFFECTS OF OPIATES

There are a variety of behavioral techniques used to assess the acute and chronic effects of opiate exposure in animals. The most common techniques will be described below. The types of data obtained from these studies range from assessments of the unconditioned effects of opiates, such as ratings of antagonist-precipitated withdrawal signs, to measures acquired from procedures involving classical and operant conditioning principles, such as place conditioning, self-administration, and drug discrimination. The measures of unconditioned effects of opiate exposure can be subjective in nature and thus require the use of procedures like blind evaluations made by observers trained to make assessments in a standardized manner or the use of automated methods to systematically analyze these effects in an objective manner (i.e., assessing ambulatory locomotor activity by automatic tabulation of the number of photobeam interruptions made). Other models of the behavioral effects of opiates involve procedures that were developed from principles of learning or conditioning. Thus, these techniques can utilize the standardized and operationalized procedures perfected through the extended use of conditioning techniques in behavioral research.

Self-Administration

Drug self-administration in animal research is a widely used model of substance abuse. For example, opiates are readily self-administered by rats (Schuster & Thompson, 1969; Weeks, 1962) and primates (Deneau et al., 1969). Self-administration is based on principles of operant conditioning. The animal learns to respond in such a way as to receive delivery of a drug. Although there are many variations in this method, probably the most common involves the animal's learning to press a lever to receive an injection of a drug through an intravenous catheter. The behavior required to receive the drug will then increase, presumably because of the positive reinforcement of the drug stimulus. Drug self-administration in general, and intravenous self-administration of opiate drugs in particular, is believed to be a valid model of the human condition of addiction not only because the animal must perform a task to receive the drug injection, analogous to a heroin addict's procuring the drug, but also because the drug is often delivered via the same route (i.e., intravenous) often used by heroin addicts. Moreover, the evidence that self-administration behavior is maintained by the drug reinforcement is strong. Pressing the lever that produced drug infusions will cease if the drug is replaced by saline or if drug delivery is no longer contingent upon lever pressing (Pickens & Thompson, 1968). Pressing the lever will resume, if the drug is available again (Stewart & Wise, 1992).

Although there are some differences between drug reinforcement and behavior established by "natural" reinforcers, such as food or water (Wise, 1987), drug self-administration behavior shares many characteristics with these other operant conditioning paradigms (Johanson, 1978; Schuster & Thompson, 1969; Thompson, 1968) as originally described by Skinner (1938). As with behavior maintained by food reinforcement in the food-deprived rat, animals will bar press to receive injections of psychoactive drugs, such as opiate drugs. The typical schedule of reinforcement used in drug self-administration is a fixed ratio 1 (FR1) where one bar press results in the programmed infusion of a unit amount of drug. Rate of bar pressing can be used as a measure of positive reinforcement, though, unlike responding maintained by food, the relation of this behavioral response to drug dose in self-administration studies can be described as an inverted-U-shaped function. That is, as the drug dose increases from low to moderate doses, the rate of bar pressing goes up to a maximal level; this process is figured in the ascending limb of the dose–response curve. As the dose is increased further, the rate of bar pressing will go down; this process is figured in the descending limb of the dose–response curve. Since, at each dose, one bar press results in a different dose of the drug infused, this function indicates, to a certain extent, that the animal is self-administering a fairly constant level of the drug.

It is necessary to understand this dose–response function in order to interpret studies that examine the effects of putative antagonist agents. If assessments are made, for example, by using doses of heroin for the ascending limb, an opiate antagonist, such as naloxone, would be predicted to decrease the behavioral response. However, if assessments are made by using heroin doses for the descending limb, naloxone would be predicted to increase the behavioral response, so that the level of responding would be more like that evoked by a lower dose. Although this finding appears counterintuitive, it has been suggested that this phenomenon indicates that the animal is attempting to compensate for the pharmacological blockade (Koob & Bloom, 1988). Rate of bar pressing is only one way to examine the relative reinforcing effects of drugs and the neuropharmacological mechanisms underlying these effects. Indeed, some have argued that rate measurements confound reinforcement with locomotor effects (Johanson & Fischman, 1989). Alternative measures that are more "rate free" include assessments of choice between two drug doses or assessments of food-reinforced behavior and drug-reinforced behavior in the same session. Another measure of drug reinforcement that is considered less affected by level of activity is the so-called progressive-ratio schedule. In this paradigm, the average number of responses required to receive the drug infusion increases after each correct response. The point at which responding levels off or is extinguished is known as the "breaking point." This measure is thought to reflect how much the animal will work to obtain the drug reinforcement. As with rate measures, the relation of the heroin dose to the breaking point resembles an inverted-U-shaped curve, and administration of the opiate antagonist, naltrexone, decreases the breaking points for heroin (Roberts & Bennett, 1993).

Drug Discrimination

Drug discrimination is another widely used procedure to assess the behavioral effects of psychoactive drugs, and, like self-administration, it is an operant conditioning procedure. In contrast to self-administration, where the drug stimulus acts as a reinforcer, in drug discrimination animals use the drug stimulus to determine which operant behavior will be reinforced. That is, animals are trained to respond in a certain way after administration of one drug stimulus and to respond in another way after administration of another drug stimulus or, more typically, its vehicle. The typical procedure involves differential lever selection in which depression of one lever results in food reinforcement after presentation of one drug stimulus and depression of another lever results in food reinforcement after presentation of the vehicle. It is believed that this discrimination behavior is established because the animal uses the interoceptive cues of the drug to learn the operant. Many drugs have been differentiated in this way, and this paradigm has become a standard assay in nonhuman behavioral pharmacology because of the high concordance between drug discrimination behavior and receptor binding studies. Moreover, drug discrimination behavior shows high pharmacological specificity, such that discrimination behavior will generalize to drugs of the same pharmacological class, but not to drugs of a different pharmacological class (e.g., Colpaert, 1986).

Once the drug exerts discriminative stimulus control of behavior, animals will show dose-related responding, such that doses that are lower than the training dose will engender vehicle-appropriate responding; and as the dose increases to the level of the training dose, more drug-appropriate responding will be seen. There are two standard ways in which the data obtained from drug discrimination studies are directly relevant as animal models of drug abuse. First, other drugs can be examined to see if the animal will generalize the discrimination behavior to the test drug. The degree to which another drug substitutes for the training drug will be evidenced by the former's ability to engender drug-appropriate responding. This type of test can be used to assess the potential abuse liability of novel drugs. An indication of a new drug's potential for abuse may be the degree to which the new compound, which may resemble an established drug of abuse in its chemical structure, leads to drug-appropriate responding that was established with a known abused substance. Second, one can examine in this paradigm other drugs that are thought to antagonize the pharmacological actions of the discriminative stimulus drug. If antagonism occurs, administration of the putative antagonist drug before the various doses of the training drug will result in a shift to the right of the dose–response function. Such a shift indicates that the antagonist drug decreases the ability of the animal to discriminate lower doses of the training drug. This type of test can be used to investigate a potential treatment agent for drug abuse because the degree to which the test agent can antagonize the discriminative stimulus effects of the training drug may indicate the antagonist's potential as a blocking agent. Consistent with these portrayals, the opiate agonist morphine is discriminated by animals; this behavior will generalize to other opiate agonists and is antagonized by opiate antagonists (Shannon & Holtzman, 1976; Teal & Holtzman, 1980).

There are other applications of drug discrimination procedures that are used to study opioidergic agents in particular. One is to use drug discrimination as an *in vivo* tool to assess the relative effects of opioidergic compounds on various opioid receptor types, which may not only vary across compounds but also across doses of one compound, as in partial agonists (Picker et al., 1993). Another use of the drug discrimination procedure is to assess the development of tolerance to the behavioral effects of morphine. Tolerance, which will be discussed in more detail below, occurs when a drug effect diminishes with drug exposure. Tolerance to the morphine discriminative stimulus occurs after chronic morphine treatment, as indicated by a shift to the right in the morphine dose–response function, wherein higher doses of morphine are then necessary to evoke drug-appropriate responding (Young et al., 1991). A further application of the drug discrimination paradigm is that morphine-treated animals can learn to discriminate the opiate antagonist naltrexone, which may be a particularly sensitive measure of opiate withdrawal (Holtzman, 1985). This application will be discussed below. Finally, drug discrimination procedures have been translated from the animal laboratory to the human laboratory (Preston & Jasinski, 1991). Such studies in humans will likely provide valuable information to help guide potential treatments for opiate abuse.

Place Conditioning

Another procedure used to assess the behavioral effects of psychoactive drugs is the place conditioning procedure. This procedure is based on classical conditioning principles whereby originally neutral cues are specifically paired with the drug effects. The degree to which the animal approaches or avoids the cues associated with the drug effects will likely reflect either the rewarding or the aversive aspects of the drug. In general, place conditioning is established by using a chamber with at least two distinctive compartments. These compartments can be made distinct by the use of some combination of visual, tactile, and olfactory cues. The animal is confined to one compartment after drug injections and is confined to another compartment after vehicle injections. After a few such pairings, the animal is allowed access to both compartments; in some cases the access is through a "neutral," or nonpaired, zone. The amount of time spent on the drug-paired side is the measure of place conditioning. If the animal spends more time on the drug-paired side after the drug pairings or compared to vehicle-treated controls, the drug is said to support a conditioned place preference that probably reflects its rewarding effects (Carr et al., 1989).

Many psychoactive drugs that are abused support place conditioning in this manner (Carr et al., 1989; Schechter & Calcagnetti, 1993). Morphine readily conditions place preferences, an effect lessened by pretreatment with opiate antagonists (e.g., Reid et al., 1989). One standard use for place conditioning is to examine the abuse liability of new compounds, an effect that would be suggested by the ability of a compound to support place conditioning. Conversely, the ability of a new compound to antagonize the establishment of place conditioning to an opiate would suggest potential pharmacological treatment agents.

Place conditioning procedures have also been used to assess the aversive, or negative, motivational effects of opiate withdrawal (Mucha, 1987). That is, when an opiate antagonist is paired with the environmental cues in morphine-exposed animals, the animals will spend less time in the drug-paired environment, presumably because of the aversive effects of precipitated opiate withdrawal (Mucha, 1987). There is a positve relation between antagonist dose and the degree of place avoidance in this paradigm, and doses much lower than those used to elicit observable withdrawal signs are effective (Mucha, 1987). This implies that the place conditioning procedure is a sensitive measure of opiate withdrawal. Place conditioning procedures have also been used to assess tolerance, the diminished effect of the drug with exposure. Chronic morphine treatment decreases the ability of morphine to support place conditioning, as evidenced by an increase in dose or in number of training trials to obtain the same level of conditioned place preference (Bechara & van der Kooy, 1992; Shippenberg et al., 1988).

The validity of the place conditioning procedure as an animal model of drug abuse has been questioned because, unlike the self-administration procedure, the animal is not required to respond in order to obtain the drug effect. Yet, classical conditioning effects in general (Siegel, 1979; Wikler, 1973) and environmental cues in particular (Marlatt & Gordon, 1985; Meyer & Mirin, 1982) are strongly related to continued drug-using behavior and to relapse to use after abstinence.

Withdrawal Assessments

Cessation of chronic opiate exposure is associated with withdrawal phenomena, which will be discussed in detail below. A more severe withdrawal syndrome occurs when a morphine-exposed animal is given an opiate antagonist; this phenomenon is known as precipitated opiate withdrawal. The classic method of assessing precipitated opiate withdrawal is through the objective measures of the frequency and/or severity of the expression of certain physical signs (e.g., Blasig et al., 1973). Such signs include wet-dog shakes, jumping, lacrimation, salivation, teeth chatters, chewing, and diarrhea. It is necessary to try to maintain standards of ratings throughout studies because the nature of these types of data is not as objective as the data obtained in the techniques described above. One way that may advance the application of these measures is the use of video and audio data collection by utilizing digital analysis with computer software programs. However, other methods of assessing opiate withdrawal are used. As mentioned above, precipitated opiate withdrawal supports place conditioning (Mucha, 1987), and morphine-exposed animals can learn to discriminate opiate antagonists

(Holtzman, 1985). Other methods of assessing opiate withdrawal are used, including disruptions of schedule-controlled behavior responses (e.g., bar pressing for food).

ACUTE EFFECTS OF OPIATES

Subjective Effects

One of the prominent features of acute opiate exposure related to its abuse potential is the ability of opiates to induce a reported sense of euphoria or well-being. In addition to, or perhaps related to, this effect is the observation that acute administration of morphine or other opiates relieves the distress of pain. Subjects report that when administered opiates, although they are still aware of pain, the pain is less disturbing (Jaffe, 1985). It is tempting to postulate that the euphoric and analgesic effects of opiates are connected, particularly since many drugs of abuse (e.g., alcohol, cocaine, sedatives) possess both properties. However, because the investigation of these two effects generally necessitates different experimental designs (see pp. 16–17 above), it is unlikely that researchers will be able to determine the degree to which the euphoric and analgesic aspects of psychoactive drugs are related.

Positive Reinforcement and Reward

In animals, many opiate drugs are known to possess the property of positive reinforcement. That is, the delivery of an opiate drug after a behavioral action such as lever pressing results in increases in this behavior. More generally, reinforcement is a construct defined by Skinner (1938) as behavior that is controlled by its consequences. In the case of positive reinforcement, the presentation of the stimulus results in an increase in behavior. In contrast, negative reinforcement occurs when the removal of the stimulus results in an increase in behavior. Negative reinforcement likely plays a role in opiate abuse since the ingestion of opiates relieves the withdrawal distress associated with opiate abstinence (Jaffe, 1985).

   Although researchers do not know the reasons that the delivery of an opiate drug tends to lead to increases in the behavior connected with obtaining it, many researchers believe that this phenomenon reflects the rewarding properties of the drug (Koob & Bloom, 1988; Wise, 1987). The concept of reward has been useful in the investigation of psychoactive drug effects. Drugs serve as positive reinforcers in the absence of a deprivation state, unlike the more typical reinforcers, such as food or water, in the deprived animal. Yet, it should be kept in mind that reward is a construct used to explain the animal's behavior and cannot be investigated in its own right. It does, nonetheless, provide guidance in designing studies of opiate abuse with animal models. While it is tempting to assume that the concepts of reward and positive reinforcement are analogous to the subjective effects of opiates reported by humans (e.g., euphoria, "high," etc.), these concepts are not interchangeable. Positive reinforcement is measured by changes in behavior. Behavior can be altered in the absence of a cognitive awareness of the reason for the behavior change. Indeed, behavioral measures are more sensitive than subjective measures, which is why translation of these techniques from the animal laboratory to the human laboratory is useful (e.g., Fischman & Foltin, 1992; Preston & Jasinski, 1991).

Other Effects

Another characteristic of many psychoactive drugs is that they have effects on locomotor activity. Since the degree of positive reinforcement is measured by quantifying behavioral performance, it is important to remember that psychoactive drugs, including opiates, can alter performance not only because of their motoric effects but also because of their reinforcing effects. In rats, low doses of morphine that can serve as positive reinforcers lead to increases in locomotor activity. Higher doses that are associated with the development of tolerance and dependence generally decrease activity levels. Thus, well-designed studies that use animal models of opiate abuse will need rigorous controls and, as some researchers argue, "rate-free" measures (e.g., Johanson & Fischman, 1989; see pp. 18–20 above), to rule out the motoric actions of drugs on performance.

Finally, the acute exposure to opiate drugs has many other physiological effects that are likely related to abuse of those drugs. For example, opiates tend to decrease heart rate, blood pressure, and body temperature and to alter gastrointestinal processes. Indeed, some antidiarrhea drugs are opiates. These effects will be discussed further, in the following section, because they relate to chronic effects of opiates, including tolerance and dependence.

CHRONIC EFFECTS OF OPIATES

Tolerance

Long-term exposure to opiates is associated with many alterations in the behavioral and other effects of opiates. In many cases, tolerance will occur, that is, there will be a diminished effect of the opiate after long-term exposure. Tolerance is also characterized by the need for an increased dose or amount in order to obtain an effect seen originally with acute exposure. Analgesic tolerance is a common effect seen with opiates. The pain-relieving effect of opiates becomes reduced over usage time, which means that the doses must be increased to maintain the analgesic effect. Tolerance also develops to many of the physiological effects of opiates, such that the original effect of an opiate in decreasing heart rate, blood pressure, or body temperature lessens with use.

One can speculate that the subjective effects of euphoria or a "high" become diminished with use because, during the course of opiate abuse, the addict usually increases the amount that he or she uses or may move to a more effective route of administration (e.g., from the intranasal to the intravenous route). This speculation cannot, however, be examined in controlled studies of human opiate abusers, except by obtaining retrospective data. Gathering self-reports of drug use patterns and subjective effects in this manner would not provide useful data because the data are based on addicts' recall over a long period of time.

It is not possible to address the issue of whether subjective effects are altered over time in animal studies; however, it is possible to examine whether certain behavioral effects, such as the positive reinforcing, rewarding, or discriminative effects of opiates, are modified over time. In self-administration studies, animals maintain a fairly stable level of drug administration throughout the course of the study. However, in many studies, the animals are allowed to self-administer the drug during discrete time periods (e.g., 2 hours) each day, which does not provide a good test of the amount that the animal would ingest in an unlimited access situation. Nonetheless, the development of tolerance to the behavioral effects of opiates has been examined by using animal models of drug discrimination and place conditioning. Researchers have found that there is development of tolerance to the discriminative stimulus effects of morphine. In a series of studies by Young and colleagues, it was shown that if morphine discrimination training is suspended (Sannerud & Young, 1987) and animals are treated with morphine doses greater than the training dose (Young et al., 1990), one will observe a shift to the right of the dose–response curve, compared to pretreatment. This effect suggests that tolerance to the behavioral effects of morphine developed because higher doses were required to evoke drug-appropriate responding after the chronic treatment. Tolerance to the place conditioning effects of morphine has also been shown. If animals are chronically treated with morphine before the onset of morphine place conditioning, one can see a shift to the right of the dose–response function for this behavior (Bechara & van der Kooy,

1992; Shippenberg et al., 1988). Again, this shift indicates that a higher dose is needed to obtain the usual behavioral effects of morphine.

Dependence

Physical dependence is another characteristic of chronic treatment with opiates. Dependence is defined as the presence of physical withdrawal signs and symptoms with the abrupt cessation of opiate use. A constellation of signs and symptoms can include physical effects such as yawning, perspiration, piloerection, hypertension, rhinorrhea, lacrimation, nausea, and tremor. Behavioral effects can be manifest as well, including agitation and restlessness. Many of these withdrawal effects are opposite to those seen with administration of an acute dose of the opiate. Much research has indicated that these opposing effects seen with withdrawal, as compared to the observed acute effects, may be due to neuronal adaptations to the chronic opiate exposure. With the removal of the opiate exposure, these neuronal adaptations are unopposed, and hyperexcitability of some neurons results (see Chapter 3 for Eric J. Nestler's detailed descriptions of these adaptive mechanisms). In addition to the neuronal adaptations, the development of dependence and its associated withdrawal effects are the consequence of conditioning factors, which will be discussed in the following section.

The Role of Conditioning in the Effects of Chronic Opiate Exposure

As discussed above, chronic morphine exposure is associated with the phenomena of tolerance and dependence. While these phenomena likely reflect neuronal alterations caused by the repeated pharmacological effects of opiates (see Chapter 3), much research has shown that there is a conditioning aspect to these phenomena as well. For example, in procedures that assess the development of tolerance to morphine, the animal is typically tested for the effect in a specific environment or test apparatus. The test apparatus and the procedures involved in testing can function as conditioned stimuli because they are paired with the drug injections. Indeed, this is another example of the role of classical conditioning in drug effects (see pp. 22–23 above). Tolerance to various effects of morphine and other drugs is greater when animals are tested in a specific environment or apparatus, compared to animals that receive drug injections in an environment that differs from the test environment. There are different explanations for the mechanism by which conditioning to drug effects occurs (Baker & Tiffany, 1985; Siegel, 1979; Wikler, 1973); nonetheless, it is well accepted that these effects play an important role in the development of tolerance to and dependence on drug use.

APPLICATIONS OF ANIMAL BEHAVIORAL DATA FOR THE TREATMENT OF OPIATE ABUSE

Detoxification

Opiate abuse can be treated by detoxification from opiates, which can involve one of a number of withdrawal-inducing strategies. Opiates can be discontinued abruptly (e.g., "cold turkey"), an uncomfortable process that can take days to accomplish. The dose of opiates can be decreased over days (e.g., methadone tapering), an approach that is less uncomfortable but takes longer to finish compared to abrupt discontinuation. Finally, opiate withdrawal can be precipitated with an opiate antagonist, such as naltrexone. The precipitated withdrawal is associated with more intense symptomatology, but is shorter lasting. Symptom discomfort and withdrawal distress associated with any of these detoxification procedures can be attenuated with certain pharmacological agents. The most commonly used agent is clonidine, an alpha-2 agonist (Gold et al., 1978; Washton & Resnick, 1980). This treatment agent was discovered through animal research (Aghajanian, 1978). Briefly, discontinuation of a chronic opiate exposure leads to enhanced firing of the locus coeruleus, a noradrenergic nucleus of cells in the brain stem. This nucleus projects to many areas of the mid- and forebrain, and enhanced firing is temporally associated with the expression of opiate withdrawal signs. Clonidine acts to shutdown the firing of locus coeruleus neurons through an autoreceptor mechanism. Pretreatment with clonidine reduces the severity of physical signs of precipitated opiate withdrawal in rats (Taylor et al., 1988; Tseng et al., 1975) and also reduces other behavioral effects of withdrawal (Kosten, 1994; Sparber & Meyer, 1978). Because clonidine reduces withdrawal through a nonopiate mechanism, it has been seen as a relatively safe adjunct to detoxification. However, clonidine does have some effects, such as its hypotensive effects, that can contraindicate its use in some addicts. Thus, it is useful to pursue the application of other potential pharmacological agents that may have fewer side effects. This avenue of investigation can begin with the use of the various animal models of opiate withdrawal (e.g., symptom ratings, place conditioning, antagonist discrimination) described above.

Maintenance

Another treatment approach for opiate abuse is to maintain the opiate addict on another opiate agonist, such as methadone. Methadone maintenance works through cross-tolerance to heroin and is thought to be effective because it alleviates withdrawal and, possibly, drug craving (Dole & Nyswander, 1967). In conjunction with supportive psychological interventions, methadone maintenance has been a useful treatment approach, as discussed in Chapter 4. While methadone maintenance has been used for decades with a fair degree of success, other potential pharmacological agents are also being evaluated. These agents include levo-alpha-acetylmethadol (LAAM), a longer-acting opiate agonist, and buprenorphine, a partial opiate agonist (Lewis, 1985). The latter has been hypothesized to be useful because an opiate abuser can begin buprenorphine treatment with low, agonistlike doses and then can have the dose increased slowly until it becomes antagonistlike. At the higher doses, buprenorphine should function as a "blocking" agent, described in the next section.

Blocking Agents

A third approach to the treatment of opiate abuse is to use a pharmacological "blocking" agent, that is, maintenance on a compound that would antagonize the reinforcing effects of opiate ingestion. To a certain extent, methadone accomplishes this effect through cross-tolerance. However, detoxified opiate abusers can be maintained on the opiate antagonist, naltrexone, which blocks the acute, presumably reinforcing, effects of heroin. If an opiate addict uses heroin while on naltrexone therapy, the effects of the drug would be attenuated. Thus, the addict may come to disassociate the drug with its reinforcing effects. In practice, however, this approach has met with limited success, in part because an addict can decide to discontinue the medication use if he or she wants to begin heroin use again. Again, this pharmacotherapy needs to be given in conjunction with psychological support in order to be effective and may only be effective for a small population of highly motivated opiate addicts.

Relapse Prevention

In addition to the use of animal models to direct and test the above described pharmacological treatment agents, the behavioral and conditioning principles derived from animal models have contributed to the development of a psychotherapy approach to treating drug and alcohol abuse (Carroll et al., 1991; Marlatt & Gordon, 1985). This style of psychotherapy is known as relapse prevention. Part of its basis was developed from studies that found that drug effects or withdrawal effects can be classically conditioned, as was described above (Siegel, 1979; Wikler, 1973). Briefly, cues in the environment that were reliably associated with drug procurement or drug use can come to elicit drug-opposing (Siegel, 1979) or drug-withdrawal-like (Wikler, 1973) effects. Thus, the sight of the place where drugs were bought can lead to drug craving and relapse in a detoxified opiate abuser. Relapse prevention helps the addict to recognize and deal with these effects as one aspect of maintaining drug abstinence.

CONCLUSIONS

Thus, there are a multitude of ways in which animal models have helped to guide treatment strategies for opiate abuse. But more research is needed at this level as well as in human laboratory and clinical trial settings to further understand the etiology of this disorder, to establish more effective treatment strategies, and to ascertain which of the many treatment approaches would be best for the different populations of opiate abusers.

ACKNOWLEDGMENTS

Support was provided by the National Institute on Drug Abuse (Grant Nos. P50-DA04060 and DA08227) and by the Abraham Ribicoff Research Facilities, Department of Mental Health, State of Connecticut.

REFERENCES

Aghajanian, G. K. (1978). Tolerance of locus coeruleus neurons to morphine and suppression of withdrawal responses by clonidine. *Nature, 276,* 186–188.

American Psychiatric Association. (1994). *Diagnostic and statistical manual of mental disorders* (4th ed.). Washington, DC: Author.

Baker, T. B., & Tiffany, S. T. (1985). Morphine tolerance as habituation. *Psychological Reviews, 92,* 78–108.

Bechara, A., & van der Kooy, D. (1992). Chronic exposure to morphine does not alter the neural tissues subserving its acute rewarding properties: Apparent tolerance is overshadowing. *Behavioral Neuroscience, 106,* 364–373.

Blasig, J., Reinhold, H. K., & Zieglegansberger, S. (1973). Development of physical dependence on morphine in respect to time and dosage and quantification of the precipitated withdrawal syndrome in rats. *Psychopharmacologia (Berlin), 33,* 19–38.

Carr, G. D., Fibiger, H. C., & Phillips, A. G. (1989). Conditioned place preference as a measure of drug reward. In J. M. Liebman & S. J. Cooper (Eds.), *The neuropharmacological basis of reward* (pp. 264–230). New York: Oxford Universty Press.

Carroll, K. M., Rounsaville, B. J., & Keller, D. S. (1991). Relapse prevention strategies for the treatment of cocaine abuse. *American Journal of Drug and Alcohol Abuse, 17,* 249–265.

Colpaert, F. C. (1986). Drug discrimination: Behavioral, pharmacological, and molecular mechanisms of discriminative drug effects. In S. R. Goldberg & I. P. Stolerman (Eds.), *Behavioral analysis of drug dependence* (pp. 161–193). New York: Academic Press.

Deneau, G., Yanagita, T., & Seevers, M. H. (1969). Self-administration of psychoactive substance by the monkey: A measure of psychological dependence. *Psychopharmacologia, 16,* 30–48.

Dole, V. P., & Nyswander, M. (1967). A medical treatment for diacetylmorphine (heroin) addiciton. *Journal of the American Medical Association, 193,* 646–650.

Fischman, M. W., & Foltin, R. W. (1992). Self-administration of cocaine by humans: choice between smoked and intravenous cocaine. *Journal of Pharmacology and Experimental Therapeutics, 261,* 841–849.

Gallup, G. G., & Suarez, S. D. (1985). Alternatives to the use of animals in psychological research. *American Psychologist, 40,* 1104–1111.

Gold, M. S., Redmond, D. E., & Kleber, H. D. (1978). Clonidine in opiate withdrawal. *Lancet, ii,* 599.

Henn, F. A., & McKinney, W.. (1987). Animal models in psychiatry. In H. Y. Meltzer (Ed.), *Psychopharmacology: The third generation of progress* (pp. 687–696). New York: Raven Press.

Holtzman, S. G. (1985). Discriminative stimulus effects of morphine withdrawal in the dependent rat: Suppression by opiate and nonopiate drugs. *Journal of Pharmacology and Experimental Therapeutics, 233,* 80–86.

Jaffe, J. H. (1985). Drug addiction and drug abuse. In L. S. Goodman & A. Gilman (Eds.), *The pharmacological basis of therapeutics* (5th ed., pp. 532–584). New York: Macmillan.

Johanson, C. E. (1978). Drugs as reinforcers. In D. E. Blackman & D. J. Sanger (Eds.), *Contemporary research in behavioral pharmacology* (pp. 325–390). New York: Plenum Press.

Johanson, C. E., & Fischman, M. W. (1989). The pharmacology of cocaine related to its abuse. *Pharmacological Reviews, 41,* 3–52.

Koob, G. F., & Bloom, F. E. (1988). Cellular and molecular mechanisms of drug dependence. *Science, 242,* 715–723.

Kosten, T. A. (1994). Clonidine attenuates conditioned aversion produced by naloxone-precipitated opiate withdrawal. *European Journal of Pharmacology, 254,* 59–63.

Lewis, J. W. (1985). Buprenorphine. *Drug and Alcohol Dependence, 14,* 363–372.

Marlatt, G. A., & Gordon, J. R. (Eds.). (1985). *Relapse prevention.* New York: Guilford Press.

Meyer, R. D., & Mirin, S. M. (1982). *The heroin stimulus: Implications for a theory of addiction.* New York: Plenum Press.

Miller, N. E. (1985). The value of behavioral research on animals. *American Psychologist, 40,* 423–440.

Mucha, R. F. (1987). Is the motivational effect of opiate withdrawal reflected by common somatic indices of precipitated withdrawal? A place conditioning study in the rat. *Brain Research, 418,* 214–220.

Pickens, R., & Thompson, T. (1968). Cocaine-reinforced behavior in rats: Effects of reinforcement magnitude and fixed-ratio size. *Journal of Pharmacology and Experimental Therapeutics, 161,* 122–129.

Picker, M. J., Yarbrough, J., Hughes, C. E., Smith, M. A., Morgan, D., & Dykstra, L. A. (1993). Agonist and antagonist effects of mixed action opioids in the pigeon drug discrimination procedure: Influence of training dose, intrinsic efficacy and interanimal differences. *Journal of Pharmacology and Experimental Therapeutics, 266,* 756–767.

Preston, K. L., & Jasinski, D. R. (1991). Abuse liability studies of opioid agonist-antagonists in humans. *Drug and Alcohol Dependence, 28,* 49–82.

Reid, L. D., Marglin, S. H., Mattie, M. E., & Hubbell, C. L. (1989). Measuring morphine's capacity to establish a place preference. *Pharmacology, Biochemistry and Behavior, 33,* 765–775.

Roberts, D. C. S., & Bennett, S. A. L. (1993). Heroin self-administration in rats under a progressive ratio schedule of reinforcement. *Psychopharmacology, 111,* 215–218.

Sannerud, C. A., & Young, A. M. (1987). Environmental modification of tolerance to morphine discriminative properties in rats. *Psychopharmacology, 93,* 59–68.

Schechter, M. D., & Calcagnetti, D. J. (1993). Trends in place preference conditioning with a cross-indexed bibliography, 1957–1991. *Pharmacology, Biochemistry and Behavior, 17,* 21–41.

Schuster, C. R., & Thompson, T. (1969). Self-administration of and behavioral dependence on drugs. *Annual Review of Pharmacology, 9,* 483–502.

Shannon, H. E., & Holtzman, S. G. (1976). Evaluation of the discriminative effects of morphine in the rat. *Journal of Pharmacology and Experimental Therapeutics, 198,* 54–65.

Shippenberg, T. S., Emmett-Oglesby, M. W., Ayesta, F. J., & Herz, A. (1988). Tolerance and selective cross-tolerance to the motivational effects of opioids. *Psychopharmacology, 96,* 110–115.

Siegel, S. (1979). The role of conditioning in drug tolerance and addiction. In J. D. Keehn (Ed.), *Psychopathology in animals: Research and clinical applications* (pp. 143–168). New York: Academic Press.

Skinner, B. F. (1938). *The behavior of organisms.* New York: Appleton-Century-Crofts.

Sparber, S. G., & Meyer, D. R. (1978). Clonidine antagonizes naloxone induced suppression of conditioned behavior and body weight in morphine-dependent rats. *Pharmacology, Biochemistry and Behavior, 9,* 319.

Stewart, J., & Wise, R. A. (1992). Reinstatement of heroin self-administration habits: Morphine prompts and naltrexone discourages reward responding after extinction. *Psychopharmacology, 108,* 79–84.

Taylor, J. R., Elsworth, J. D., Garcia, E. J., Grant, S. J., Roth, R. H., & Redmond, D. E. Jr. (1988). Clonidine infusions into the locus coeruleus attenuate behavioral and neurochemical changes associated with naloxone-precipitated withdrawal. *Psychopharmacology, 96,* 121–134.

Teal, A. H., & Holtzman, S. G. (1980). Stimulus effects of morphine in the monkey: Quantitative analysis of antagonisms. *Journal of Pharmacology and Experimental Therapeutics, 12,* 587–593.

Thompson, T. (1968). Drugs as reinforcers: Experimental addiction. *International Journal of the Addictions, 3,* 199–206.

Tseng, L. F., Loh, H. H., & Wei, E.T. (1975). Effects of clonidine on morphine withdrawal signs in the rat. *European Journal of Pharmacology, 30,* 93–99.

Washton, A. M., & Resnick, R. B. (1980). Clonidine for opiate detoxification: Outpatient clinical trial. *American Journal of Psychiatry, 137,* 1121.

Weeks, J. R. (1962). Experimental morphine addiction: Method for automatic intravenous injections in unrestrained rats. *Science, 138,* 143–144.

Wikler, A. (1973). Dynamics of drug dependence. *Archives of General Psychiatry, 28,* 611–616.

Wise, R. A. (1987). Intravenous drug self-administration: A special case of positive reinforcement. In M. A.. Bozarth (Ed.), *Methods of assessing the reinforcing properties of abused drugs* (pp. 117–141). New York: Springer.

Young, A. M., Kapitsolpoulos, G., & Makhay, M. M. (1991). Tolerance to morphine-like stimulus effects of mu opioid agonists. *Journal of Pharmacology and Experimental Therapeutics, 257,* 795–805.

Young, A. M., Sannerud, C. A., Steigerwald, E. S., Doty, M. D., Lipinski, W. J., & Tetrick, L. (1990). Tolerance to morphine stimulus control: Role of morphine maintenance dose. *Psychopharmacology, 102,* 59–67.

Chapter 3

BASIC NEUROBIOLOGY
OF OPIATE ADDICTION

Eric J. Nestler, M.D., Ph.D.

The mechanisms by which opiates induce addiction have long been a subject of great interest. Two prominent features of opiate addiction have been described: (1) tolerance, characterized by a diminishing drug effect after repeated administration, and (2) dependence, revealed by a withdrawal syndrome after abrupt discontinuation of opiate exposure. Opiates induce both physical and psychological dependence. Opiates are physically addicting in that discontinuation of opiate exposure leads to a number of characteristic physical signs and symptoms that compose the opiate abstinence syndrome. Opiates are also psychologically addicting in that the drugs are acutely reinforcing, with escalating drug seeking seen with repeated drug exposure. The traditional distinction between physical and psychological addiction is artificial because both are mediated by the brain, possibly even by similar neural mechanisms, as will be seen below.

Although many regions of the central nervous system are opiate responsive, certain well-characterized regions have provided particularly useful model systems for the study of the cellular and molecular mechanisms underlying the acute and chronic actions of opiates on the nervous system. Three model systems will be discussed here: (1) the locus coeruleus, (2) the mesolimbic dopamine system, and (3) the dorsal root ganglion–spinal cord. In these systems, the cellular and molecular actions of opiates can be understood within a functional context, making it possible to relate these actions to specific behavioral aspects of opiate tolerance, dependence, and withdrawal. Before considering the specific signal transduction pathways through which opiates regulate neuronal function in these regions acutely and chronically, an overview of the signal transduction pathways of the brain will be presented.

OVERVIEW OF SIGNAL TRANSDUCTION PATHWAYS

When a neurotransmitter binds to its receptor on the surface of a neuron, the effects evoked in the neuron may be mediated by a number of distinct mechanisms. However, with the exception of neurotransmitter receptors that also function as ion channels (e.g., most glutamate and gamma-aminobutyric acid [GABA] receptors), the responses elicited by ligand binding of most other types of neurotransmitter receptors are mediated initially by a class of membrane-bound proteins known as guanine nucleotide-binding proteins, or G proteins, which mediate the effects of receptor activation on a diverse range of neuronal processes (see Figure 3.1) (reviewed in Nestler & Duman, 1994). Numerous types of G proteins have been found in the brain. Each is a heterotrimer composed of single a, b, and g subunits. Distinct a subunits confer functional activity on the different types of G proteins, which appear to share common bg subunits, although multiple forms of b and g subunits also exist. Activation of a G protein-linked receptor by ligand binding causes a conformational change in its associated G protein. In some cases, the activated G protein directly activates (e.g., "gates") specific types of ion channels (e.g., K^+ or Ca^{2+} channels) and thereby elicits some of the electrophysiological effects of the original neurotransmitter stimulus. In other cases, the actions of G proteins are mediated by the generation of second messengers in the brain, such as cyclic AMP, cyclic GMP, calcium, nitric oxide, and metabolites of phosphatidylinositol (Figure 3.1) (Nestler & Duman, 1994).

The mechanism by which G proteins regulate neuronal cyclic AMP levels is now well established. Binding of ligands to certain receptors activates G proteins known as Gs, which, in turn, activate adenylyl cyclase, the enzyme that catalyzes the synthesis of cyclic AMP. Other ligands acting through different receptors activate G proteins known as Gi, which inhibit adenylyl cyclase and decrease cellular cyclic AMP levels. In addition to Gs and Gi, the brain contains other forms of G proteins. Go, which does not have a prominent effect on adenylyl cyclase, appears to mediate some of the effects of some neurotransmitter receptors on ion channels mentioned above. Gq is a G protein that mediates the ability of some neurotransmitter receptors in some cell types to activate the enzyme phospholipase C, which leads to the activation of the phosphatidylinositol cycle. In other circumstances, this action is mediated via subtypes of Gi.

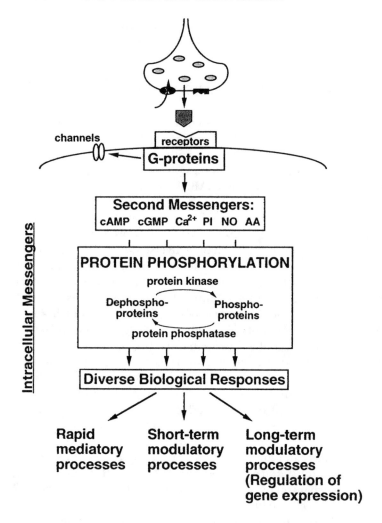

FIGURE 3.1. Schematic illustration of the role played by intracellular messenger systems in synaptic transmission in the brain. Most types of neurotransmitters produce diverse types of physiological responses in target neurons through a complex cascade of intracellular messengers. These intracellular messenger pathways consist of coupling factors (called G proteins), second messengers (e.g., cyclic AMP [cAMP], cyclic GMP [cGMP], Ca^{2+}, nitric oxide [NO], and the metabolites of phosphatidylinositol [PI] and arachidonic acid [AA]), and protein phosphorylation (involving the phosphorylation of phosphoproteins by protein kinases and their dephosphorylation by protein phosphatases). The figure illustrates three major roles subserved by these intracellular messengers. Intracellular messenger pathways mediate the actions of some neurotransmitters in activating or inhibiting the neurotransmitters' target ion channels. In addition, intracellular messengers mediate most of the other actions on the target neurons by the neurotransmitters. Some intracellular messengers are relatively short lived and involve modulation of numerous types of neuronal processes; others are relatively long lived and are achieved through

Following the generation of second messengers, physiological responses of neurons are mediated largely by changes in protein phosphorylation (Figure 3.1) (Nestler & Greengard, 1994). This process is accomplished in most cases by the activation of specific second messenger-dependent protein kinases, for example, cyclic AMP-dependent protein kinase, cyclic GMP-dependent protein kinase, calcium-dependent protein kinases, and so on. Activation of these protein kinases results in the phosphorylation of a specific array of substrate proteins for each enzyme. In some cases, extracellular stimuli alter the phosphorylation of neuronal proteins by influencing the activity of specific protein phosphatases, the enzymes that dephosphorylate proteins. By either mechanism, a change in the phosphorylation state of the substrate proteins alters their function so as to lead to many of the physiological responses of the original neurotransmitter stimulus. Virtually every type of neuronal protein, and consequently every type of neural process, is now known to be regulated by phosphorylation. Thus, protein phosphorylation is a central regulatory mechanism in neurons, affecting neurotransmitter synthesis, neurotransmitter release, generation of synaptic potentials, electrical excitability of neurons, axoplasmic transport, neuronal shape and motility, elaboration of dendritic and axonal processes, and development and maintenance of differentiated characteristics of neurons. Regulation of many of these processes reflects protein phosphorylation-mediated changes in neuronal gene expression.

OVERVIEW OF OPIATE-REGULATED SIGNAL TRANSDUCTION PATHWAYS

Opioid Receptors

The identification of opioid receptors in the 1970s represented a major advance in our understanding of the molecular substrates of addiction. Three subtypes of opioid receptor (mu, delta, and kappa; μ, δ, κ) have been identified on the basis of differential ligand binding (see Johnson & Fleming, 1989; Loh & Smith, 1990; Pasternak, 1988). Morphine-like opiates preferentially bind to the μ opiate receptor, whereas the

the regulation of gene expression in the target neurons. The figure is drawn to illustrate the amplification that intracellular messenger systems can give to neurotransmitter action. Thus, a single event of a neurotransmitter binding to its receptor at the first messenger level can act through the second, third, fourth, and so on messenger levels to produce an increasingly wider array of physiological effects. From Nestler (1994). Copyright 1994 by Elsevier Science. Reprinted by permission.

benzomorphan opiates preferentially bind to the κ receptor. Of the endogenous opioid peptides, β-endorphin has the greatest affinity for μ receptors, enkephalins for δ receptors, and dynorphin for κ receptors. However, despite these rank orders of affinity, there do not appear to be separate endogenous opioid systems in the brain that match certain peptides with receptor types, and the differences in affinity are not so great as to be exclusive. Thus, *in vivo,* the determinants of which peptide stimulates which receptor depends not only on affinity but also on the proximity of the various peptides. It has also been difficult to assign a particular physiological role to a particular receptor system, with analgesia and physical dependence apparently involving more than one receptor type. In contrast, there does appear to be some receptor specificity with respect to psychological addiction to opiates, with μ and δ receptors implicated in mediating the reinforcing actions of opiates and κ receptors mediating their aversive actions (Koob, 1992; Self & Nestler, 1995).

In recent years, distinct μ, δ, and κ opioid receptors have been cloned (Evans et al., 1992; Reisine, 1993). Each is a member of the G protein-coupled receptor superfamily characterized by seven transmembrane domains; the opioid receptors are most closely homologous to somatostatin receptors. The messenger RNAs for the three known opioid receptors are expressed in the brain in a pattern that closely follows the distribution of μ, δ, and κ opioid receptor binding. Work is now under way to define the ligand-binding domains of the receptors and to further characterize their molecular properties.

There have been numerous claims over the years, based on classical pharmacological-binding studies, that multiple subtypes for the μ, δ, and κ receptors exist in the brain (e.g., Pasternak, 1988). Indeed, considerable work has been invested in identifying and characterizing these binding variants. However, the molecular basis of these variants remains uncertain, since molecular-cloning studies have, to date, failed to identify subtypes of the μ, δ, or κ receptor.

Postreceptor Signaling Pathways

A summary of known opioid receptor-regulated signal transduction pathways is shown schematically in Figure 3.2. In most systems, opioid receptors are coupled to the Gi and Go type of G protein and thereby inhibit adenylyl cyclase and regulate specific K^+ and Ca^{2+} channels. Opiate inhibition of adenylyl cyclase has been documented in numerous regions of the central nervous system and in several cultured cell lines (Childers, 1991; Johnson & Fleming, 1989). This effect can be medi-

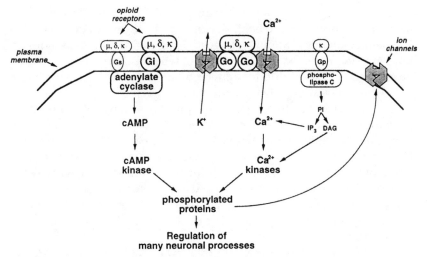

FIGURE 3.2. Schematic illustration of opiate-regulated signal transduction pathways. Opiates produce their effects in target neurons via interactions with three major classes of receptor, called μ, δ, and κ opiate receptors. There are two major signal transduction pathways through which each of these receptors has been shown to influence target neuron functioning. First, opiates, via coupling to a pertussis toxin-sensitive G protein (presumably Gi), inhibit adenylate cyclase and thereby reduce cellular cyclic AMP levels, the activity of cyclic AMP-dependent protein kinase, and the phosphorylation state of numerous substrate proteins for the protein kinase. Such substrate proteins include ion channels (as shown in the figure) and many other types of neuronal proteins known to be regulated by cyclic AMP-dependent phosphorylation (see text). Through this action, therefore, opiates induce many and diverse types of effects in target neurons. Second, opiates, via coupling to Gi and/or Go, increase the conductance of certain types of K⁺ channels and decrease the conductance of voltage-dependent Ca²⁺ channels. In most cases, the opiate-regulated K⁺ channel appears to be identical to the inward-rectifying channel regulated by several other types of neurotransmitter receptors (e.g., δ2-dopaminergic, α2-adrenergic, and 5-HT1a-serotonergic receptors), also via coupling with a pertussis toxin-sensitive G protein. Regulation of these channels has direct effects on the electrical properties of the target neurons. Such regulation also leads to decreases in intracellular Ca²⁺ levels and, consequently, to decreases in the activity of calcium-dependent protein kinases (both Ca²⁺/calmodulin-dependent protein kinases and protein kinase C) and the phosphorylation state of numerous types of substrate proteins for these protein kinases. As with regulation of the cyclic-AMP system, opiate-induced changes in calcium-dependent protein phosphorylation leads to many changes in neuronal function.

In addition to these prominent actions of opiates on signal transduction pathways, which have been observed in many tissues by many laboratories, two other actions have been reported (see text). In dorsal root ganglion–spinal cord co-cultures, opiates (via μ, δ, and κ receptors) have been shown to activate adenylate cyclase apparently via coupling with Gs. There is growing evidence to support the physiological importance of this novel opiate action. In addition, opiates have been reported to stimulate the phosphatidylinositol system in a variety of cell types. Such regulation presumably occurs via opiate inhibition or activation of phospholipase C, which catalyzes the breakdown of phosphatidylinositol (PI) into inositol triphosphate (IP3) and diacylglycerol (DAG). Based on our knowledge of the PI system from other studies, one would expect that opiate-induced changes in IP3

ated by μ, δ, or κ receptors, depending on the cell type. In a number of cell types, opiates have been shown to activate an inward-rectifying K^+ channel and/or to inhibit voltage-dependent Ca^{2+} channels; both actions are also mediated via Gi and Go subtypes of G proteins and would be expected to exert inhibitory effects on neuronal activity (for review, see Harris & Nestler, 1993; North, 1979).

In at least one system, namely the dorsal root ganglion–spinal cord preparation, activation of μ, δ, or κ opioid receptors has been shown to result in stimulation of adenylyl cyclase, apparently via coupling to Gs (Crain & Shen, 1990). There are also isolated reports of opiate regulation of second messengers in addition to cyclic AMP, particularly the phosphatidylinositol system: μ, δ, and κ receptor agonists have been reported to stimulate phosphatidylinositol turnover in a variety of experimental preparations (e.g., Barg et al., 1993; Okajima et al., 1993; Smart et al., 1994).

The fact that opiates regulate adenylyl cyclase, Ca^{2+} channels, and phosphatidylinositol turnover indicates that opiates also produce prominent changes in cyclic AMP-dependent and calcium-dependent protein phosphorylation in specific target neurons. Indeed, opiate regulation of protein phosphorylation has been demonstrated in a growing number of experimental systems (Childers, 1991; Guitart & Nestler, 1989; Nestler et al., 1993). As discussed above, such opiate regulation of protein phosphorylation would be expected to mediate the effects of opiates on diverse aspects of neuronal function: for example, on the conductances of specific ion channels, as well as on the sensitivity of various neurotransmitter receptors, neurotransmitter synthesis and release, axonal transport, and, ultimately, gene expression.

CHRONIC ADAPTATIONS IN SIGNAL TRANSDUCTION PATHWAYS AS THE BASIS OF OPIATE TOLERANCE, DEPENDENCE, AND WITHDRAWAL

Opioid Receptors

The discovery of opioid receptors raised the exciting possibility that aspects of opiate addiction might be mediated by alterations in these

---

and DAG levels exert multiple effects on target neurons. Changes in IP3 levels would lead to changes in cellular Ca^{2+} levels (by altering the release Ca^{2+} from intracellular stores) and consequent changes in calcium-dependent protein kinase activity. Changes in DAG would lead to changes in the activity of protein kinase C. Further studies are needed to establish the occurrence and functional importance of opiate regulation of the PI system. From Harris and Nestler (1993). Copyright 1993 by CRC Press. Reprinted by permission.

endogenous receptors. However, over 15 years of research has failed to identify consistent changes in the number of opiate receptors, or changes in their affinity for opiate ligands, under conditions of opiate addiction (see below). It is important to emphasize, however, that these studies have relied exclusively on ligand-binding techniques to assess the effect of opiate treatments on receptors, since opioid receptors have been cloned only recently. It may well prove to be true that a more complete analysis of opiate receptors will reveal important changes in receptor function associated with opiate addiction.

Based on the structure of the known opioid receptors, one form of receptor regulation that would be expected is receptor phosphorylation. Many G protein-coupled receptors are known to be regulated by phoshorylation, with such phosphorylation mediating either heterologous or homologous forms of desensitization. These mechanisms are best established for the β-adrenergic receptor (Lefkowitz, 1993). Activation of the receptor, which is coupled to Gs, results in activation of the cyclic AMP pathway; among the substrates for cyclic AMP-dependent protein kinase is the receptor itself. Such phosphorylation of the receptor functionally uncouples it from Gs. This is a form of heterologous desensitization since activation of the cyclic AMP pathway by any receptor system could produce this type of opioid receptor desensitization. Simultaneously, agonist binding to the receptor induces a conformational change in the receptor that renders it a good substrate for β-adrenergic receptor kinases (or βARKs). Compared to the cyclic AMP-dependent enzyme, βARKs phosphorylate the receptor on distinct amino acid residues. Phosphorylation of the receptor by ARKs triggers its binding to another protein, β-arrestin, which then impedes the ability of the receptor to couple to its Gs. This cascade results in homologous desensitization since only those receptors occupied by an agonist would undergo desensitization. Similar mechanisms have been established for certain other G protein-coupled receptors, and several βARK-like enzymes (termed G protein receptor kinases, or GRKs) have been cloned. There has been indirect evidence to support the notion that opioid receptors are also regulated via phosphorylation (Harada et al., 1989; Werling et al., 1989). Moreover, each of the cloned opioid receptors contains specific serine residues that represent putative sites of phosphorylation. Recently, there have been reports showing direct phosphorylatron of opioid receptors (e.g., Pei et al., 1995).

Chronic exposure to agonists leads to many types of receptor regulation in addition to receptor phosphorylation. These other types of changes, which are also best characterized for the β-adrenergic receptor, include receptor sequestration and recycling within cells and altered levels of expression of receptors at the messenger RNA and protein levels (Duman & Nestler, 1994). The absence of specific probes for the opioid receptors until very recently has made the documentation of such phenomena virtually impossible. However, numerous receptor-binding studies have been carried out to investigate changes induced by chronic opiate exposure. These studies are reviewed elsewhere (Harris & Nestler, 1993; Johnson & Fleming, 1989; Loh & Smith, 1990) and only selected examples are given here. Long-term incubation of cultured cell lines with D-ala, D-leu enkephalin (DADLE) or diprenorphine results in down-regulation of opioid receptors as evidenced by a decrease in maximal specific binding. These and other studies have provided compelling evidence that, in cultured cell lines, opioid receptors can be modified by chronic opiate exposure. However, it remains unclear whether these results can be extended to predict changes in opioid receptors in the intact central nervous system. For example, in one study, chronic administration of etorphine to rats resulted in regional changes in binding, but these changes failed to correlate with the induction of behavioral tolerance (Tao et al., 1987). Many other studies have failed to detect changes in opiate binding induced by chronic opiate exposure (Harris & Nestler, 1993).

Inconsistent findings obtained with ligand-binding studies make it difficult to attribute opiate tolerance and dependence to changes in opiate receptors per se. Now that opioid receptors have at long last been cloned, it will be possible to investigate opiate regulation of opioid receptors by use of more specific probes (cDNAs, antibodies) to determine whether, for each type of opioid receptor, chronic exposure to opiates results in altered expression, phosphorylation, and so forth, of the receptor and whether such alterations are related to opiate tolerance, dependence, and withdrawal in specific neuronal cell types.

Postreceptor Signal Transduction Pathways

In contrast to the difficulty of establishing consistent effects of chronic opiate exposure on opioid receptors, studies of the chronic effects of opiates on postreceptor signal transduction pathways have been more fruitful. The first studies of such postreceptor mechanisms of opiate addiction were carried out in cultured cell lines. Acutely, opiates were found to decrease cellular levels of cyclic AMP in neuroblastoma–glioma cells (Sharma et al., 1975). Chronic exposure was found to result in substantial increases in adenylyl cyclase activity in this system. This compensatory up-regulation of adenylyl cyclase was proposed to represent the biochemical equivalence of tolerance and dependence. However, the physiological significance of these findings has remained unclear until recently.

More recently, similar types of mechanisms have been identified in specific regions of the central nervous system. As will be seen below, it now appears that chronic exposure to opiates produces long-term changes in levels of specific G protein subunits and in the individual proteins that comprise the cyclic AMP system in a number of opiate-responsive neurons in the central nervous system. Increasing evidence indicates that such postreceptor adaptations play an important role in opiate tolerance, dependence, and withdrawal.

OPIATE ACTION IN THE LOCUS COERULEUS

The locus coeruleus (LC) is located on the floor of the fourth ventricle in the anterior pons (see Figure 3.3). It contains the major noradrenergic nucleus in the brain, with widespread projections to both the brain and spinal cord. This diffuse innervation allows the LC to regulate the animal's general state of arousal, attention, and autonomic tone. An important role for the LC in opiate physical dependence and withdrawal has been established at both the behavioral and electrophysiological levels: overactivation of LC neurons is both necessary and sufficient for producing many of the behavioral signs of withdrawal (Aghajanian, 1978; Koob et al., 1992; Maldonado & Koob, 1993; Nestler, 1992; Nestler et al., 1993; Rasmussen et al., 1990). Indeed, it was this knowledge of the LC's role in physical opiate dependence that led to the introduction of clonidine, an α2-adrenergic agonist that produces effects on the LC similar to those of morphine (Aghajanian, 1978), as the first non-

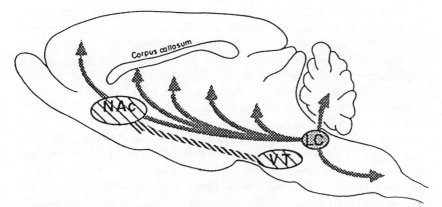

FIGURE 3.3. Schematic illustration of the location of the locus coeruleus (LC), ventral tegmental area (VT), and nucleus accumbens (NAc) in the rat brain. From Nestler et al. (1994). Copyright 1994 by American Psychiatric Press. Reprinted by permission.

opiate treatment for opiate withdrawal used clinically (Gold et al., 1978). It is now known that overactivation of LC neurons during withdrawal arises from both extrinsic and intrinsic sources. The extrinsic source involves a hyperactive excitatory glutamatergic input to the LC from the nucleus paragigantocellularis (Akaoka & Aston-Jones, 1991; Rasmussen & Aghajanian, 1989). The intrinsic source involves intracellular adaptations in signal transduction pathways coupled to opioid receptors in the LC neurons.

MECHANISMS OF ACUTE AND CHRONIC OPIATE ACTION ON LOCUS COERULEUS NEURONS

Acutely, opiates inhibit LC neurons via activation of an inward-rectifying K^+ channel and inhibition of an inward Na^+ current (Aghajanian & Wang, 1986; Alreja & Aghajanian, 1993; North et al., 1987). Both actions are mediated via pertussis toxin-sensitive G proteins (i.e., Gi or Go). Opiates directly activate the K^+ channel via Gi or Go proteins. In contrast, inhibition of the Na^+ current appears to be indirect, through Gi-mediated inhibition of cyclic AMP formation and reduced cyclic AMP-dependent protein kinase activity (Alreja & Aghajanian, 1993). Biochemical studies have confirmed that opiates acutely inhibit adenylyl cyclase activity and cyclic AMP-dependent protein phosphorylation in the LC (Guitart & Nestler, 1989; Nestler, 1992) (Figure 3.4 top).

Chronically, LC neurons develop tolerance to these acute inhibitory actions of opiates, as neuronal activity recovers toward preexposure levels (Aghajanian, 1978; Christie et al., 1987). Abrupt cessation of opiate treatment, for example, via administration of an opioid receptor antagonist, causes a marked increase in neuronal firing rates above preexposure levels both *in vivo* and in isolated slice preparations (Aghajanian, 1978, Kogen et al., 1992; Rasmussen et al., 1990). Given the role of G proteins and the cyclic AMP pathway in the acute electrophysiological actions of opiates on LC neurons, long-term adaptations in intracellular messenger proteins along this pathway have been studied to determine whether they could be involved in the tolerance, dependence, and withdrawal observed in these neurons. Chronic opiate exposure has been shown to increase LC levels of Gi and Go, adenylyl cyclase, cyclic AMP-dependent protein kinase, and several phosphoprotein substrates for the protein kinase (Guitart & Nestler, 1989; Nestler, 1992). One of these substrates, tyrosine hydroxylase, is the rate-limiting enzyme in the biosynthesis of norepinephrine. This up-regulation of the cyclic AMP pathway occurs in the absence of alterations in several other major protein kinases in this brain region.

The up-regulated cyclic AMP pathway is thought to contribute to the reduced ability of opiates to inhibit the activity of LC neurons, and thus to account, at least in part, for opiate tolerance. In addition, these compensatory adaptations appear to contribute to the intrinsic hyperexcitability of LC neurons seen during withdrawal (Kogan et al., 1992; Nestler, 1992; Nestler et al., 1993) (Figure 3.4 bottom). This scheme is similar to one proposed earlier based on studies of neuroblastoma–glioma cells (Sharma et al., 1975). While there are likely other mechanisms of opiate dependence in the LC and elsewhere, up-regulation of the cyclic AMP pathway represents one example in which some of the behavioral manifestations of opiate dependence can be attributed directly to molecular and cellular adaptations in specific neurons. Related work, to be discussed below, has suggested that similar types of adaptations may underlie the long-term actions of opiates in other regions of the central nervous system.

MOLECULAR MECHANISMS OF OPIATE ACTION

One of the central questions raised by these studies concerns the precise molecular mechanisms by which chronic opiate administration leads to up-regulation of the G protein/cyclic AMP system in the LC. Recent evidence indicates that many of the intracellular adaptations occur at the protein and messenger RNA level (Nestler et al., 1993). Although there are many mechanisms by which levels of proteins and mRNAs can be modified in a neuron, the most widely investigated involves the regulation of gene expression.

Neurotransmitter regulation of gene expression is now known to occur via second messenger-dependent phosphorylation and/or induction of a class of proteins referred to as transcription factors—that is, proteins that bind to specific DNA sequences (called response elements) in the promoter regions of genes and that thereby increase or decrease the rate at which those genes are transcribed (Hyman & Nestler, 1993; Morgan & Curran, 1991). Two general types of mechanisms appear to be involved. In the first, protein kinases, activated in response to a first- and second-messenger stimulus, phosphorylate and activate transcription factors that are already present in the cell. CREB (cyclic AMP response element binding) proteins function in this manner. CREB proteins consist of a family of related transcription factors that mediate many of the effects of cyclic AMP (and probably of calcium), and of those neurotransmitters that act through cyclic AMP (and calcium), on

ACUTE OPIATE ACTION IN THE LC

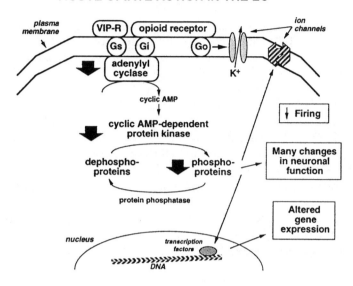

CHRONIC OPIATE ACTION IN THE LC

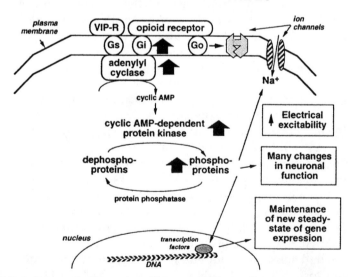

FIGURE 3.4. Schematic illustration of the mechanisms of acute and chronic opiate action in the locus coeruleus. Top panel: Opiates acutely inhibit locus coeruleus neurons by increasing the conductance of a K^+ channel (stippled) via coupling with a pertussis toxin-inhibitable G protein (perhaps Go), and by decreasing the conductance of a nonspecific cation channel (striped) via coupling with Gi (the inhibitory G protein) and the consequent inhibition of the cyclic AMP pathway (downward bold arrows) and reduced phosphorylation of the channel or a closely

gene expression. Alternatively, protein kinases, through the phosphory-lation and activation of CREB or a CREB-like protein, stimulate the expression of a family of transcription factor genes referred to as im-mediate early genes, for example, c-fos, c-jun, and zif268. The newly synthesized immediate early gene products would return to the nucleus where they would regulate the expression of other target genes. Figure 3.5 illustrates the potential role played by these mechanisms in medi-ating the addictive actions of opiates in the LC and elsewhere in the nervous system.

There have to date been a few studies aimed at identifying the specific transcription factors through which opiates might regulate the expression of G proteins and the cyclic AMP system in the LC. In 1990, it was demonstrated that, acutely, opiates decrease levels of c-fos ex-pression in the LC and that such decreased expression persists with chronic opiate administration (Hayward et al., 1990). In contrast, c-fos expression is induced severalfold during naltrexone-precipitated opi-ate withdrawal. Similar regulation of c-jun was observed in this study. These investigations indicate that decreased levels of c-fos (and relat-ed transcription factors) might play a role in triggering and in main-taining some of the intracellular adaptations to chronic morphine and that increased levels of the transcription factors might be involved in the recovery of these adaptations during withdrawal. Induction of c-fos during opiate withdrawal was also observed in a number of other regions of the central nervous system, suggesting that this transcrip-tion factor probably mediates some of the effects of opiates on gene expression in a number of neuronal cell types.

More recently, opiate regulation of CREB has been studied in the LC (Guitart et al., 1992). Acute morphine administration was found to decrease the phosphorylation state of CREB, an effect that became

---

associated protein. Inhibition of the cyclic AMP pathway, via decreased phosphory-lation of numerous other proteins, would affect many processes in the neuron; in addition to reducing firing rates, for example, it would initiate alterations in gene expression via regulation of transcription factors. Bottom panel: Chronic adminis-tration of opiates leads to a compensatory up-regulation of the cyclic AMP path-way (upward bold arrows), which contributes to opiate dependence in the neurons by increasing their intrinsic excitability via increased activation of the nonspecific cation channel. In addition, up-regulation of the cyclic AMP pathway presumably would be associated with persistent changes in transcription factors that maintain the chronic morphine-treated state. Chronic opiate administration also leads to a relative decrease in the degree of activation of the K^+ channel owing to tolerance, the mechanism of which is unknown. Also shown in the figure are VIP-R, or vasoac-tive intestinal polypeptide receptor (VIP is a major activator of the cyclic AMP path-way in the LC), and Gs, the stimulatory G protein that activates adenylate cyclase. From Nestler (1992). Copyright 1992 by Oxford University Press. Reprinted by per-mission.

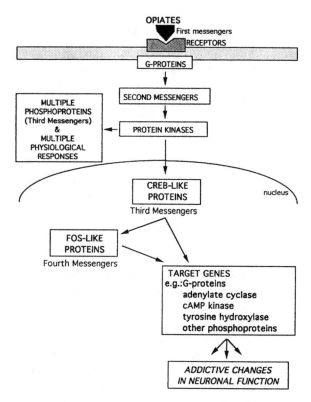

FIGURE 3.5. Schematic illustration of the intracellular messenger pathways through which opiates and other extracellular signals regulate gene expression in target neurons. CREB-like transcription factors refer to those that are expressed constitutively and that are by extracellular agents primarily through changes in their degree of phosphorylation. Transcription factors that are fos-like refer to those that are expressed at very low levels under basal conditions and that are regulated by extracellular agents primarily through induction of the expression of the transcription factors (presumably via CREB-like proteins). Both types of mechanisms could contribute to the addictive actions of opiates and other drugs of abuse. From Nestler (1992). Copyright 1992 by Oxford University Press. Reprinted by permission.

attenuated after chronic exposure to the opiate. In contrast, acute precipitation of opiate withdrawal increased CREB phosphorylation in this brain region. This regulation of CREB phosphorylation is consistent with the known effects of acute and chronic opiates and of opiate withdrawal on the activity of the cyclic AMP system in the LC. Chronic opiate exposure has also been shown to increase the total amount of CREB in the LC (Widnell et al., 1994). Studies are now needed to relate altered CREB phosphorylation and total amount to the altered levels of expression of specific G proteins and of protein constituents of the cyclic AMP pathway in this brain region.

These studies of opiate regulation of transcription factors, while preliminary, highlight the utility of the LC as a model system in which to study transcription factor regulation: a system in which specific target genes have been identified and in which changes in those genes have been shown to be physiologically important. Through increasingly mechanistic studies of this system, it will be possible to delineate the precise molecular steps by which opiates regulate the expression of specific intracellular messenger proteins and, as a result, induce aspects of tolerance, dependence, and withdrawal in these neurons.

EXTRINSIC FACTORS IN WITHDRAWAL ACTIVATION OF THE LOCUS COERULEUS

The above discussion of opiate addiction in the LC focuses on factors that are intrinsic to LC neurons. However, extrinsic factors also contribute importantly to opiate dependence and withdrawal exhibited by the LC. Thus, lesions of the PGi, a region in the rostral medulla that provides a major excitatory input to the LC (Ennis & Aston-Jones, 1988), partially attenuates the severalfold withdrawal activation of LC neurons *in vivo* (Rasmussen & Aghajanian, 1989). Intracerebroventricular or intracoerulear administration of glutamate receptor antagonists produces a similar effect (Akaoka & Aston-Jones, 1991; Rasmussen & Aghajanian, 1989), consistent with the view that the PGi input to the LC is mediated by an excitatory amino acid, presumably glutamate. Based on the twofold withdrawal activation of LC neurons observed in brain slices *in vitro*, and the partial ($\approx 50\%$) reduction in withdrawal activation induced by PGi lesions or kynurenic acid *in vivo*, it would appear that intrinsic and extrinsic factors contribute about equally to the overall withdrawal activation of LC neurons observed in the intact animal. Of course, this leaves unanswered the resulting question, namely, the location and nature of the changes that underlie the role of the PGi in withdrawal activation of LC neurons. Such changes could conceivably occur (1) in nerve terminals within the LC that are derived from the PGi, (2) in PGi cell bodies, and/or (3) in any afferents that innervate the PGi (e.g., spinal regions). Indeed, chronic opiate-induced up-regulation of the cyclic AMP system, similar to that observed in the LC, has been observed in dorsal root ganglion–spinal cord cultures (see below) and, in preliminary studies, in the PGi itself (Nestler, 1992). Further studies are needed to investigate the role played by these changes in the actions of the PGi on the LC during opiate withdrawal.

Such knowledge of the role of excessive glutamatergic activation of the LC during withdrawal may explain, at least in part, the ability of glutamate receptor antagonists to attentuate opiate withdrawal upon systemic administration (Rasmussen et al., 1991). Although glutamate receptor antagonists available for clinical use are still very limited, there are preliminary reports that agents (e.g., dextromethorphan) that decrease glutamate function in the brain attentuate the severity of opiate withdrawal syndromes in people (Koyuncuoglu & Saydam, 1990). A role for glutamate in the long-term actions of opiates on the nervous system is indicated further by the findings that administration of competitive and noncompetitive NMDA glutamate receptor antagonists can attenuate the development of physical opiate dependence as well as reduce the tolerance that develops to the antinociceptive effects of opiates (Tiseo et al., 1994; Trujillo & Akil, 1990).

Inhibitors of nitric oxide synthetase (NOS), the enzyme that generates nitric oxide, have been shown to similarly reduce development of opiate tolerance (Kolesnikov et al., 1993). The rationale for this experiment is the evidence, stated above, that NMDA glutamate antagonists attenuate opiate tolerance and that the generation of nitric oxide in the nervous system can be stimulated upon activation of NMDA glutamate receptors (Duman & Nestler, 1994). Nitric oxide then functions as a second messenger in regulating a variety of intracellular processes.

While these studies highlight potential approaches to the development of new treatments for opiate tolerance and physical dependence, they must be viewed with caution. Glutamatergic neurotransmission occurs at a large fraction of all synapses in the brain, such that the above observations may indicate the requirement for multiple, intact neural networks in the development and expression of opiate tolerance and dependence and not a specific role for glutamate in these phenomena per se.

OPIATE ACTION IN THE MESOLIMBIC DOPAMINE SYSTEM

Increasing evidence indicates that the mesolimbic dopamine system — consisting of dopaminergic neurons in the ventral tegmental area (VTA) and their projection regions, most notably the nucleus accumbens (NAc) — plays an important role in mediating the reinforcing actions of opiates on brain function (see Figure 3.3). Animals will self-administer opiates directly into the VTA and NAc and will develop conditioned place preference after such local drug administration (Koob, 1992; Self & Nestler, 1995; Wise, 1990). Moreover, lesions of the VTA and NAc attenuate the systemic self-administration of opiates. Other regions of the mesolimbic dopamine system have been similarly implicated in opiate reinforcement, including the ventral pallidum, which receives a major input from the NAc. Similar types of experiments have implicated these same brain structures in the reinforcing actions of cocaine and amphetamine. It is also known that virtually any drug abused by humans, including opiates, cocaine, amphetamine, ethanol, nicotine, and 9-tetrahydrocannabinol, causes increased dopamine release in the NAc after acute administration (Chen et al., 1990; DiChiara & Imperato, 1988). These findings strongly implicate the VTA-NAc mesolimbic dopamine pathway as a neural substrate of drug reward mechanisms in general. It should be noted that while opiates do exert rewarding effects via the mesolimbic dopamine system, there are also non-dopaminergic mechanisms of opiate reward (Koob, 1992).

Much less is known about the electrophysiological actions of opiates on the mesolimbic dopamine system compared to the LC, in part because the VTA and NAc are much more heterogeneous brain regions. Nevertheless, a number of studies have investigated opiate action in the VTA and NAc. Both regions contain high levels of μ, δ, and κ opiate receptors. Acute systemic administration of opiates to rats excites dopaminergic neurons of the VTA. Studies in brain slices *in vitro* have shown that such activation represents an indirect effect of the opiates: opiates, apparently via activation of μ receptors, directly inhibit GABA-ergic neurons within the VTA and thereby reduce the inhibitory influence of these cells on the dopaminergic neurons (Johnson & North, 1992). Opiates are primarily, but not exclusively, inhibitory in the NAc after systemic administration. Opiates can inhibit NAc neurons directly as well as indirectly via actions on the VTA (Hakan & Hendrikson, 1989). Presumably, opiate activation of the VTA increases dopaminergic transmission to the NAc, which is inhibitory to most cells in that brain region. In contrast to these acute actions of opiates on the VTA and NAc, virtually nothing is known about the electrophysiological responses of these neurons to chronic opiate exposure.

There have been numerous studies of opiate-induced changes in levels of neurotransmitters and their receptors as possible mediators of the long-term effects of opiates in the VTA and NAc. However, as stated earlier in this chapter, it has been difficult to identify changes in opioid receptors in the brain, including the mesolimbic dopamine system, in response to chronic opiate administration. Opiate-induced adaptations in other neurotransmitter receptors have similarly not been consistently observed in this neural pathway. In contrast, there are numerous reports that chronic opiate exposure can alter extracellular levels of dopamine in the VTA-NAc pathway as determined by *in vivo* microdialysis (e.g., Acquas et al., 1990). Such changes in dopamine levels could be involved in chronic opiate-induced alterations in drug reward mechanisms. The molecular mechanisms underlying such changes in dopamine levels remain unknown but could be related to opiate regulation of tyrosine hydroxylase in the VTA and NAc (Beitner-Johnson & Nestler, 1991; see below).

ADAPTATIONS IN G PROTEINS AND THE CYCLIC AMP PATHWAY IN THE NAc

Chronic opiate exposure induces similar adaptations in G proteins and the cyclic AMP pathway in the NAc as seen in the LC, with decreased levels of Gi and increased levels of adenylyl cyclase and cyclic AMP-dependent protein kinase activity observed in the NAc (Terwilliger et al., 1991). The physiological significance of these intracellular adaptations cannot be understood fully until the functional effects of chronic opiates on NAc neuronal activity are established. Nevertheless, recent studies suggest that such intracellular changes may be functionally important and relevant to drug reward mechanisms. First, chronic exposure to cocaine or ethanol produces changes in G proteins, adenylyl cyclase, and cyclic AMP-dependent protein kinase equivalent to those observed in response to chronic morphine, whereas chronic exposure to several drugs without reinforcing properties fails to produce these changes (Nestler et al., 1993). Second, administration of agents that activate or inhibit Gi/Go or cyclic AMP-dependent protein kinase directly into the NAc has been shown recently to regulate the acute reinforcing properties of opiates and cocaine as measured by drug self-administration (Self & Nestler, 1995). These findings provide the first direct evidence that adaptations in G proteins and the cyclic AMP pathway following chronic opiate (or cocaine or alcohol) exposure may represent part of the pathophysiological mechanisms underlying long-term, drug-induced changes in drug reward mechanisms (e.g., drug craving) mediated via the NAc.

ADAPTATIONS IN THE VENTRAL TEGMENTAL AREA

Chronic morphine, cocaine, and alcohol administration have also been shown to regulate many of the same proteins in the VTA (Beitner-Johnson et al., 1992; Nestler et al., 1993). Among these proteins are tyrosine hydroxylase and glial fibrillary acidic protein (the major intermediate filament protein in astrocytes), both of which are up-regulated by drug treatment, and several neurofilament proteins (the major intermediate filament protein in neurons), which are down-regulated by drug treatment. As would be expected, this down-regulation in neurofilaments is associated with impaired axoplasmic transport from the VTA to the NAc. Together, these findings, particularly the reciprocal regulation of glial and neurofilament proteins, would suggest that chronic morphine administration is associated with prominent structural and functional changes in VTA dopamine neurons, perhaps even changes that resemble neural insult or injury. Further work is needed to define the physiological consequences of these various biochemical adaptations in the VTA, as well as to relate those changes to specific behavioral features of drug addiction.

OPIATE ACTIONS IN THE DORSAL ROOT GANGLION AND SPINAL CORD

The dorsal root ganglion (DRG) and spinal cord play an important role in the analgesic effects of opiates. These regions contain high levels of μ, δ, and κ opioid receptors, and complex electrophysiological effects of opiates have been described on these neurons. Much of this work has been performed by Crain and by Attali and Vogel and their colleagues on cultures of DRG and spinal cord neurons *in vitro*. Acutely, the most prominent effect of opiates on DRG neurons is inhibition of the cells via a μ, δ, and κ receptor-induced increase in the conductance of K^+ channels, and a κ receptor-induced decrease in the conductance of voltage-dependent Ca^{2+} channels (Attali et al., 1989; Crain & Shen, 1990; Shen & Crain, 1989). These actions are mediated via Gi and/or Go. Acute opiates also inhibit adenylyl cyclase in DRG–spinal cord cultures (Makman et al., 1988), an action that may further contribute to the acute electrophysiological (and other) effects of opiates on these cells.

Neurons in DRG–spinal cord co-cultures develop tolerance to the acute inhibitory effects of opiates with chronic exposure to the drug. Such tolerance could be explained, at least in part, by an up-regulation of the cyclic-AMP system that occurs in the cultures in response to chronic opiate exposure, similar to that observed in the LC and NAc. Chronic opiates decrease levels of Gi (Attali & Vogel, 1989) and increase levels of adenylyl cyclase (Makman et al., 1988) and cyclic AMP-dependent protein kinase (Terwilliger et al., 1991) in these cells.

Chronic exposure of DRG–spinal cord co-cultures to opiates was found to reveal an excitatory effect of opiates on the cells (Crain & Shen, 1990). This excitatory effect appears to be due to loss of the inhibitory effects of opiates (tolerance as mentioned above) and to supersensitization of a direct excitatory effect of opiates on these cells. This excitatory effect appears to represent a novel mechanism of opiate action, namely, opiate receptor coupling to Gs and to the activation of adenylyl cyclase. It will be very interesting in future studies to identify the precise type of opioid receptor that mediates this effect and to identify whether such excitatory responses to opiates are seen elsewhere in the nervous system. Supersensitization of this response in chronic opiate-treated cultures could be explained by up-regulation of the cyclic AMP system observed earlier. There is also evidence that the excitatory effect of opiates on Gs and adenylyl cyclase can be modulated by GM1 ganglioside (a type of membrane lipid) under control conditions and that such modulation, perhaps via changes in levels of the ganglioside, is altered in the opiate-addicted state (Crain & Shen, 1992; Shen & Crain, 1990).

GENERAL ROLE FOR AN UP-REGULATED CYCLIC AMP SYSTEM IN OPIATE ADDICTION

In addition to the LC, NAc, and DRG, chronic opiate exposure has been shown to up-regulate components of the cyclic AMP system in some other discrete regions of the central nervous system, including the amygdala and thalamus (Terwilliger et al., 1991) as well as striatum under certain experimental conditions (Tjon et al., 1994). These findings indicate that up-regulation of adenylyl cyclase and cyclic AMP-dependent protein kinase may represent a common mechanism by which a number of opiate-sensitive neurons adapt to chronic morphine and thereby develop aspects of opiate tolerance, dependence, and/or withdrawal. It is interesting that neurons of the LC, which contribute to physical dependence in the animal, and neurons of the NAc, which contribute to the reinforcing actions of opiates in the animal, show similar biochemical adaptations to chronic opiates. This supports the view that similar biochemical mechanisms mediate both physical and psychological aspects of drug addiction depending on the neuronal cell type involved. The findings emphasize that the distinction between physical and psychological dependence is arbitrary: both are due to changes in brain function mediated via biochemical adaptations in specific neuronal cell types that lead to alterations in the functional state of these neurons and in the particular behavioral parameters subserved by the neurons.

ROLE OF G PROTEINS IN OPIATE ADDICTION

An important question raised by these studies concerns the differential effects that chronic opiate exposure has on the expression of inhibitory G proteins. As noted above, chronic opiate treatment increases levels of Gi and Go in the LC, but decreases levels of Gi in the NAc and DRG-spinal cord co-cultures. Chronic morphine has also been reported to increase levels of these G proteins in the amygdala (Terwilliger et al., 1991) and to alter levels of various G protein subunits in striatal neurons and other brain cells in culture (Van Vliet et al., 1991; Vogel et al., 1990). It has been proposed (Terwilliger et al., 1991) that these differential responses account for the phenomena of homologous and heterologous desensitization observed in these various systems, with increased levels of Gi and Go leading to homologous desensitization and with decreased levels leading to heterologous desensitization.

CONCLUSIONS

The studies described in this chapter support the view that through the investigation of signal tranduction pathways it will be possible to learn a great deal about the biochemical and molecular mechanisms by which opiates and other drugs of abuse induce changes in brain function that underlie addiction. Studies of the LC have provided the clearest indication to date of some of the specific biochemical mechanisms involved in opiate addiction. Adaptations in G proteins and the cyclic AMP second messenger and protein phosphorylation system have been shown to play an important role in mediating opiate tolerance, dependence, and withdrawal in this cell type. There are indications that similar mechanisms may be involved in a number of other opiate-responsive neurons, including neurons in the mesolimbic dopamine system, a system that plays a critical role in the rewarding properties of opiates.

It will be important in future studies to identify the precise molecular pathways through which chronic opiate treatments produce alterations in intracellular messenger pathways in their target neurons. Given the preliminary evidence that such alterations are mediated, at least in part, at the level of gene expression, opiate regulation of transcription factors would appear to represent the ultimate mechanism by which addictive changes are induced in the brain (see Figure 3.5). Studies are needed, therefore, to characterize the effects of acute and chronic drug treatment on specific types of transcription factors in opiate-responsive brain regions. Eventually, it will be necessary to provide direct evidence for a causal role of a particular factor in mediating changes in brain function associated with addiction. While this is a particularly difficult challenge in an *in vivo* setting, recently developed tools in molecular biology (e.g., involving the use of antisense oligonucleotides or transgenic and gene knock-out animals) make these types of studies feasible for the first time.

One of the major advantages of the LC and DRG–spinal cord systems, as discussed above, is the relative ease with which it has been possible to relate biochemical and molecular phenomena to electrophysiological changes known to reflect opiate tolerance, dependence, and withdrawal. In contrast, our relative lack of knowledge of the influence of chronic opiates on VTA and NAc neurons has made less straightforward the assessment of the functional significance of adaptations in G proteins and the cyclic AMP system in these other brain regions. Clearly, studies that attempt to correlate biochemical and electrophysiological regulation of these cells are needed. Eventually, the role played by specific biochemical changes in a given brain region in mediating aspects of drug addiction can be tested in various animal models. A related line of investigation concerns identification of specific genes that modify an individual's responsiveness to opiates and other drugs of abuse after acute and chronic administration. Among such genes are probably those that contribute to an individual's vulnerability to drug addiction.

These studies of the molecular neurobiology of drug addiction have a number of potential implications. A better understanding of the mechanisms underlying drug addiction will lead to the development of pharmacological agents that prevent or reverse the actions of the drugs on specific target neurons. Such drugs could be used not only to treat physical abstinence syndromes but also to reduce the craving for abused substances. Such latter actions by pharmacological agents would represent a revolutionary step in our battle against drug addiction. Moreover, identification of some of the genetic factors that predispose individuals to drug abuse would greatly advance our understanding of drug addiction, as well as its eventual treatment and prevention.

ACKNOWLEDGMENTS

This work was supported by U.S. Public Health Service Grant Nos. DA08220, DA07359, DA00203, and DA04060, and by the Abraham Ribicoff Research Facilities, Connecticut Mental Health Center, State of Connecticut Department of Mental Health.

REFERENCES

Acquas, E., Carboni, E., & DiChiara, G. (1990). Profound depression of mesolimbic dopamine release after morphine withdrawal in dependent rats. *European Journal of Pharmacology, 193*, 133–134.

Aghajanian, G. K. (1978). Tolerance of locus coeruleus neurones to morphine and suppression of withdrawal response by clonidine. *Nature, 267*, 186–188.

Aghajanian, G. K., & Wang, Y. Y. (1986). Pertussis toxin blocks the outward currents evoked by opiate and 2-agonists in locus coeruleus neurons. *Brain Research, 371*, 390–394.

Akaoka, A., & Aston-Jones, G. (1991). Opiate withdrawal-induced hyperactivity of locus coeruleus neurons is substantially mediated by augmented excitatory amino acid input. *Journal of Neuroscience, 11*, 3830–3839.

Alreja, M., & Aghajanian, G. K. (1993). Opiates suppress a resting sodium-dependent inward current in addition to activating an outward potassium current in locus coeruleus neurons. *Journal of Neuroscience, 13*, 3525–3532.

Attali, B., Saya, D., Nah, S., & Vogel, Z. (1989). Kappa opiate agonists inhibit Ca^{++} influx in rat spinal cord-dorsal root ganglion cocultures. *Journal of Biological Chemistry, 264*, 347–353.

Attali, B., & Vogel, Z. (1989). Long-term opiate exposure leads to reduction of the ai-1 subunit of GTP-binding proteins. *Journal of Neurochemistry, 53*, 1636–1639.

Barg, J., Belcheva, M. M., Rowinski, J., & Coscia, C.J. (1993). K-Opioid agonist modulation of [3H]thymidine incorporation into DNA: Evidence for the involvement of pertussis toxin-sensitive G protein-coupled phosphoinositide turnover. *Journal of Neurochemistry, 60*, 1505–1511.

Beitner-Johnson, D., Guitart, X., & Nestler, E. J. (1992). Neurofilament proteins and the mesolimbic dopamine system: Common regulation by chronic morphine and chronic cocaine in the rat ventral tegmental area. *Journal of Neuroscience, 12*, 2165–2176.

Beitner-Johnson, D., & Nestler, E. J. (1991). Morphine and cocaine exert common chronic actions on tyrosine hydroxylase in dopaminergic brain reward regions. *Journal of Neurochemistry, 57*, 344–347.

Chen, J., Paredes, W., Li, J., Smithe, D., Lowinson, J., & Gardener, E. L. (1990). 9-Tetrahydrocannabinol produces naloxone-blockable enhancement of presynaptic basal dopamine efflux in nucleus accumbens of conscious, freely-moving rats as measured by intracerebral microdialysis. *Psychopharmacology, 102*, 156–162.

Childers, S. (1991). Opioid receptor-coupled second messenger systems. *Life Science, 48*, 1991–2003.

Christie, M. J., Williams, J. T., & North, R. A. (1987). Cellular mechanisms of opioid tolerance: Studies in single brain neurons. *Molecular Pharmacology, 32*, 633–638.

Crain, S. M., Crain, B., & Makman, M. H. (1987). Pertussis toxin blocks depressant effects of opioid, monoaminergic and muscarinic agonists on dorsal-horn network responses in spinal cord–ganglion cultures. *Brain Research, 400*, 185–190.

Crain, S. M., & Shen, K. F. (1990). Opioids can evoke direct receptor-mediated excitatory effects on sensory neurons. *Trends in Pharmacological Sciences, 11,* 77–81.

Crain, S. M., & Shen, K. F. (1992). After chronic opioid exposure sensory neurons become supersensitive to the excitatory effects of opioid agonists and antagonists as occurs after acute elevation of GM1 ganglioside. *Brain Research, 575,* 13–24.

DiChiara, G., & Imperato, A. (1988). Drugs abused by humans preferentially increase synaptic dopamine concentrations in the mesolimbic system of freely moving rats. *Proceedings of the Nationall Academy of Sciences of the United States of America, 85,* 5274–5278.

Duman, R. S., & Nestler, E. J. (1994). Signal transduction pathways for catecholamine receptors, In F. E. Bloom & D. J. Kupfer (Eds.), *Psychopharmacology: Fourth generation of progress* (pp. 303–320). New York: Raven Press.

Ennis, M., & Aston-Jones, G. (1988). Activation of locus coeruleus from nucleus para-gigantocellularis: A new excitatory amino acid pathway in brain. *Journal of Neuroscience, 8,* 3644–3657.

Evans, C. J., Keith, D. E. Jr., Morrison, H., Magendzo, K., & Edwards, R. H. (1992). Cloning a delta opioid receptor by functional expression. *Science, 258,* 1952–1955.

Gold, M. S., Redmond, D. E., & Kleber, H. D. (1978). Clonidine in opiate withdrawal. *Lancet, ii,* 599–602.

Guitart, X., & Nestler, E. J. (1989). Identification of morphine and cyclic AMP-regulated phosphoproteins (MARPPs) in the locus coeruleus and other regions of rat brain. Regulation by acute and chronic morphine. *Journal of Neuroscience, 9,* 4371–4387.

Guitart, X., Thompson, M., Greenberg, M. E., & Nestler, E. J. (1992). Regulation of CREB phosphorylation by acute and chronic morphine in the rat locus coeruleus. *Journal of Neurochemistry, 58,* 1168–1171.

Hakan, R. L., & Hendrikson, S. J. (1989). Opiate influences on nucleus accumbens neuronal electrophysiology: Dopamine and non-dopamine mechanisms. *Journal of Neuroscience, 9,* 3538–3546.

Harada, H., Ueda, H., Wada, Y., Katada, T., Ui, M., & Satoh, M. (1989). Phosphorylation of m-opioid receptors: A putative mechanism of selective uncoupling of receptor–Gi interaction, measured with low-Km GTPase and nucleotide-sensitive agonist binding. *Neuroscience Letters, 100,* 221–226.

Harris, H. W., & Nestler, E. J. (1993). Opiate regulation of signal transduction pathways, In R. P. Hammer Jr. (Ed.), *The neurobiology of opiates* (pp. 301–332). Boca Raton, FL: CRC Press.

Hayward, M. D., Duman, R. S., & Nestler, E. J. (1990). Induction of the c-fos proto-oncogene during opiate withdrawal in the locus coeruleus and other regions of rat brain. *Brain Research, 525,* 256–266.

Hyman, S. E., & Nestler, E. J. (1993). *The molecular foundations of psychiatry.* Washington, DC: American Psychiatric Press.

Johnson, S. M., & Fleming, W. W. (1989). Mechanisms of cellular adaptive sensitivity changes: Applications to opioid tolerance and dependence. *Pharmacological Reviews, 41,* 435–488.

Johnson, S. W., & North, R. A. (1992). Opioids excite dopamine neurons by hyperpolarization of local interneurons. *Journal of Neuroscience, 12*, 483–488.

Kogan, J. H., Nestler, E. J., & Aghajanian, G. K. (1992). Elevated basal firing rates and enhanced responses to 8-Br-cAMP in locus coeruleus neurons in brain slices from opiate-dependent rats. *European Journal of Pharmacology, 211*, 47–53.

Kolesnikov, Y., Pick, C. G., Ciszewska, G., & Pasternak, G. W. (1993). Blockade of tolerance to morphine but not to k opioids by a nitric oxide synthase inhibitor. *Proceedings of the National Academy of Sciences of the United States of America, 90*, 5162–5166.

Koob, G. F. (1992). Drugs of abuse: Anatomy, pharmacology and function of reward pathways. *Trends in Pharmacological Sciences, 13*, 177–184.

Koob, G. F., Maldonado, R., & Stinus, L. (1992). Neural substrates of opiate withdrawal. *Trends in Neurosciences, 15*, 186–191.

Koyuncuoglu, H., & Saydam, B. (1990). Treatment of heroin addicts with dextromethorphan: A double-blind comparison of dextromethorphan with chlorpromazine. *International Journal of Clinical Pharmacology, Therapy and Toxicology, 28*, 147–152.

Lefkowitz, R. J. G. (1993). Protein-coupled receptor kinases. *Cell*, 74409–74412.

Loh, H. H., & Smith, A. P. (1990). Molecular characterization of opioid receptors. *Annual Review of Pharmacology and Toxicology, 30*, 123–147.

Makman, M. H., Dvorkin, B., & Crain, S. M. (1988). Modulation of adenylate cyclase activity of mouse spinal cord–ganglion explants by opioids, serotonin and pertussis toxin. *Brain Research, 445*, 303–313.

Maldonado, R., & Koob, G. F. (1993). Destruction of the locus coeruleus decreases physical signs of opiate withdrawal. *Brain Research, 605*, 128–138.

Morgan, J. I., & Curran, T. (1991). Stimulus-transcription coupling in the nervous system. *Annual Review of Neuroscience, 14*, 421–452.

Nestler, E. J. (1992). Molecular mechanisms of drug addiction. *Journal of Neuroscience, 12*, 2439–2450.

Nestler, E. J. (1994). Molecular neurobiology of drug addiction. *Neuropsychopharmacology, 11*, 77–87.

Nestler, E. J., & Duman, R. S. (1994). G-proteins and cyclic nucleotides in the nervous system, In G. J. Siegel, R. W. Albers, B. W. Agranoff, & P. Molinoff (Eds.), *Basic neurochemistry: Molecular, cellular, and medical aspects* (5th ed., pp. 429–448). Boston: Little, Brown.

Nestler, E. J., Fitzgerald, L. W., & Self, D. W. (1994). Neurobiology of substance abuse. In *APA annual review of psychiatry* (Vol. 14, pp. 51–81). Washington, DC: American Psychiatric Press.

Nestler, E. J., & Greengard, P. (1994). Protein phosphorylation and the regulation of neuronal function. In G. J. Siegel et al. (Eds.), *Basic neurochemistry: Molecular, cellular and medical aspects* (5th Ed., pp. 449–474). New York: Raven Press.

Nestler, E. J., Hope, B. T., & Widnell, K. L. (1993). Drug addiction: A model for the molecular basis of neural plasticity. *Neuron, 11*, 995–1006.

North, R. A. (1979). Minireview: Opiates, opioid peptides and single neurones. *Life Sciences, 24*, 1527–1546.

North, R. A., Williams, J. T., Suprenant, A., & Christie, M. J. (1987). m and a receptors belong to a family of receptors that are coupled to potassium channels. *Proceedings of the National Academy of Sciences of the United States of America, 84,* 5487–5491.

Okajima, F., Tomura, H., & Kondo, Y. (1993). Enkephalin activates the phospholipase C/Ca^{2+} system through cross-talk between opioid receptors and P2-purinergic or bradykinin receptors in Ng 108-15 cells. *Biochemical Journal, 290,* 241–247.

Pasternak, G. W. (1988). Multiple morphine and enkephalin receptors and the relief of pain. *Journal of the American Medical Association, 259,* 1362–1367.

Pei, G., Kieffer, B. L., Lefkowitz, R. J., & Freedman, N. J. (1995). Agonist-dependent phosphorylation of the mouse delta-opioid receptor: Involvement of G protein-couples receptor kinases but not protein knase C. *Molecular Pharmacology, 48,* 173–177.

Rasmussen, K., & Aghajanian, G. K. (1989). Withdrawal-induced activation of locus coeruleus neurons in opiate-dependent rats: Attenuation by lesions of the nucleus paragigantocellularis. *Brain Research, 505,* 346–350.

Rasmussen, K., Beitner-Johnson, D., Krystal, J. H., Aghajanian, G. K., & Nestler, E. J. (1990). Opiate withdrawal and the rat locus coeruleus: Behavioral, electrophysiological, and biochemical correlates. *Journal of Neuroscience, 10,* 2308–2317.

Rasmussen, K., Krystal, J. H., & Aghajanian, G. K. (1991). Excitatory amino acids and morphine withdrawal: Differential effects of central and peripheral kynurenic acid administration. *Psychopharmacology, 105,* 508–512.

Reisine, T., & Bell, G. I. (1993). Molecular biology of opioid receptors. *Trends in Neurosciences, 16,* 506–510.

Self, D. W., & Nestler, E. J. (1995). Molecular mechanisms of drug reinforcement and addiction. *Annual Review of Neuroscience, 18,* 463–495.

Sharma, S. K., Klee, W. A., & Nirenberg, M. (1975). Dual regulation of adenylate cyclase accounts for narcotic dependence and tolerance. Proceedings of the National Academy of Sciences of the United States of America, 72, 3092–3096.

Shen, K. F., & Crain, S. M. (1989). Dual opioid modulation of the action potential duration of mouse dorsal root ganglion neurons in culture. *Brain Research, 49,* 227–242.

Shen, K. F., & Crain, S. M. (1990). Cholera toxin-A subunit blocks opioid excitatory effects on sensory neuron action potentials indicating mediation by Gs-linked opioid receptors. *Brain Research, 525,* 225–231.

Smart, D., Smith, G., & Lambert, D. G. (1994). m-Opioid receptor stimulation of inositol (1,4,5) trisphosphate formation via a pertussis toxin-senstive G protein. *Journal of Neurochemistry, 62,* 1009–1014.

Tao, P. L., Law, P. Y., & Loh, H. H. (1987). Decrease in delta and mu opioid receptor binding capacity in rat brain after chronic etorphine treatment. *Journal of Pharmacology and Experimental Therapeutics, 240,* 809–816.

Terwilliger, R. Z., Beitner-Johnson, D., Sevarino, K. A., Crain, S. M., & Nestler, E. J. (1991). A general role for adaptations in G-proteins and the cyclic AMP system in mediating the chronic actions of morphine and cocaine on neuronal function. *Brain Research, 548,* 100–110.

Tiseo, P. J., Cheng, J., Pasternak, G. W., & Inturrisi, C. E. (1994). Modulation of morphine tolerance by the competitive N-methyl-D-aspartate receptor antagonist LY274614: Assessment of opioid receptor changes. *Journal of Pharmacology and Experimental Therapeutics, 268,* 195–201.

Tjon, G. H. K., De Vries, T. J., Ronken, E., Hogenboom, F., Wardeh, G., et al. (1994). Repeated and chronic morphine administration causes differential long-lasting changes in dopaminergic neurotransmission in rat striatum without changing its δ- and κ-opioid regulation. *European Journal of Pharmacology, 252,* 205–212.

Trujillo, K. A., & Akil, H. (1990). Inhibition of morphine tolerance and dependence by the NMDA receptor antagonist MD-801. *Science, 251,* 85–87.

Van Vliet, B. J., Wardeh, G., Mulder, A. H., & Schoffelmeer, A. N. M. (1991). Reciprocal effects of chronic morphine administration on stimulatory and inhibitory G-protein a subunits in primary cultures of rat striatal neurons. *European Journal of Pharmacology, 208,* 341–342.

Vogel, A., Barg, J., Attali, B., & Simantov, R. (1990). Differential effect of μ, δ, and κ ligands on G protein a subunits in cultured brain cells. *Journal of Neuroscience Research, 27,* 106–111.

Werling, L. L., McMahon, P. N., & Cox, B. M. (1989). Selective changes in m opioid receptor properties induced by chronic morphine exposure. *Proceedings of the National Academy of Sciences of the United States of America, 86,* 6393–6397.

Widnell, K. L., Russell, D. S., & Nestler, E. J. (1994). Regulation of cAMP response element binding protein in the locus coeruleus in vivo and in a locus coeruleus-like (CATH.a) cell line in vitro. *Proceedings of the National Academy of Sciences of the United States of America, 91,* 10947–10951.

Wise, R. A. (1990). The role of reward pathways in the development of drug dependence. In D. J. K. Balfour (Ed.), *Psychotropic drugs of abuse* (pp. 23–57). Oxford: Pergamon Press.

Part II

OPTIMIZING TRADITIONAL TREATMENTS

Section A

REFINING THE USE
OF PHARMACOTHERAPY

Chapter 4

NEW DEVELOPMENTS IN METHADONE TREATMENT AND MATCHING TREATMENTS TO PATIENTS

Susan M. Stine, M.D., Ph.D.

Methadone maintenance has been the primary pharmacotherapy for chronic opioid dependence since its introduction by Dole and Nyswander (1965, 1968). Although levo-alpha-acetylmethadol (LAAM), a long-acting congener of methadone, has been used experimentally since the 1970s for maintenance treatment, it was only recently approved by the U.S. Food and Drug Administration (FDA) for maintenance therapy and is now available for general use in opioid treatment programs (see Chapter 11). More recently, buprenorphine has been studied in clinical trials as a maintenance therapy in opioid-dependent patients and shows considerable promise as an alternative to methadone maintenance (see Chapter 12). These new substitution therapy agents are considered elsewhere in this volume. Methadone however, remains the most thoroughly used and studied medication, and its optimal use is still being refined, especially with respect to its use with specific psychosocial services and additional biological treatments in defined subpopulations of opiate-dependent patients. Because of its relative familiarity and reliable track record for more than 30 years, the use of methadone in combination with adjunctive treatments provides a model for the use of adjunctive therapies with the newer opiate pharmacotherapies, such as LAAM and buprenorphine. This chapter will review methadone treatment and focus on new information about the pharmacology of methadone and the progress in matching methadone treatment and adjunctive services to specific subpopulations.

BRIEF DESCRIPTION OF METHADONE MAINTENANCE TREATMENTS

Methadone is an orally effective, long-acting agonist at the μ-opioid receptor, and maintenance therapy with methadone is designed to support patients with opioid dependence for months or years while the patient engages in counseling and other therapy to change the opioid-dependent lifestyle. Experience with methadone has shown it to be both safe and effective. While patients in methadone maintenance show physiological signs of opioid tolerance, there are minimal side effects, and the patients' general health and nutritional status improve. Further, investigators have shown that criminal behavior decreases in as much as 85% of maintenance patients while employment among maintenance patients typically ranges from 40 to 80%.

Methadone maintenance programs are strictly licensed and regulated by the FDA and the Drug Enforcement Administration. To be eligible for methadone maintenance, a person must be at least 18 years of age and must be physiologically dependent on heroin or other opioids for a period of at least 1 year. The occasional applicant who has been using opioids for very brief periods of time or who has no past or current history of opioid dependence with physiological features must be carefully screened out. This screening can be done in a variety of ways that include observing the patient over a 12- to 24-hour period for the signs and symptoms of opioid withdrawal; using a naloxone challenge test; or obtaining information from independent observers, such as family members or probation officers, or from other treatment programs. Urine drug tests are also important as a screening device, though they are not proof of physiological dependence.

Most clinics have a highly structured behavioral mode of treatment. A typical program is described by Kosten et al. (1982). The major emphasis of methadone maintenance programs is on rehabilitation. Explicit program goals include teaching clients real-life problem solving and enabling some program members to give up methadone. Many methadone programs are hierarchically structured, and rule making and rule enforcing are managed through a clearly defined "chain of command." Small counseling groups are the major rehabilitative structure. These small groups engage and maintain addicts in treatment. However, because the clients' dependency needs are met in the small-group setting, such a setting may paradoxically impede full return to the community. Problems with such programs therefore include (1) monitoring psychiatric disorders in the client population since deviant behaviors and affective symptoms are routinely identified in the small group as a reflection of socially determined individual problems and (2) development of more adequate structures to help to prepare patients for withdrawal from methadone, graduation from the program, and the loss of small-group and organizational supports.

Although many treatment clinics are hierarchically organized, clinics design their own rules and treatment programs within the guidelines set by state and federal agencies, and these rules vary widely. Many clinics are open only 6 days per week, thus giving all patients at least one take-home dose of methadone weekly; others are open 7 days per week and require a patient to "earn" any take-home privileges by compliance with the clinic rules and abstinence from abusable substances (including alcohol). All clinics must obtain urine toxicologies on patients, but the frequency varies from two to three times per week to one time per month. Despite evidence that patients on higher (more than 60 mg/day) doses of methadone are more successful in maintaining drug-free urines (Ball & Ross, 1991), some clinics and states have set upper limits on the dose of methadone. Some clinics have limits of 30 or 40 mg, daily doses that are clearly too low for many patients. In general, patients should be dosed on an individual basis such that they have little chance of achieving an opioid effect from illicit drugs. Finally, psychosocial services, which are essential for optimal response to pharmacological treatment, vary widely across clinics. In view of the length of time (30 years) that methadone has been available as a treatment, it is remarkable that the advances in defining elements of program efficacy have been achieved so recently.

IMPORTANCE OF DOSE

When administered in adequate oral doses, a single dose of methadone in a stabilized patient usually lasts between 24 and 36 hours, without creating euphoria or sedation. Narcotic cross-tolerance, or "blockade," is an essential therapeutic property of this medication: in sufficient doses, methadone "blocks" the narcotic effects of normal street doses of short-acting narcotics, such as heroin. Treatment staff have often tended to minimize the maintenance dose for several reasons. First, staff members have had preconceived notions that abstinence was an achievable goal for the majority of addicts; second, they have thought that lower doses were less toxic and easier to withdraw (or "detox") from; and finally, they have believed that less diversion would occur if doses were lower. Patients themselves also continued to resist adequate dosages based on mythologies that methadone "rots the bones," decreases libido, and is more difficult to "kick" than heroin (Goldsmith et al., 1984; Rosenblum et al., in press).

Nevertheless, scientific knowledge is now available to suggest that the original dosage protocol studied by Dole and Nyswander (1965) works best and that low doses are appropriate for only a limited number of patients. A series of large-scale studies have emerged and have shown that patients maintained on doses of 60 mg/day or more had better treatment outcomes than those maintained on lower doses (Ball & Ross, 1991; Caplehorn & Bell, 1991; Hartel, 1989–1990; Hartel et al., 1988, 1989). These studies confirm that dosages below 60 mg appear inadequate for most patients. This is especially important at the beginning of treatment, when patients may experiment with heroin to test the effectiveness of the medication. These studies also confirm that medical decisions should not be based on public biases but on scientific knowledge and clinical evaluation. Low doses of methadone are rarely therapeutic; in fact, they prevent the effective treatment of narcotic addiction. The effectiveness of methadone was even greater for patients on a 70-mg dose and was still more pronounced for patients on 80 mg/day or more. A very influential survey reported on a 3-year study of six methadone programs in three Northeastern cities (U.S. General Accounting Office, 1990). This report showed that patients reduced their use of intravenous heroin by 71% when compared with the preadmission level, thus confirming the effectiveness of this treatment. Most important, however, this study revealed that opiate use was directly related to methadone dose levels. In patients on doses of about 71 mg/day, no heroin use was detected, whereas those patients on doses below 46 mg were 5.15 times more likely to use heroin than those receiving higher doses (Ball & Ross, 1991). Caplehorn and Bell (1991) reported similar results and demonstrated that patients on methadone treatment in Australia who received higher doses remained in treatment longer. Finally, in a review of 24 methadone treatment programs throughout the nation, the U.S. General Accounting Office (1990) concluded that "sixty milligrams of methadone is the lowest dose to stop heroin use and low dose maintenance (20 to 40 milligrams) is inappropriate."

SPECIFIC PHARMACOLOGICAL ISSUES AND DRUG INTERACTIONS

There are many diverse factors that may, in theory, significantly modify the pharmacological effectiveness of methadone. Three factors that have been demonstrated to significantly modify the disposition of methadone, and thus potentially its pharmacological effectiveness, will be discussed. These factors include: (1) chronic diseases, such as chronic liver disease, chronic renal disease, and possibly other diseases; (2) drug interactions, including interactions of methadone with rifampin and phenytoin in humans, possibly with ethanol and disulfiram, and also, by inference from animal studies, interactions of methadone with phenobarbital, diazepam, desipramine, and other drugs, as well as with estrogen steroids; and (3) altered physiological states—in particular, pregnancy. These factors have been reviewed in detail by Kreek (1986).

Chronic liver disease is the most common medical problem. There is biochemical evidence of chronic liver disease in 50–60% of all heroin addicts entering methadone maintenance treatment. Methadone itself is not hepatotoxic. Chronic hepatic dysfunction observed in methadone-maintained patients is primarily of two etiological types: (1) sequelae of earlier acute infection with hepatitis B virus or one of the non-A and non-B viruses; and (2) alcohol-induced liver disease, including fatty liver, alcoholic hepatitis, and alcohol cirrhosis. The liver may play a central role in several aspects of methadone disposition, including not only methadone metabolism and clearance but also storage and subsequent release of unchanged methadone. In a study by Kreek et al. (1978), unchanged methadone persisted in the liver for up to 6 weeks, and methadone disposition was significantly altered only in a patient subgroup with moderately severe but compensated cirrhosis. Although no studies of methadone disposition and effects have been conducted in patients with severe or uncompensated chronic liver disease or in acute fulminant forms of liver disease, methadone use has been well characterized in milder disease and used successfully in these patients. Very severe liver disease or abrupt changes in hepatic status in patients with these conditions may cause significant alterations in methadone disposition with concomitant clinical symptoms. To facilitate proper selection and subgroup classification of patients with chronic liver disease, a liver function test, the stable-isotope-labeled [^{13}C]aminopyrine breath test, has been modified and validated in methadone-maintained patients (Kreek et al., 1981).

With respect to the effect of drug interactions, the clinical efficacy of methadone has been shown to be significantly altered in humans by several pharmacological agents frequently used in this population. The antituberculosis drug, rifampin, is a major example of this phenomenon. Twenty-one of 30 methadone-maintained patients in a special tuberculosis clinic developed mild to severe narcotic withdrawal symptoms when rifampin was added to their therapeutic regimens (Kreek, 1986). Urinary excretion of pyrrolidine, the major metabolite of methadone, increased 150% during rifampin treatment, and a lowering of plasma levels of methadone was observed.

A second clinically important drug interaction with methadone that has been documented is the development of signs and symptoms of narcotic withdrawal within 2–3 days after initiation of phenytoin treatment for seizures (Finelli 1976; Tong et al., 1981). This drug reaction is due to enhanced metabolism of methadone during phenytoin administration. Similar observations have been made for phenobarbital and carbamazepine (Bell et al., 1987).

The widely used medication for gastric acidity called cimetidine, a histamine H_2 receptor antagonist that has recently been marketed over the counter, has been shown to inhibit cytochrome P-450 (Bauman & Kimelblatt, 1982) and to reduce hepatic blood flow (Freely et al., 1981). This medication has been reported to increase morphine toxicity and also to decrease metabolism of methadone. Because of the over-the-counter availability of this medication, methadone program staff should educate methadone patients about this interaction. This effect interestingly has also been proposed as a therapeutic intervention to increase the duration of methadone action (discussed later in this chapter).

With the increasing number of HIV-infected patients in methadone maintenance programs, potential interactions between methadone and antiviral agents used in the treatment of HIV are particularly important to define. A study of possible interactions between methadone and zidovudine (AZT) conducted at Montefiore Medical Center (Bronx, New York) has shown that serum levels of methadone are not affected by this drug, which is used to treat HIV infection, but that some patients who receive methadone maintenance treatment may show a potentially toxic increase in serum levels of AZT (Friedland et al., 1992). Although the mechanism through which the blood levels of AZT were increased in these patients was not ascertained in this study, Friedland and his team determined that neither AZT metabolism nor excretion was altered. These authors caution against making changes in the dosage of AZT for HIV-positive patients who are taking methadone, but the authors do suggest careful clinical monitoring for signs of dose-related AZT toxicity in such patients.

Alcohol is used to excess by 20–50% of methadone-maintained patients (Kreek et al., 1978; Kreek, 1981a, 1981b). It was shown that ethanol has a biphasic effect on drug metabolism. When ethanol is present in large amounts, drug metabolism is inhibited; yet when ethanol is no longer present, following chronic administration of large amounts of this agent, drug metabolism is accelerated. Ethanol does not prevent the hepatic uptake of methadone (Kreek, 1981a). Possible effects of chronic methadone treatment on ethanol elimination have been studied in rats (Wendell & Kreek 1979; Kreek, 1981a). Chronic treatment with methadone alone caused an acceleration in ethanol disappearance rates that were significantly higher than the accelerated elimination rates observed in animals treated on a chronic basis with ethanol.

Disulfiram (Antabuse) is the only pharmacological agent that has been shown thus far to have significant deterrent effects on recidivism following detoxification from ethanol. This agent is an important therapeutic tool for the subpopulation with comorbid alcohol and opiate dependence, but this agent also interacts with methadone metabolism. The ratio of urinary excretion of methadone to its major pyrrolidine metabolite was significantly lowered during concomitant disulfiram administration. These findings suggest that the N-demethylation of methadone may be enhanced. Although the mean plasma levels of methadone were lower during concomitant disulfiram administration, these levels were not significantly different from the methadone levels observed during methadone treatment alone, and therefore the findings do not present a practical problem for treatment in most cases. These pharamacokinetic interactions are summarized in Table 4.1.

TABLE 4.1. Pharmacokinetic Interactions with Methadone

Pharmacological agent	Effect on methadone	Clinical signs and symptoms	Comments
Rifampin Phenytoin Phenobarbital Carbamazepine	Increases methadone metabolism.	Has withdrawal signs.	
Cimetidine	Decreases methadone metabolism.	Increases sedation and other opiate effects.	Can be used in patients with low-trough methadone levels to prolong action (must also consider cimetidine effects on other concurrent medications).
Zidovudine (AZT)	Has no effect on methadone, but methadone may increase AZT levels.	Possibly increases toxicity of AZT.	Close clinical monitoring of AZT needed.
Disulfiram	May decrease methadone levels, but not significantly.	Not clinically problematic.	

The third type of influence reviewed by Kreek (1986) that may alter the pharmacological effectiveness of methadone is that of altered physiological states. For example, during pregnancy the effectiveness of methadone seems to be reduced. Binding of methadone to plasma proteins during late pregnancy does not account for all the changes in plasma levels of methadone observed. These findings have suggested that methadone metabolism may be altered in late pregnancy possibly owing to a predominant effect of progestins on hepatic drug metabolism. This phenomenon is discussed further by Chang (Chapter 10, this volume).

USEFULNESS OF METHADONE BLOOD LEVELS

Given the above identified influences on methadone metabolism and the evidence for the importance of dose, it might be expected that measurement of methadone levels in the blood would be useful in clinical management. Kreek (1973, 1991) did use blood plasma levels to establish doses and stated that methadone doses should never be used for social rewards or punishment (Kreek, 1973, 1991), a method that is often part of the behavioral management of patients in methadone programs. Also, it was recommended that all doses be determined individually, because of differences in metabolism, body weight, and maintenance of appropriate methadone blood levels throughout the 24-hour period. This method, however, is expensive, and blood levels are not widely used in clinical management. Nevertheless, the identification of an ideal therapeutic blood level or range and the clinical usefulness of blood levels in clinical management of methadone is an issue still under active investigation. Dole (1980) specified a therapeutic range of 100–1,000 ng/ml. Most studies support the standard that patients who take daily doses of methadone that exceed 80 mg/day and who maintain an average plasma concentration of about 400 ng/ml show little drug use and can have a good psychosocial response to treatment (Inturrusi & Verebely, 1972; Kreek, 1973; Tennant et al., 1983).

For most patients, determination of actual drug levels may not be necessary. Some individuals, however, have inadequate plasma concentrations despite high methadone doses (Tennant, 1987) and appear to metabolize methadone in an aberrant fashion. The clinical significance of this observation is not as clear since some complaints of withdrawal symptoms have been found to be unrelated to oral dose and plasma concentration (Blake & Distasio, 1973; Goldstein 1971; Horns et al., 1975; Kreek 1973). Further, although some studies (e.g., Tennant et al., 1983) have shown a correlation between "poor performance" in methadone treatment and lower-trough methadone levels, other studies dispute this finding. For example, Bell et al. (1987) reported that a trough level of 100 ng/ml is adequate for effective maintenance and that performance in treatment was independent of serum level above this threshold. However, these same authors confirmed the usefulness of serum levels as an intervention for some patients and also confirmed the special problems seen in patients who were concomitantly using enzyme-inducing drugs such as phenobarbital, phenytoin, and carbamazepine. A separate pharmacokinetic study (Nilsson et al., 1983), comparing eight treatment failures to an unselected group of 12 inpatients on methadone, revealed a smaller volume of distribution and high fluctuation of methadone in the later part of the 24-hour dosage interval in the group of treatment failures. These authors proposed that this fluctuation increased the likelihood of an initial "high" as well as a later shortened "straight" period and prolonged withdrawal period, thus increasing relapse risk in more than one way (Nilsson et al., 1983). These authors state that the solution lies in the use of either a shorter dosage interval or a longer-acting drug such as LAAM.

Another strategy to increase the duration of action of methadone is the use of cimetidine coadministration. As mentioned above, cimetidine, an H_2 blocker used to treat ulcers by reducing gastric acid secretion, prolongs the half-life of several medications through inhibition of the cytochrome P-450 enzyme system in the liver (Brunton, 1990; Sedman, 1984), resulting in an increased duration of action. This effect may lead to a more continuous prevention of opiate withdrawal symptoms in patients on maintenance treatment, leading to increased treatment compliance and reduced illicit opiate use. If cimetidine is used in this way, its concurrent action on other medications used by the patients, such as ketoconazole, penicillin, anticoagulants, benzodiazepines, and others (Sedman, 1984), must be considered.

The small number of patients (n's for these reports range between 12 and 48) studied in the above reports about the importance of blood levels prevents the acceptance of any of the above-cited studies as definitive. However, the studies serve in the aggregate to emphasize the importance of the issue for the optimal use of methadone, especially in some patients with complaints of withdrawal symptoms while on relatively high methadone doses.

IDENTIFYING POPULATION CHARACTERISTICS, PROGRAM CHARACTERISTICS, AND REFINING GOALS OF METHADONE TREATMENT

One of the major accomplishments over the last several years has been the reexamination of methadone programs with respect to specific patient characteristics as well as to treatment components and outcomes. Only two prospective studies of methadone efficacy that used random assignment have been reported before the 1980s. The first (Dole et al., 1969) used a relatively narrow range of outcome measures (relapse, employment, and crime) and did not describe the psychosocial treatment available to the control group but overwhelmingly supported the efficacy of methadone (Dole et al., 1969). A second controlled prospective study in Hong Kong (Newman & Whitehall, 1979) randomly assigned 100 heroin-addicted volunteers to either methadone or a placebo and provided a broad range of supportive services to all. After 32 weeks, only 10% of the controls remained in treatment, whereas 76% of the methadone group continued and had less than half as many convictions for criminal activity than the control patients did. Both of these studies agreed in that they found that methadone treatment was effective. Although these early studies did not attempt to make distinctions between patient subclasses and program characteristics, it was clear that methadone is a useful treatment when administered to patients who are chronic narcotic addicts, who are actively addicted, and who are living in an environment in which narcotics are readily available. However, no evidence is available that maintenance under these conditions leads to permanent discontinuation of narcotic addiction. Rather than cure opiate dependence itself, methadone maintenance appears to provide control over personal and social problems associated with opiate dependence. The importance of defining specific outcome measures and specific components of methadone treatment has only recently become clear.

The most extensive and complete review of methadone treatment is found in a study that was carried out by the National Institute on Drug Abuse (NIDA) (Cooper et al., 1983), which sponsored a series of meetings that examined many aspects of methadone treatment, including outcome. Several large-scale studies had been completed and were reviewed, particularly those of Sells (1979) and McLellan et al. (1982). These studies confirmed that methadone-treated patients showed significant gains when compared with addicts not in treatment, the initial positive findings of Dole and Nyswander (1965). Reductions of illicit drug use, reductions in crime, and increased rates of employment are examples of documented improvements seen in methadone programs. These findings were further supported in a study by Ball et al. (1983) of treated and untreated addicts in Baltimore and Philadelphia. The treated addicts reported significant reductions in criminal activity compared to the rates they reported prior to treatment. The reports were also verified by comprehensive arrest, penal, hospital, and other institutional data. Consequently, these studies not only confirmed previously reported benefits of methadone but also gave matching subpopulations access to elements of treatment other than the pharmacological agent itself.

Although an important beginning, the above studies in general rely on historical controls or on patient self-reports. Independent measures such as police records, urine test results, or documentation of employment are available in some studies (e.g., Ball et al., 1983) but not in others. A second NIDA review (Grabowski et al., 1984) made an advance by attempting to further define specific patient characteristics, particularly with respect to the behavioral problems demonstrated by addicts and ways to manage them. Most participants in this review felt that many of these problems originated from drug-seeking behavior, which is, of course, a characteristic of the addiction syndrome. Such problems include fabricating stories to obtain controlled substances, buying or selling illicit drugs, attempting to falsify urine samples to avoid loss of take-home methadone doses, or attempting to divert methadone at the pharmacy window. A serious problem reported by many programs was loitering. The most common motive for loitering appeared to be social contact, but a considerable amount of drug dealing was also observed to take place (Hunt et al., 1984). Persistent loitering was felt to serve as a nidus for the development of other behavioral problems, such as arguments or fights. Loitering was also noted to be frightening to people who happened to be in the vicinity of the program and who were not familiar with the personalities and lifestyles of addicts. Threats, disruptive behavior, fighting, or even carrying weapons were reported occasionally. These problems were thought to be related to the addiction itself, to personality disorders or other psychiatric problems, or to socioenvironmental circumstances. Participants in the NIDA conference (Grabowski et al., 1984) that reviewed these problems were in reasonably good agreement that effective control of these disorders requires a combination of support and structure involving specified rules that include suspension of those who display serious behavioral problems (see also the earlier program description in Kosten, 1982).

Because of the above evidence, further attention was focused on behavioral treatments, especially as they apply to patients who demonstrate a poor response to methadone therapy. One serious problem that occurs with some maintenance patients is persistent drug use in spite of methadone doses that are more than sufficient to suppress withdrawal symptoms and that also provide some degree of cross-tolerance to injected opioids (thus reducing or eliminating the "reward" of using street opioids). Special behavioral interventions or contracts may have to be used with patients who continue to use opiates despite treatment with adequate doses of methadone and the achievement of adequate blood levels as described above. In these cases, some recommend raising the methadone dose to the highest allowable levels (80–100, or even 120, mg/day). Sometimes this intervention is combined with a treatment contract that states that the patient must accomplish certain behaviors within a specified period of time or face suspension from the program (Bigelow et al., 1984). When these behavioral contracts include a decrease in methadone dose in response to problematic behaviors (as described further in Chapter 8), this intervention conflicts not only with pharmacological issues but also with the more purely medical choice of dose advocated by Kreek (1986). Goals to be achieved can include giving drug-free urine specimens, keeping all counseling appointments, and demonstrating proof that job-seeking behavior is occurring. Selectivity in choosing patients for contracts is important, as is choosing realistic goals. A recent study shows that 50–60% of carefully selected patients who were given a treatment contract succeeded in achieving the specified goals within the allotted time (Dolan et al., 1985). Those who fail a contract can be offered the option of transferring to another methadone program or of entering another treatment modality, such as a therapeutic community or narcotic antagonist (naltrexone) treatment.

Although major refinements in behavioral aspects of treatment have been made, little work is available that measures the level of physiological dependence on opioids prior to methadone treatment and then relates this to dose and outcome. Methadone treatment outcome data derive from approved programs that are periodically inspected for compliance with the FDA requirements for maintenance treatment. The FDA mandates current physiological dependence in addition to other characteristics that signify long-term addiction, but the regulations do not define criteria that quantify degrees of dependence. McLellan et al. (1983) showed that the amount of drugs used and the length of the drug dependence did not relate to treatment outcome. There is, however, one study of 37 consecutive applicants to methadone maintenance that has shown that high naloxone challenge scores were found to predict poor program retention and elevated symptoms of depression at a 3-month follow-up (Jacobson & Kosten, 1989). Thus, although information on this point is sketchy, and the data available point to features other than levels of physiological dependence as major determinants of outcome, the role of physiological dependence nevertheless merits further investigation.

ADDITION OF SERVICES TO METHADONE TREATMENT

As the effective use of methadone has become more clearly delineated, one specific question of importance for clinicans and clinical researchers is the efficacy of counseling services as an adjunct to methadone for opiate addicts. The need for services has been questioned by some, leading to the promotion of methadone medication alone as a means of saving funds and including more patients in treatment. In order to examine this study, McLellen et al. (1990) completed a prospective random assignment study of different levels of services within a methadone maintenance program. In this study, voluntary patients, at the beginning of their methadone maintenance treatment, were randomly assigned to different types and amounts of treatment service over 6 months. All patients received initial physical examinations, laboratory testing, and a short AIDS education program and were assigned to three levels of care. Level I patients received methadone maintenance (blocking doses of 60 mg or more) without additional counseling except on an emergency basis. Level II patients received the same methadone stabilization but also received regular counseling by a trained rehabilitation specialist. Level III patients received the same services as Level II patients but were also provided family therapy, employment, counseling, and regular medical and psychiatric care as needed. The analysis by McLellan's group revealed significant differences in the amounts of improvement shown by patients at these three levels. Those patients in Level I showed some improvement in drug use, as well as modest improvements in employment, but no other changes. Interestingly, the family and psychiatric problems of Level I patients actually worsened, though not significantly. The simple addition of a counselor to this level of services (i.e., Level II) was associated with significantly enhanced improvement in most areas; and the additional services rendered by the family therapists, physicians, employment specialists, and social workers for Level III patients produced still more changes. Methadone alone, therefore, has some effects in uncomplicated patients. Most important, however, substantial numbers of patients with additional disorders will not respond without the addition of other services. In conclusion, this study supported the hypothesis that the efficacy of methadone treatment can be enhanced by additional services, such as counseling or psychotherapy (although specific differentiation among these services, such as the specific effect of psychotherapy, was not directly attempted).

Another example of a more intensive treatment is a day treatment program. To examine the hypothesis that a structured day treatment approach with methadone-maintained patients is more effective than standard treatment, we conducted an open pilot study that compared patients admitted to the Veterans Administration (VA) day treatment program between 1990 and 1992 ($n = 99$) to a patient sample matched for gender (male) and admitted to the inner-city methadone maintenance program at the Addiction Prevention Treatment Foundation in New Haven, Connecticut, during 1992 (n = 89). The comparison was based on the following: (1) illicit substance use during the first 3 months of treatment, (2) retention in treatment, and (3) employment status at discharge. The inner-city site offered only weekly therapeutic contacts. A significantly smaller percentage of urines tested positive for illicit substances during the first 3 months of treatment (M = 21.1%) at the VA day treatment program than at the inner-city methadone maintenance program site (M = 55.0%), $t(159)$ = 6.10, p < .0001. Both sites had comparable retention rates, but minorities seemed to have a higher risk of dropping out at the inner-city site (75% of dropouts versus 45% of initial population), while minority dropouts from the VA site were proportional to the minority representation in the initial population (35%). Prospects for patients' becoming employed after participation in the VA day treatment program were also found to be improved: 49% of patients who were unemployed at admission to the day treatment program were employed at discharge compared to only 4% of patients who were unemployed at admission and who became employed after treatment at the inner-city site (χ^2 = 38.43, p < .0001). These results appear to warrant a randomized clinical trial investigating the efficacy of day treatment for an unemployed, inner-city, methadone maintenance program population. This pilot study directly led to the ongoing Project Methadone Match study described by Avants et al., (Chapter 8, this volume).

MISCELLANEOUS ADDITIONAL NEW TREATMENT APPROACHES

Changing patient needs dictate that new and innovative approaches must be designed and studied. Since the 1980s, a few such innovations have been attempted in addition to the fundamental developments already addressed in this chapter. For instance, the Beth Israel Medical Center in New York City operated an "interim," or waiting list, clinic in 1989 as a research project (Lowinson et al., 1992). This interim maintenance was designed to reduce HIV-risk behaviors by providing immediate methadone treatment to eligible applicants on a waiting list for comprehensive methadone treatment. A study of the 301 patients showed that heroin use was reduced from 63% at admission to 29% after 1 month. Cocaine use was not significantly reduced. The controls on the waiting list showed no reduction in the use of either substance. In 1989 the FDA guidelines originally proposed for interim methadone maintenance heightened the debate concerning the appropriate use of methadone since many treatment providers believed that those entering methadone maintenance treatment in the 1990s were most in need of comprehensive service. Opponents of interim treatment referred to a study at the VA Medical Center in Philadelphia that showed that minimal or low-threshold treatment did not reduce illicit drug use significantly (McLellan et al., 1988).

One special group of methadone patients who may actually specifically benefit from less-intense treatment are those who have been stable in treatment for years and who exhibit no dependence characteristic or psychosocial deficit except for the continuing need for methadone itself. Because there are many patients in continuous treatment who function on an extremely high level, the medical maintenance model was established. In this model, patients report once every 4 weeks, submit a urine specimen, and receive a prescription for a 4-week supply of methadone in tablet form directly from the physician in charge of their treatment. Medical maintenance has been established in New York, Baltimore, and Chicago (Novick et al., 1988).

Several other models for innovative approaches have also been proposed, such as two models now being developed at the Albert Einstein College of Medicine in the Bronx, as reviewed by Lowinson et al., 1992. One of these models is designed to provide culturally sensitive, family-centered treatment. Another model attempts to mobilize intensive resources to newly admitted patients, who presumably have the greatest need of such resources; this program is designed to integrate the patient more fully into the treatment system.

PSYCHOTHERAPY

A futher goal of current research, is to refine the focus of treatment beyond simple intensity differences in order to identify specific treatment modalities. One category of specific treatment is psychotherapy, and a current concern is identifying the type of therapy and type of patients who will benefit from it. For example, patients with coexisting psychiatric disorders respond poorly to drug counseling but may show significant improvement with the addition of professional psychotherapy. Other work has studied the efficacy of professional psychotherapy with nonpsychotic addicts when psychotherapy is added to routine counseling services in a methadone program. Two major studies were completed in this area, and their results varied. One study showed no difference in outcome when interpersonal psychotherapy was added to drug counseling in a full-service methadone treatment program (Rounsaville et al., 1983). This study, although well designed, did not succeed in engaging many patients in the psychotherapy, and it also had a high dropout rate. The recruitment methods that were used suggested that some patients who did participate were probably unusually resistant to treatment since they were referred to the research project as a last resort before being discharged from the program for showing little improvement.

A second study of psychotherapy had a higher recruitment rate, fewer dropouts, and a larger total number of subjects (Woody et al., 1983). This study provided good evidence that professional psychotherapists can provide additional benefits to those benefits obtained with paraprofessional drug counselors. One of the most interesting findings from this work emerged when outcome was assessed for those classified as low-, mid-, or high-severity patients on the basis of the number and intensity of their psychiatric symptoms as rated by standard assessments, such as the Beck Depression Inventory (Beck, 1972) or the Symptom Checklist 90 (SCL-90) (Derogatis, 1970). Low-severity patients made considerable and approximately equal progress with the additional psychotherapy or with counseling alone. Mid-severity patients had better outcomes with the additional psychotherapy than with counseling alone, but counseling was associated with numerous significant improvements. High-severity patients made little progress with counseling alone, but made considerable progress if they had the additional psychotherapy. Psychiatric comorbidity was also found to predict response. Patients with only antisocial personality disorder showed little response to the additional therapy, but others, especially those with depression or with antisocial personality and depression, had a good response. It was also found that there was considerable variation in outcome among therapists, with some achieving consistently better outcomes than others did (Luborsky et al., 1985). Those therapists who had the best results were noted as having the best doctor–patient relationships and also as being the most successful in conforming to the specifications of their particular school or therapy.

The overall results of these studies, and of other similar but less comprehensive ones (Abrams, 1979; Connett, 1980; LaRosa et al., 1974; Resnick et al., 1980; Stanton et al., 1982; Willett, 1973), indicate that professional psychotherapy can probably make a valuable contribution to ongoing treatment services, particularly if it is targeted to that segment of the nonpsychotic addict population with moderate to high levels of psychiatric symptoms. The therapy program is not always simple to apply to this population (Rounsaville et al., 1983; Stanton et al., 1982; Woody et al., 1983); the program must be well integrated into the overall drug rehabilitation program and must also employ skilled therapists who relate well to opioid addicts.

PSYCHIATRIC COMORBIDITY

The issue of psychotherapy is particularly relevant to the large subgroup of methadone patients with psychiatric comorbidity. An inability to treat the psychiatric disorders of the opiate-dependent patient has contributed to poor treatment response and sometimes premature termination from therapy.

Psychiatric Disorders

Studies have been performed that describe the types of psychiatric problems seen in opiate addicts. These studies found that addicts can have almost every psychiatric illness that occurs in nonaddicts. A comprehensive evaluation of psychiatric disorders in addicts was completed by Rounsaville et al. (1982b) in a sample of 533 opiate addicts. In that study, depression was the most frequently diagnosed illness, with about 60% of the sample having had some form of depression at least once. Alcoholism was the next most common problem, followed by antisocial personality and anxiety disorders. Schizophrenia, other types of personality disorders, mania, and hypomania occurred with a much lower frequency. Eighty-five percent of the patients were found to have had a psychiatric disorder in addition to opiate dependence at some time in their lives. Symptoms not systematically studied in the above report but seen regularly are (1) acute situational reactions that involve intense but transient feelings of anger, anxiety, or depression; (2) psychiatric disorders complicated by medical conditions such as hepatitis; and (3) illnesses or injuries that produce chronic pain, such as pancreatitis, sickle cell anemia, or trauma resulting in nerve root irritation. Rounsaville et al. (1982b) also found that untreated addicts had similar types of psychiatric illnesses in relatively similar proportions to patients who were in treatment. However, treated addicts were less likely to have a current psychiatric illness. This finding could be interpreted as indicating that concurrent psychiatric illness serves as a motivator to seek treatment.

Depression

Depression, which was reported to be the most commonly diagnosed psychiatric disorder in opiate addicts, was studied in greater detail. The course of the depression seen in methadone-maintained patients was found by Rounsaville et al. (1982a) to be improved by methadone treatment. A substantial reduction in symptoms of depression occurred within the first month of treatment, but the amount of depression that remained was still substantially greater than that observed in nonaddicted controls. This group also found that the types of depression seen were generally of mild to moderate intensities, even if they were diagnosed as major depressive disorder, and were usually not of the severely retarded and psychotic types that are commonly seen on psychiatric inpatient units. Furthermore, those addicts who remained depressed beyond the initial 1-month period usually improved within 6 months even without specific antidepressant treatment. It was also found that some patients who were not initially depressed at program intake became depressed at some later point.

In conclusion, the emerging picture of the types of depression experienced by addicts has been described. These types of depression usually fit the criteria for major depressive disorder, but other types of depression are also seen. Although types of depression are very common at program intake, they often improve within the first month of treatment and are of mild to moderate intensity. Furthermore, these types of depression usually improve without specific antidepressant treatment, but recovery may take 4–6 months or longer. Depression tends to recur; new episodes are often precipitated by situational factors, such as the loss of an important relationship, an arrest, or job difficulties.

Antisocial Personality Disorder

Personality disorders have also been found at high rates among persons with substance use disorders in treatment settings, and though they have not been as well studied as Axis I disorders (with the exception of antisocial personality disorder), in general, they are associated with poorer outcomes than are Axis I disorders (Kosten et al., 1989; Rounsaville et al., 1987). It should be mentioned that no specific "addictive personality" has been identified, although if it were it would be classified as a personality disorder. Persons with substance use disorders often have traits similar to people with dependent personality disorder but those traits are probably caused by the substance use itself. The closest thing to a predictor for substance abuse that an "addictive personality" would be appears to be antisocial personality disorder, since it has been associated with such a wide range of substance use disorders. This finding has been especially strong with opiate dependence.

Antisocial personality disorder has been recognized as one of the most difficult disorders to treat, and it has been stated that a correctional facility may be the only means of controlling some antisocial patients (Widiger & Frances, 1986). For substance abuse (as well as for depression and anxiety), social failure and conditions of confinement may be useful in motivating the patient, and behavioral therapy has been proven to be useful in structured environments (Leibowitz et al., 1986). The law enforcement system usually first identifies opiate addicts as deviant. Most often they are defined as needing help, not punishment. Nevertheless entry into the mental health system also labels the addict as socially deviant (Friedson, 1966). Once the patient has entered treatment, the new label of methadone maintenance patient classifies the addict as having a long standing and severe addiction, often with several failures at opiate detoxification (Kleber, 1970; Lofchie & Muskelly, 1972).

The evolution of the methadone clinic structure has resulted in an almost ideal treatment setting for the special needs of the patient with antisocial personality disorder. The counselors use the label "antisocial personality" to segregate the patient diagnosed as such from the community that supported the patient's addiction. Within the rehabilitation setting, such an addict is confronted, not as if the addict suffered from a morally neutral disability, but as if the addict pursued a stigmatized, a morally and legally unacceptable, lifestyle, which has an identified cost that is beyond the addict's tolerance. The group norm is to expect improvement; and failures, such as "dirty urines," can result in dismissal from the program. The group also emphasizes a value system regarding the addicted and "straight" lifestyles. The group atmosphere does not condone failure or manipulation. Responsibility for one's actions is made tangible as a step toward self-respect and a straight lifestyle.

Control of patient behavior is an organizational task that takes two broad forms. First, the external boundaries of the organization must be protected by explicit rules. Second, impulsive behavior by a patient in the treatment phase of the organization must be controlled. Impulsive behavior in the treatment phase of this organization is controlled by a clear "chain of command." A patient cannot expect the group counselors to excempt him or her from the program's rules. Any exception and any major boundary decision, such as dismissal of a person from the program, must be cleared with the whole staff of the organization at the weekly meeting. This rigid structural feature helps deflect a patient's aggression away from a group counselor and toward the organization. This deflection has two benefits. First, it reduces the counselor's need for defensiveness. Second, it enables the counselor to help the group members look at the social and intrapsychic sources of the patient's rage and frustration. The major task of the group, however, is to enlist the stigmatized patient's cooperation in recognizing and dealing with the problem and attempting to behave as normally as possible. Most group members do not come to the program for psychological problems and will resist any effort by the group or its leader to explicitly characterize their group interactions as symptomatic of individual psychopathology (LaRosa et al., 1974; Willett, 1973). The model of rehabilitation is, therefore, generally an educational and inspirational one rather than a model focused on intrapsychic change.

Psychotropic Medications

Recent developments in methadone treatment have also included widespread use of psychotropic drugs other than tricyclic antidepressants for addicts with psychiatric disorders. Evidence for the efficacy of these psychotropic medications has been reviewed by Ciccone et al. (1980) and Kleber (1983). Agents studied include antianxiety agents, lithium, and disulfiram. Each of these medications may be helpful for addicts with the specific disorder for which the drugs have been found helpful in other, nonaddict populations. Kleber (1983), however, advised a conservative approach to using benzodiazepines, and many clinicians have also noted that diazepam, and also quite possibly alprazolam (R. Millman, personal communication, 1985), has a significant abuse potential with this population and should be prescribed sparingly or not at all.

METHADONE TREATMENT AND HIV INFECTION

As described in detail by O'Connor and Selwyn (Chapter 11, this volume), infection rates among intravenous drug abusers in New York are high, yet the infection rate in the group of intravenous drug users in treatment is low. Methadone treatment is one of the most helpful means of reducing the risk of AIDS, provided that programs of quality are expanded (Cooper, 1989).

In addition to risk reduction or prevention of infection, there is also need for treatment of an increasing number of existing HIV-positive opiate-dependent patients. Inner-city HIV-positive drug abusers have need of extensive medical and social services (London et al., 1995), which are most effectively delivered on-site (Selwyn et al., 1993). Wherever feasible, the psychosocial intervention should include mechanisms for ensuring that on-site services are used appropriately. Where on-site delivery of medical and social services is not possible, it is essential that there be interventions for improving patients_ compliance with medical regimens (e.g., keeping appointments, taking antiretroviral medications and prophylaxes to fight pneumosystis carinii pneumonia and tuberculosis) and for connecting patients to community social service resources. Compliance with medical regimens has the potential to improve the quality and quantity of life, and thus affects motivation for changing high-risk behaviors.

The importance of support to insure compliance with HIV treatment is illustrated well by a recent study by Wall et al. (1995). In that study, 27 HIV-positive patients with identified treatment compliance problems were randomly assigned to (1) a group that received 8 weeks of weekday supervised therapy and dispensing of AZT or (2) a group that received the usual care of the clinic. Adherence was assessed by self-report, erythrocyte mean corpuscular volume (MCV), Medication Event Monitoring Systems (MEMS), and pill counts. The high-intervention group demonstrated significantly higher MCV levels and higher (but nonsignificant) results on the other outcome measures. The most interesting finding was that these group differences did not apply to weekends (when there was no intervention difference) and did not persist on 1-month follow-ups. Thus, HIV-positive patients would seem to require ongoing intensive support to assure good medication compliance.

The interactions observed among HIV infection, AIDS, and methadone treatment, have led to the development of many specialized programs to provide research and to deliver services in an attempt to manage the high numbers of infected patients. Special issues in the concurrent management of methadone and medications for HIV (which can have pharmacokinetic interactions, as mentioned previously in this chapter) are an example of the integration of medical services required by this HIV-infected population. Risk reduction education by staff with special training in HIV spectrum disease, distribution of condoms, and assistance with referrals to infectious disease clinics are further examples of such integrated services. Primary medical care, including T-cell monitoring and prescriptions for AZT and other HIV medications, is provided along with prophylaxis for *Pneumocystis carinii* pneumonia (PCP) and other opportunistic infections. Tuberculosis case management projects and the provision of medications for prevention and treatment have developed in response to an increase in tuberculosis, especially treatment-resistant tuberculosis, within this group (Albert Einstein College of Medicine, 1989; Joseph & Springer, 1990). Another example of the specific methadone programs for HIV infection developed by hospitals is the program at St. Clare's Hospital in New York City, a special methadone clinic specifically designed for patients with HIV infection and AIDS (Lowinson et al., 1992).

SUMMARY: PATIENT-PROGRAM MATCHING

Methadone therapy taken as a whole is a striking success story in the treatment of a chronic and severely impaired population of opiate patients. Patient–program matching is a concept that promises to create considerable enhancement of this excellent therapy. The heterogeneity of methadone patients, as described earlier, provides ample justification for studies of patient–program matching as does the tremendous variability among methadone programs themselves, in regard to dose policies, ancillary services, quality of treatment facilities, and the levels of discipline imposed. Although counseling services, psychotherapy, social work, vocational counseling, and other aspects of drug rehabilitation services vary widely among programs, recent progress in identifying patients who require these services promises to increase the efficient economical use of scarce resources in the current climate of fiscal austerity and managed care.

Some specific pharmacological and psychosocial considerations mentioned in this chapter (antidepressant drugs, psychotherapy, disulfiram, contingency contracting) represent important advances in matching patients to treatments, and other special treatments for subgroups are continually being developed. The sophistication gained in the finer points of methadone treatment matching will also be an essential starting point for similar refinements in the clinical use of the newer pharmacological agents described in this volume.

REFERENCES

Abrams, J. (1979). A cognitive behavioral versus nondirective group treatment program for opioid addicted persons: An adjunct to methadone maintenance. *International Journal of the Addictions, 14,* 503–511.

Ball, J. C., & Ross, A. (1991). *The effectiveness of methadone maintenance treatment.* New York: Springer-Verlag.

Ball, J. C., Shaffer, J. W., & Nurco, D. N. (1983). The day to day criminality of heroin addicts in Baltimore: A study in the continuity of offense rates. *Drug and Alcohol Dependence, 12,* 114–119.

Bauman, J. H., & Kimelblatt, B. J. (1982). Cimetidine as an inhibitor of drug metabolism: Therapeutic implications and reviews of the literature. *Drug Intelligence and Clinical Pharmacy, 16*(5), 380–386.

Beck, A. T. (1972). Screening depressed patients in family practice. *Postgraduate Medicine, 52,* 81–85.

Bell, J., Seres, V., Bowron, P., Lewis, J., & Batey, R. (1987). The use of serum methadone levels in patients receiving methadone maintenance. *Clinical Pharmacology and Therapeutics, 43,* 623–629.

Bigelow, B. E., Stitzer, M. D., & Leibsan, I. (1984). The role of behavioral contingency management in drug abuse treatment. In J. Grabowski, M. L. Stitzer, & J. C. Henningfield (Eds.), *Behavioral intervention techniques in drug abuse treatment* NIDA Research Monograph No. 46, pp. 36–52). Rockville, MD: U.S. Government Printing Office.

Blake, D. A., & Distasio, C. (1973). A comparison of levels of anxiety, depression, and hostility with methadone plasma concentrations in opioid dependent patients receiving methadone on a maintenance dosage schedule. In *Proceedings of the Fifth National Conference on Methadone Treatment.* New York: National Association for the Prevention of Addiction to Narcotics.

Brunton, L. (1990). Agents for control of gastric acidity and treatment of peptic ulcers. In A. G. Goodman, T. W. Rall, A. S. Nies, & P. Taylor (Eds.), *The pharmacological basis of therapeutics* (8th ed., pp. 896–897).

Caplehorn, J. R. M., & Bell, J. (1991). Methadone dosage and retention of patients in maintenance treatment. *Medical Journal of Australia, 154,* 195–199.

Ciccone, P. E., O'Brien, C. P., & Khatami, M. (1980). Psychotropic agents in opiate addiction: A brief review. *International Journal of the Addictions, 15*(4), 449–513.

Connett, G. (1980). Comparison of progress of patients with professional and paraprofessional counselors in a methadone maintenance program. *International Journal of the Addictions, 15,* 585–589.

Cooper, J. R., Alterman, F., Brown, B. J., & Czechowicz, D. (Eds.). (1983). *Research on the treatment of narcotic addiction.* Rockville, MD: U.S. Government Printing Office.

Cooper, J. R. (1989). Methadone treatment and acquired immunodeficiency syndrome. *Journal of the American Medical Association, 262,* 1664–1668.

Derogatis, L. R. (1970). Dimensions of outpatient neurotic pathology: Comparison of a clinical vs. an empirical assessment. *Journal of Consulting and Clinical Psychology, 34*(2), 164–171.

Division of Substance Abuse of the Albert Einstein College of Medicine of Yeshiva University. (1989). *Annual report.* New York: Author.

Dolan, M. P., Black, J. L., Penk, W. E., Robinowitz, R., & Deford, H. A. (1985). Contracting for treatment termination to reduce drug use among methadone maintenance treatment failures. *Journal of Consulting and Clinical Psychology, 53*(4), 549–551.

Dole, V. P. (1980). Addictive behavior. *Scientific American, 243,* 136–143.

Dole, V. P., & Nyswander, M. E. (1965). A medical treatment for diacetylmorphine (heroin) addiction. *Journal of the American Medical Association, 193,* 646–650.

Dole, V. P., & Nyswander, M. E. (1968). Successful treatment of 750 criminal addicts. *Journal of the American Medical Association, 206,* 2708–2710.

Dole, V. P., Robinson, J. W., Orraca, J., Towns, E., Seargy, P., & Caine, E. (1969). Methadone treatment of randomly selected criminal addicts. *New England Journal of Medicine, 280,* 1372–1375.

Finelli, P. F. (1976). Phenytoin and methadone tolerance. *New England Journal of Medicine, 294,* 227.

Freely, J., Wilkinson, G. R., & Wood, A. J. J. (1981). Reduction of liver blood flow and propranolol metabolism by cimetidine. *New England Journal of Medicine, 304,* 692–695.

Friedland, A., Schwartz, E., Brechbuhl, A. B., Kahl, P., Miller, M., & Selwyn, P. (1992). Pharmacokentic interactions of zidovudine and methadone in intravenous drug using patients with HIV infection. *Journal of Acquired Immune Deficiency Syndromes, 5,* 619–626.

Friedson, E. (1966). Sociology and rehabilitation. American Sociological Association, Washington, D.C. M. D. Sussman (ed.), pp. 711–799.

Goldstein, A. (1971). Blind dosage comparison and other studies in large methadone program. *Journal of Psychedelic Drugs, 4,* 177–180.

Goldsmith, D. S., Hunt, D. E., Lipton, D. S., & Strug, D. L. (1984). Methadone folklore: Beliefs about side effects and their impact on treatment. *Human Organization, 43*(4), 330–340.

Grabowski, J., Stitzer, M. L., & Henningfield, J. E. (Eds.). (1984). *Behavioral intervention techniques in drug abuse treatment* (NIDA Research Monograph No. 46). Rockville, MD: U.S. Government Printing Office.

Hartel, D. (1989–1990). Cocaine use, inadequate methadone dose increase risk of AIDS for IV drug users in treatment. *NIDA Notes, 5*(1), 16–17.

Hartel, D., Selwyn, P. A., Schoenbaum, E. E., Friedland, G. H., Feingold, A. R., Alderman, M. H., & Klein, R. S. (1988, June). *Methadone maintenance treatment and reduced risk of AIDS and AIDS-specific mortality in intravenous drug users* [Abstract 8526]. 4th International Conference on AIDS, Stockholm, Sweden.

Hartel, D., Schoenbaum, E. E., Selwyn, P. A., Friedland, G. H., Feingold, A. R., Alerman, M. H., & Klein, R. S. (1989, June). *Temporal patterns of cocaine use and AIDS in intravenous drug users in methadone maintenance* [Abstract]. 5th International Conference on AIDS, Stockholm, Sweden.

Horns, W. H., Rado, M., & Goldstein, A. (1975). Plasma levels and symptoms complaints in patients maintained on daily dosage of methadone hydrochloride. *Clinincal Pharmacology and Therapeutics, 17,* 636–649.

Hunt, D., Lipton, D. S., Goldsmith, D. S., & Stug, D. L. (1984). Problems in methadone treatment: The influence of reference groups. In J. Grabowski, M. L. Stitzer, & J. E. Henningfield (Eds.), *Behavioral intervention techniques in drug abuse treatment* (NIDA Research Monograph No. 46, pp. 8–12). Rockville, MD: U.S. Government Printing Office.

Inturrusi, C. E., & Verebey, K. (1972). The levels of methadone in the plasma in methadone maintenance. *Clinincal Pharmacology and Therapeutics, 13,* 633–637.

Jacobson, L. K., & Kosten, T. R. (1989). Naloxone challenge as a biological predictor of treatment outcome in opiate addicts. *American Journal of Drug and Alcohol Abuse, 15*(4), 355–366.

Joseph, H., & Springer, E. (1990). Methadone maintenance treatment and the AIDS epidemic. In *The effectiveness of drug abuse treatment: Dutch and American perspectives* (pp. 261–274). Malabar, FL: Robert E. Krieger.

Kleber, H. D. (1970). The New Haven methadone maintenance program. *International Journal of the Addictions, 5*(3), 449–463.

Kleber, H. D. (1983). Concomitant use of methadone with other psychoactive drugs in the treatment of opiate addicts with other DSM-III diagnoses. In J. R. Cooper, F. Altman, G. S. Brown, & D. Czechowicz (Eds.), *Research on the treatment of narcotic addiction (pp. 119–149)*. Rockville, MD: U.S. Government Printing Office.

Kosten, T. R., Astrachan, B. M., Riordan, C. E., & Kleber, H. D. (1982). The organization of a methadone maintenance program. *Journal of Drug Issues* (Fall), 333–342.

Kosten, T. A., Kosten, T. R., & Rounsaville, B. J. (1989). Personality disorders in opiate addicts show prognostic specificity. *Journal of Substance Abuse Treatment, 6*(3), 163–168.

Kreek, M. G. (1973). Plasma and urine levels of methadone. *New York State Journal of Medicine, 73,* 2773–2777.

Kreek, M. J. (1978). Medical complications in methadone patients. *Annals of the New York Academy of Sciences, 311,* 110–134.

Kreek, M. J., Oratz, M., & Rothschild, M. A. (1978). Hepatic extraction of long- and short-acting narcotics in the isolated perfused rabbit liver. *Gastroenterology, 75,* 88–94.

Kreek, M. J., Schoeller, D., Wong, W., & Klein, P. (1981). Identification of cirrhosis by the ^{13}C-aminopyrine breath test (ABT) in methadone maintained patients. *Gastroenterology, 80,* 1338.

Kreek, M. J. (1981a). Metabolic interactions between opiates and alcohol. *Annals of the New York Academy of Sciences, 362,* 36–49.

Kreek, M. J. (1981b). Medical management of methadone-maintained patients. In J. H. Lowinson & P. Ruis (Eds.), *Substance abuse: Clinical problems and perspectives* (pp. 660–673). Baltimore: Williams & Wilkins.

Kreek, M. J. (1986). *Factors modifying the pharamacological effectiveness of methadone* (NIDA Monograph, DHHS Pub No. [ADM] 87-1281). Rockville, MD: National Institute on Drug Abuse.

Kreek, M. J. (1991, February). *Methadone maintenance for harm reduction.* Presentation at the International Symposium on Addiction and AIDS, Vienna, Austria.

LaRosa, J. C., Lipsius, J. H., & LaRosa, J. H. (1974). Experiences with a combination of group therapy and methadone maintenance in the treatment of heroin addiction. *International Journal of the Addictions, 9,* 605–617.

Libowitz, M., Stone, M., & Turkat, I. (1986). Treatment of Personality Disorders. In A. Frances & R. Hales (Eds.), *Psychiatry update: The American Psychiatric Association annual review* (Vol. 5, pp. 356–393). Washington, DC: American Psychiatric Press.

Lofchie, S. H., & Muskelly, T. E. (1972, March). Indices of social efficacy for methadone maintenance in a medium sized city. In *Proceedings of the Fourth National Conference of Methadone Maintenance* (pp. 159–162).

London, J., Miller, M., Sorensen, J. L., Delucchi, K., Dilley, J., Dotson, J., Schwartz, B., & Okin, R. (1995). *Problems of HIV-infected substance abusers entering case management.* Paper presented at the 57th annual scientific meeting of the College on Problems of Drug Dependence, Scottsdale, Arizona.

Lowinson, J. H., Marion, I. J., Joseph, H., & Dole, V. P. (1992). Methadone maintenance. In J. H. Lowinson, P. Ruiz, R. B. Millman, & J. G. Langrod (Eds.), *Substance abuse: A comprehensive textbook* (pp. 550–561). Baltimore: Williams & Wilkins.

Luborsky, L., McLellan, A. T., Woody, G. E., O'Brien, C. P., & Auerbach, A. (1985). Therapist success and its determinants. *Archives of General Psychiatry, 42,* 602–611.

McLellan, A. T., Arndt, I. O., Woody, G. E., & O'Brien, C. P. (1990). *Three levels of service provision in methadone maintenance.* Paper presented at the Committee of Problems of Drug Dependence Conference, Richmond, Virginia.

McLellan, A. T., Luborsky, L., O'Brien, C. P., Woody, G. E., & Druley, K. A. (1982). Is treatment for substance abuse effective? *Journal of the Americann Medical Association, 247,* 1423–1428.

McLellan, A. T., Luborsky, L., Woody, G. E., Druley, K. A., & O'Brien, C. (1983). Predicting response to alcohol and drug abuse treatments: Role of psychiatric severity. *Archives of General Psychiatry, 40,* 620–625.

McLellan, A. T., Woody, G. E., Luborsky, L., & Goehl, L. (1988). Is the counselor an "active ingredient" in substance abuse rehabilitation? An examination of treatment success among four counselors. *Journal of Nervous and Mental Disease, 176,* 423–430.

Newman, R. G., & Whitehall, W. B. (1979). Double-blind comparisons of methadone and placebo maintenance treatments of narcotic addicts in Hong Kong. *Lancet, 8141,* 485–488.

Nilsson, M. I., Gronbladh, L., Widerlov, E., & Anggard, E. (1983). Pharmacokinetics of methadone in methadone maintenance treatment: Characterization of therapeutic failures. *European Journal of Clinical Pharmacology, 25,* 497–501.

Novich, D. M., Ochshorn, M., Ghail, V., Croxson, T. S., Mercer, W. D., Chiorazzi, N., & Kreek, M. J. (1989). Natural killer activity and lymphocyte subsets in perenteral heroin abusers and long term methadone maintanance patients. *Journal of Pharmacology and Experimental Therapeutics, 250,* 606–610.

Novick, D. M., Pascarelli, E. F., & Joseph, H. (1988). Methadone maintenance patients in general medical practice: A preliminary report. *Journal of the American Medical Association, 259,* 3299–3302.

Resnick, R. B., Washton, A. M., Stone-Washton, N., et al. (1980). Psychotherapy and naltrexone in opioid dependence. In L. S. Harris (Ed.), *Problems of drug dependence* (NIDA Research Monograph Series No. 34, DHHS publication [ADM] 81-1058, pp. 109–115). Rockville, MD: National Institute on Drug Abuse.

Rosenblum, A. R., Magura, S., & Joseph, H. (1995). Ambivalence towards methadone among intravenous drug users. *Journal of Psychoactive Drugs, 27*(2), 151–159.

Rounsaville, B. J., Glazer, W., Wilber, C. H., Weissman, M. M., & Kleber, H. D. (1983). Short-term interpersonal psychotherapy in methadone-maintained opiate addicts. *Archives of General Psychiatry, 40,* 630–636.

Rounsaville, B. J., Dolinsky, Z. S., Babor, T. F., & Meyer, R. E. (1987). Psychopathology as a predictor of treatment outcome in alcoholics. *Archives of General Psychiatry, 44*(6), 505–513.

Rounsaville, B. J., Weissman, M. M., Crits-Christoph, K., Wilber, C., & Kleber, H. D. (1982a). Diagnosis and symptoms of depressions in opiate addicts. *Archives of General Psychiatry, 39,* 151–156.

Rounsaville, B. J., Weissman, M. M., Kleber, H. D., & Wilber, C. H. (1982b). The heterogeneity of psychiatric diagnosis in treated opiate addicts. *Archives of Genearl Psychiatry, 39,* 161–166.

Sedman, A. J. (1984). Cimetidine-drug interactions. *American Journal of Medicine, 76,* 109–114.

Selwyn, P. A., Budner, N. S., Wasserman, W. C., & Arno, P. S. (1993). Utilization of on-site primary care services by HIV-seropositive and seronegative drug users in a methadcone maintenance program. *Public Health Reports, 108,* 492–500.

Sells, S. B. (1979). Treatment effectiveness. In R. L. Dupont, A. Goldstein, & J. O'Donnell (Eds.), *Handbook on drug abuse* (pp. 105–118). Rockville, MD: National Institute on Drug Abuse.

Stanton, M. D., Todd, T. C., & Associates. (1982). *The family therapy of drug abuse and addiction.* New York: Guilford Press.

Tennant, F. S. Jr. (1987). Inadequate plasma concentrations in some high dose methadone maintenance patients. *American Journal of Psychiatry, 144,* 1349–1350.

Tennant, F. S. Jr., Rawson, R. A., Cohen, A., Tarver, A., & Clabough, D. (1983). Methadone plasma levels and persistent drug abuse in high dose methadone patients. *Substance and Alcohol Actions/Misuse, 4,* 369–374.

Tong, T. G., Pond, S. M., Kreek, M. J., Jaffery, N. F., & Benowitz, N. L. (1981). Phenytoin induced methadone withdrawal. *Annals of Internal Medicine, 94,* 349–351.

United States General Accounting Office. (1990). *Methadone maintenance: Some treatment programs are not effective. Greater federal oversight needed* (Publication No. GAO/HRD-90-104). Washington DC: U.S. Government Printing Office.

Wall, T. L., Sorensen, J. L., Batki, S. L., Delucchi, K. L., London, J. A., & Chesney, M. A. (1995). Adherence to zidovudine (AZT) among HIV-infected methadone patients: A pilot study of supervised therapy and dispensing compared to usual care. *Drug and Alcohol Dependence, 37,* 261–269.

Wendell, G. D., & Kreek, M. J. (1979). Effects of chronic methadone treatment on rate of ethanol elimination in the rat in vivo. [Abstract of the 10th Annual NCA/AMSA/RSA Medical-Scientific Conference of the National Alcoholism Forum, Washington, DC]. *Alcoholism, 3,* 220.

Widiger, T. A., & Frances, A. (1986). Personality disorders. In J. A. Talbatl, R. E. Haber, & S. C. Yudofsky (Eds.), *The American Psychiatric Press textbook of psychiatry* (pp. 621–648). Washington, DC: American Psychiatric Press.

Wilkinson, W., & Williams, S. (1991). Personal communications. St. Clare's Hospital, New York City.

Willett, E. A. (1973). Group therapy in a methadone treatment program: An evaluation of changes in interpersonal behavior. *International Journal of the Addictions, 8,* 33–39.

Woody, G. E., Luborsky, L., McLellan, A. T., O'Brien, C. P., Beck, A. T., Blaine, J., Hermer, I., & Hole, A. (1983). Psychotherapy for opiate addicts: Does it help? *Archives of General Psychiatry, 40,* 639–645.

Chapter 5

USE OF PHARMACOLOGICAL AGENTS IN OPIATE DETOXIFICATION

Marc Rosen, M.D.

Opioid addiction is, in many ways, a physical problem. Addicts become physically addicted to opiates, and in the later stages of addiction, become preoccupied with relieving the physical symptoms of withdrawal. Addicts become highly attuned to their bodily signals that withdrawal is coming. A heroin addict spends most of his or her waking life procuring, using, and withdrawing from heroin, using three times a day, 7 days a week, 52 weeks a year, for years.

DISCOVERY OF OPIATE WITHDRAWAL SIGNS

Up through the 1950s, many of the medications used to treat heroin withdrawal were largely ineffective, and in some cases the cure was worse than the disease. Numerous ineffective treatments have been used, including thorazine, barbiturates, and electroshock therapy. One method used belladonna and laxatives, based on the incorrect theory that narcotics needed to be "rinsed" from the bodily tissues in which they were stored. Commenting on these methods, two researchers said: "The knockout feature of these treatments . . . doubtless had the effect of holding until cured many patients who would have discontinued a withdrawal treatment before being cured and the psychological effect of doing something for patients practically all the time has a tendency, by allaying apprehension to hold them even though what is done is harmful" (Kolb & Himmelsbach, 1938; Kleber, 1981).

Federal prisoners addicted to narcotics were sent to the prison in Lexington, Kentucky, until the 1960s. The contributions of the Lexington researchers to our understanding of opiate dependence have been reviewed elsewhere (Jasinski, 1977). An important contribution was the development of standardized ratings of opiate withdrawal severity, such as the Himmelsbach rating scale (Himmelsbach, 1939). This scale was developed by assigning point values to a number of observer-rated signs of withdrawal severity after opiate maintenance was discontinued in dependent subjects. Another methodology developed at Lexington, the suppression study (Himmelsbach, 1934), examined whether a drug suppressed the withdrawal caused by discontinuation of maintenance morphine (Himmelsbach & Andrews, 1943). A modification of this method, the substitution study, involves a 1-day substitution of the medication to be tested for maintenance morphine in dependent individuals; an effective medication will suppress the emergence of morphine withdrawal signs (Fraser & Isbell, 1960; Jasinski et al., 1985). More recently, attempts have been made to test opiate detoxification agents by determining whether pretreatment with the agent attenuates naloxone-precipitated withdrawal in people made dependent on acute (Sullivan et al., 1994) or chronic (Rosen et al., 1996) doses of maintenance opiate. Naloxone-precipitated opiate withdrawal is now recognized as involving psychological, in addition to physical, symptoms (Kanof et al., 1992; Strain et al., 1992).

METHODS OF DETOXIFICATION

Opioid Substitution, Stabilization, and Taper

The simplest approach to detoxification is to substitute a prescribed opioid for the heroin that the addict is dependent on, and then to gradually lower the dose of the prescribed opioid. The prescribed opioid commonly is methadone (Senay et al., 1981; Silsby & Tenant, 1974; Wilson et al., 1974). Because of methadone's relatively long duration of action (Olsen et al., 1977), withdrawal from it is more gradual and has a lesser peak severity than with heroin withdrawal. A typical detoxification procedure would be to verify that an addict is dependent on opioids (by some combination of observed withdrawal, a withdrawal response to naloxone, or evidence of heavy opioid use). The addict is then given an appropriate dose of methadone, which treats the withdrawal symptoms. The addict is monitored for oversedation from the methadone, or undermedication of withdrawal symptoms. For an intravenous user of street heroin admitted to the hospital, a starting methadone dose of 25 mg is usually well tolerated. The methadone dose is then gradually lowered over the next several days; for a starting methadone dose of 25 mg, a taper over 7 days is typical. Methadone maintenance, as opposed to methadone stabilization, induces a high degree of opiate dependence and is associated with prolonged withdrawal symptoms. A controlled study of detoxification from a mean dose of 31 mg of methadone found that a 10% dose decrease per week was associated with more withdrawal symptoms and interrupted treatment than there was with detoxification at 3% per week (Senay et al., 1977). Although there is wide variability in long-term abstinence rates after methadone detoxification, the rates appear to be quite low (Cushman & Dole, 1973).

The same principles of methadone stabilization and discontinuation apply to detoxification by using the longer-acting opioid agonist levo-alpha-acetylmethadol (LAAM). However, LAAM dosing needs to account for the accumulation of LAAM and its metabolites with repeated dosing (Blaine et al., 1981) and the metabolistes' long duration of action. The withdrawal from LAAM has a delayed onset, relative to methadone discontinuation, but a similar time course (Fraser & Isbell, 1952; Sorensen et al., 1982).

Buprenorphine is a partial μ-agonist with an extremely high receptor affinity (Gal, 1989; Lewis, 1985; Neal, 1984). Several clinical findings suggest that buprenorphine dissociation from opiate receptors occurs slowly. Naloxone's reversal of respiratory suppression by buprenorphine takes 3 hours (Gal, 1989), buprenorphine blockade of the effects of exogenous hydromorphone doses continues for 3 days after buprenorphine discontinuation (Rosen et al., 1994), and the withdrawal syndrome after buprenorphine discontinuation is relatively mild and gradual. There have only been two inpatient studies of abrupt buprenorphine discontinuation. An early study (Jasinski et al., 1978) found a mild, delayed withdrawal syndrome after discontinuation of a daily subcutaneous buprenorphine dose of 8 mg daily in three volunteers. A later study (Fudala et al., 1990) of 15 addicts who completed detoxification from a daily sublingual buprenorphine dose of 8 mg found no significant physiological or observer-reported evidence of opiate withdrawal. There were complaints by subjects, which included sleep disturbance, that showed no meaningful change from days 1–3 off of buprenorphine and that then peaked sharply at day 5. Despite more promising initial reports, spontaneous withdrawal from buprenorphine appears to be associated with high relapse rates (Bickel et al., 1988; Resnick et al., 1992).

Nonopioids: Clonidine

Another approach avoids the difficulties of prescribing an opioid to an addict. It involves using the antihypertensive clonidine to treat opiate withdrawal symptoms when the addict stops using the opiates. Clonidine suppresses many of the physical signs of opiate withdrawal but is less effective against many of the more subjective complaints during withdrawal: lethargy, restlessness, and dysphoria (Jasinski et al., 1985). Clonidine's side effects of low blood pressure (Rudd & Blaschke, 1985), sedation, and blurry vision make it unpleasant to take and unlikely to be abused by addicts. Clonidine is ineffective in addicts for detoxification from maintenance methadone doses higher than 30 mg. In outpatients, an additional risk in addicts cross-addicted to alcohol or sedatives is that clonidine may mask autonomic signs of withdrawal without preventing withdrawal seizures. Although clonidine is not approved by the U.S. Food and Drug Administration for opiate detoxification, it is widely used.

Clonidine's efficacy in the treatment of opiate withdrawal is controversial. A study comparing single doses of clonidine to placebo in addicts after methadone discontinuation showed clonidine attenuation of subjective symptoms such as nervousness and irritability and of Weak Opiate Withdrawal Scale subject ratings of opiate withdrawal (Gold et al., 1980). In this paradigm, clonidine may show efficacy because of the contrast with the preceding symptomatic withdrawal period. A study comparing placebo to dynorphin in withdrawing opiate addicts reported placebo effecting an approximately 20% reduction of subject-rated withdrawal and reported somewhat less attenuation in observer-rated withdrawal (Wen & Ho, 1982). A study comparing clonidine to placebo substitution in morphine-stabilized patients found that clonidine attenuated many autonomic symptoms of withdrawal, but had small affect on subjects' withdrawal distress (Jasinski et al., 1985).

A large study of 49 methadone-maintained outpatients undergoing detoxification from a maintenance dose of 20 mg compared abrupt methadone discontinuation and clonidine substitution to tapering of the maintenance methadone dose by 1mg/day (Kleber et al., 1985). Both outpatient groups had statistically equivalent 40% detoxification completion rates. However, the clonidine-treated group had more symptoms during the first 2 weeks of detoxification (Rounsaville et al., 1985). Clonidine-treated subjects who did not complete the detoxification showed a discrepancy between lower observer ratings of opiate withdrawal severity and higher subject ratings (Kosten et al., 1985). A randomized clinical trial comparing clonidine, guanfacine, and methadone taper in controlling heroin withdrawal (San et al., 1990) found less severe withdrawal symptoms initially in the methadone group.

OPIATE ANTAGONISTS

By as yet unknown mechanisms, the administration of opiate antagonists to dependent subjects reverses opiate dependence and accomplishes a detoxification. Administration of naloxone in dependent monkeys causes a desensitization to subsequent naloxone doses (Krystal et al., 1989). Repeated naloxone administration has been used to complete detoxification of low-dose methadone maintenance patients (Resnick et al., 1977) and has also been used, in combination with clonidine, to accomplish rapid detoxification (Riordan & Kleber, 1980). An inpatient study (Charney et al., 1982) of combined clonidine–naltrexone detoxification found a rapid diminution of withdrawal after the first day of naltrexone; this diminution was more rapid than when clonidine alone was used in a historical control group (Charney et al., 1981). Clonidine–naltrexone detoxification requires a careful titration of (1) the level of dependence of the subjects, (2) the doses of naltrexone administered, and (3) the doses of clonidine used. In the Charney study (1982) of methadone-dependent inpatients, the initial naltrexone dose was 1 mg and was gradually increased with successive doses given 4 hours apart. A study of outpatients given a mean naltrexone dose of 20.9 mg required that subjects be sedated with a mean of 1.22 mg of clonidine and 75.4 mg of diazepam, which produced a state of being "rousable" (Brewer et al., 1988). Transitioning opiate-dependent addicts with naloxone to opiate antagonist maintenance in 1 day is theoretically possible. Loimer has reported the efficacy, but not the clinical feasibility, of single-day "detoxifications" by using high-dose naloxone infusions under barbiturate (Loimer et al., 1990) and benzodiazepine (Loimer et al., 1991) anesthesia. After the naloxone infusions, subjects were able to tolerate further antagonist doses without precipitation of withdrawal.

NONPHARMACOLOGICAL ASPECTS

Neuroticism, as measured by the Eysenck Personality Questionnaire, and the degree of distress that a client expects predict subsequent levels of opiate withdrawal severity (Phillips et al., 1986). In the aforementioned study of clonidine and methadone detoxification from methadone maintenance (Rounsaville et al., 1985), six of the nine subscales on the Symptom Checklist 90 (SCL-90) (Derogatis, 1977) indicated more psychological distress in patients who failed to complete detoxification. The authors note that the "best predictor of detoxification failure was a high level of psychological symptoms at the onset of the study." Involving patients in their treatment appears to improve outcome. Subjects on open methadone maintenance have fewer withdrawal symptoms than patients on double-blinded dosing schedules (Senay et al., 1977). Methadone maintenance patients who are told their dose-reduction schedule complain of fewer symptoms (Stitzer et al., 1992).

PROTRACTED ABSTINENCE PHENOMENON

Chronic use of opioids causes neurobiological alterations that persist for months after discontinuation of the opiates (Satel et al., 1993). This "protracted withdrawal" has been implicated in such clinically crucial phenomena as the difficulty of detoxifying from methadone maintenance (Senay et al., 1977), high rates of relapse after abstinence (Dole, 1972), and drug craving (Mirin et al., 1976).

Up to 9 months after detoxification, opiate addicts manifest abstinence symptoms of weight gain, increased basal metabolic rate, decreased temperature, increased respiration, increased blood pressure, and decreased erythrocyte sedimentation rate (Himmelsbach, 1942). A controlled study (Eisenman et al., 1969; Martin & Jasinski, 1969) examined seven drug-free ex-addicts who were (1) admitted to a research ward, (2) readdicted to morphine, and (3) detoxified under supervision. They showed significant increases over baseline for 6–9 weeks after detoxification in Himmelsbach abstinence scale ratings, blood pressure, body temperature, and pupillary size. Respiratory rate and urinary epinephrine were elevated for 17 weeks. Some of the parameters described in the abstinence studies showed a biphasic response in which abnormalities during the first 4–9 weeks after detoxification reverted afterward for several months to values more consistent with intoxication. The exact neurobiological basis for these changes has not been defined, although preclinical research has shown supersensitivity during abstinence in dopaminergic (Lal & Puri, 1972; Gianutsos et al., 1974), cholinergic (Glick & Cox, 1977), and opioid systems (Brase et al., 1976; Goldberg & Schuster, 1969).

SUMMARY

The medications for treating and detoxifying opioid addicts are powerful agents that interrupt the cycle of intoxication and withdrawal. A literature review suggests several potential new directions in the study of detoxification. One is to develop nonabusable medications that do not have clonidine's drawbacks of undesirable side effects and questionable efficacy against subjective withdrawal distress. Another clinical need is for agents to ease the transition from opioid agonist to antagonist treatment. Finally, there may be a role for pharmacotherapy in ameliorating any long-term abstinence symptoms that contribute to relapse.

REFERENCES

Bickel, W. K., Stitzer, M. L., Bigelow, G. E., Liebson, I. A., Jasinski, D. R., & Johnson, R. E. (1988). A clinical trial of buprenorphine: comparison with methadone in the detoxification of heroin addicts. *Clinical Pharmacology and Therapeutics, 43,* 72–78.

Blaine, J. D., Thomas, D. B., Barnett, G., Whysner, J. A., & Renault, P. F. (1981). Levo-alpha acetylmethadol (LAMM): Clinical utility and pharmaceutical development. In J. Lowinson & P. Ruiz (Eds.), *Substance abuse: Clinical problems and perspectives* (pp. 360–388). Baltimore: Williams & Wilkins.

Brase, D. A., Iwamoto, E. T., Loh, H. H., & Way, E. L. (1976). Reinitiation of sensitivity to naloxone by a single narcotic injection in post-addict mice. *Journal of Pharmacology and Experimental Therapeutics, 197,* 317–325.

Brewer, C., Hussein, R., & Bailey, C. (1988). Opioid withdrawal and naltrexone induction in 48–72 hours with minimal drop-out using a modification of the naltrexone-clonidine technique. *British Journal of Psychiatry, 153,* 340–343.

Charney, D. S., Sternberg, D. E., Kleber, H. D., Heninger, G.R., & Redmond, E. (1981). The clinical use of clonidine in abrupt withdrawal from methadone. *Archives of General Psychiatry, 38,* 1272–1277.

Charney, D. S., Riordan, C. E., Kleber, H. D., Murburg, M., Braverman, P., Sternberg, D. E., Heninger, G. R., & Redmond, E. (1982). Clonidine and naltrexone: A safe, effective, and rapid treatment of abrupt withdrawal from methadone therapy. *Archives of General Psychiatry, 39,* 1327–1332.

Cushman, P., & Dole, V. P. (1973). Detoxification of methadone maintenance patients. *Journal of the American Medical Association, 226,* 747–751.

Derogatis, L. R. (1977). *The SCL-90 manual I: Scoring, administration, and procedures from the SCL-90-R.* Baltimore: Clinical Psychometrics Research.

Dole, V. P. (1972). Narcotic addition, physical dependence and relapse. *New England Journal of Medicine, 286*(18), 988–992.

Eisenman, A. J., Sloan, J. W., Martin, W. R., Jasinski, D. R., & Brooks, J. W. (1969). Catecholamine and 17-hydroxycorticosteroid excretion during a cycle of morphine dependence in man. *Journal of Psychiatric Research, 7,* 19–28.

Fraser, H. F., & Isbell, H. (1952). Actions and addiction liabilities of alpha-acetylmethadols in man. *Journal of Pharmacology and Experimental Therapeutics, 105,* 458–465.

Fraser, H. F., & Isbell, H. (1960). Human pharmacology and addiction liabilities of phenazocine and levophenacylmorphan. *Bulletin of Narcotics, 12,* 15–23.

Fudala, P. J., Jaffe, J. H., Dax, E. M., & Johnson, R. E. (1990). Use of buprenorphine in the treatment of opioid addiction: 2. Physiologic and behavioral effects of daily and alternate-day administration and abrupt withdrawal. *Clinical Pharmacololgy and Therapeutics, 47,* 525–534.

Gal, T. J. (1989). Naloxone reversal of buprenorphine-induced respiratory depression. *Clinical Pharmacology and Therapeutics, 45,* 66–71.

Gianutsos, G., Hynes, M. D., Puri, S. K., Drawbaugh, R. B., & Lal, H. (1974). Effect of apomorphine and nigrostriatal lesions on aggression and striatal dopamine turnover during morphine withdrawal: Evidence for dopaminergic supersensitivity in protracted abstinence. *Psychopharmacologia, 34,* 37–44.

Glick, S., & Cox, R. D. (1977). Changes in sensitivity to operant effects of dopaminergic and cholinergic agents following morphine withdrawal in rats. *European Journal of Pharmacology, 42,* 303–306.

Gold, M. S., Pottash, A. C., Sweeney, D. R., & Kleber, H. D. (1980). Opiate withdrawal using clonidine. *Journal of the American Medical Association, 243*(4), 343–346.

Goldberg, S. R., & Schuster, C. R. (1969). Nalorphine: Increased sensitivity of monkeys formerly dependent on morphine. *Science, 166,* 1548–1549.

Himmelsbach, C. K. (1934). Addiction liability of codeine. *Journal of the American Medical Association, 103,* 1420.

Himmelsbach, C. K. (1939). Studies of certain addiction characteristics of: (a) dihydromorphine (paramorphan), (b) dihydrodesoxymorphine-D (desmorphine), (c) dihydrodesoxycodeine-D (desocodeine), (d) dihydromorphinone (metopon). *Journal of Pharmacology and Experimental Therapeutics, 67,* 239–249.

Himmelsbach, C. K. (1942). Clinical studies of drug addiction: physical dependence, withdrawal and recovery. *Archives of Internal Medicine, 69,* 766–772.

Himmelsbach, C. K., & Andrews, H. L. (1943). Studies on the modification of the morphine abstinence syndrome by drugs. *Journal of Pharmacology and Experimental Therapeutics, 77,* 17–23.

Jasinski, D. R. (1977). Assessment of the abuse potential of morphine-like drugs (methods used in man). In W. R. Martin (Ed.), *Drug addiction I* (Vol. 45, Handbook of Experimental Pharmacology Series; pp. 197–258). Heidelberg: Springer-Verlag.

Jasinski, D. R., Hevnick, J. S., & Griffith, J. D. (1978). Human pharmacology and abuse potential of the analgesic buprenorphine. *Archives of General Psychiatry, 35,* 601–616.

Jasinski, D. R., Johnson, R. E., & Kocher, T. R. (1985). Clonidine in morphine withdrawal: Differential effects on signs and symptoms. *Archives of General Psychiatry, 42*(11), 1063–1066.

Kanof, P. D., Handelsman, L., Aronson, M. J., Ness, R., Cochrane, K. J., & Rubinstein, K. J. (1992). Characteristics of naloxone-precipitated opiate withdrawal in human opioid-dependent subjects. *Journal of Pharmacology and Experimental Therapeutics, 260*(1), 355–363.

Kleber, H. D. (1981). Detoxification from narcotics. In J. H. Lowinson & P. Ruiz (Eds.), *Substance abuse: Clinical problems and perspectives.* Baltimore: Williams & Wilkins.

Kleber, H. D., Riordan, C. E., Rounsaville, B. J., Kosten, T. R., Charney, D. S., Gaspari, J., Hogan, I., & O'Connor, C. (1985). Clonidine in outpatient detoxification from methadone maintenance. *Archives of General Psychiatry, 42*(4), 391–394.

Kolb, L., & Himmelsbach, C. K. (1938). Clinical studies of drug addiction: 3. A critical review of the withdrawal treatments with method of evaluating abstinence syndromes. *Public Health Reports, 128*(1).

Kosten, T. R., Rounsaville, B. J., & Kleber, H. D. (1985). Comparison of clinician ratings to self reports of withdrawal during clonidine detoxification of opiate addicts. *American Journal of Drug and Alcohol Abuse, 11*(1–2), 1–10.

Krystal, J. H., Walker, M. W., & Heninger, G. R. (1989). Intermittent naloxone attenuates the development of physical dependence on methadone in rhesus monkeys. *European Journal of Pharmacology, 160,* 331–338.

Lal, H., & Puri, S. K. (1972). Morphine withdrawal aggression: Role of dopaminergic stimulation. *Drug Addiction, 1,* 301–310.

Lewis, J. W. (1985). Buprenorphine. *Drug and Alcohol Dependence, 14,* 363–372.

Loimer, N., Lenz, K., Schmid, R., & Presslich, O. (1991). Technique for greatly shortening the transition from methadone to naltrexone maintenance of patients addicted to opiates. *American Journal of Psychiatry, 148,* 933–935.

Loimer, N., Schmid, R., Lenz, K., Presslich, O., & Grunberger, J. (1990). Acute blocking of naloxone-precipitated opiate withdrawal symptoms by methohexitone. *British Journal of Psychiatry, 157,* 748–752.

Martin, W. R., & Jasinski, D. R. (1969). Physiological parameters of morphine dependence in man-tolerance, early abstinence, protracted abstinence. *Journal of Psychiatric Research, 7,* 9–17.

Mirin, S. M., Meyer, R. E., & McNamee, B. H. (1976). Psychopathology and mood during heroin use: Acute vs. chronic effects. *Archives of General Psychiatry, 33,* 1503–1508.

Neil, A. (1984). Affinities of some common opioid analgesics towards four binding sites in mouse brain. *Naunyn-Schmeideberg's Archives of Pharmacology, 328,* 24–29.

Olsen, G. D., Wendel, H. A., Livermore, J. D., Leger, R. M., Lynn, R. K., & Gerber, N. (1977). Clinical effects and pharmacokinetics of racemic methadone and its optical isomers. *Clinical Pharmacology and Therapeutics, 21*(2), 147–157.

Phillips, G. T., Gossop, M., & Bradley, B. (1986). The influence of psychological factors on the opiate withdrawal syndrome. *British Journal of Psychiatry, 149,* 235–238.

Resnick, R. B., Galanter, M., Pycha, C., Cohen, A., Grandison, P., & Flood, N. (1992). Buprenorphine: An alternative to methadone for heroin dependence treatment. *Psychopharmacology Bulletin, 28*(1), 109–113.

Resnick, R. B., Kestenbaum, R. S., Washton, A. W., & Poole, D. (1977). Naloxone-precipiated withdrawal: a method for rapid induction onto naltrexone. *Clinical Pharmacology and Therapeutics, 21,* 409–413.

Riordan, C. E., & Kleber, H. D. (1980). Rapid opiate detoxification with clonidine and naloxone. *Lancet, 1,* 1079–1080.

Rosen, M. I., McMahon, T. J., Hameedi, F. A. Pearsall, H. R., Woods, S. W., Kreek, M. J., & Kosten, T. R. (1996). Effect of clonidine pretreatment on naloxone-precipitated opiate withdrawal. *Journal of Pharmacology and Experimental Therapeutics, 276*(3). 1128–1135.

Rosen, M. I,, Wallace, E. A., McMahon, T. H., Pearsall, H. R., Woods, S. W., Price, L. H., & Kosten, T. R. (1994). Buprenorphine: Duration of blockade of effects of intramuscular hydromorphone. *Drug and Alcohol Dependence, 35,* 141–149.

Rounsaville, B. J., Kosten, T. R., & Kleber, H. D. (1985). Success and failure at outpatient opioid detoxification: Evaluating the process of clonidine and methadone-assisted withdrawal. *Journal of Nervous and Mental Disease, 173*(2), 103–110.

Rudd, P., & Blaschke, T. F. (1985). Antihypertensive agents and the drug therapy of hypertension. In A. G. Gillman, L. S. Goodman, T. W. Rall et al. (Eds.), *The pharmacological basis of therapeutics* (7th ed.). New York: Macmillan.

San, L., Cami, J., Peir, J. M., Mata, R., & Porta, M. (1990). Efficacy of clonidine, guanfacine and methadone in the rapid detoxification of heroin addicts: A controlled clinical trial. *British Journal of Addictions, 85*(1), 141–147.

Satel, S. L., Kosten, T. R., Schuckit, M. A., & Fischman, M. W. (1993). Should protracted withdrawal from drugs be included in DSM-IV? *American Journal of Psychiatry, 150,* 695–704.

Senay, E. D., Dorus, W., & Showalter, C. V. (1981). Short-term detoxification with methadone. *Annals of the New York Academy of Sciences, 362,* 203–216.

Senay, E. C., Dorus, W., Goldberg, F., & Thornton, W. (1977). Withdrawal from methadone maintenance: Rate of withdrawal and expectation. *Archives of General Psychiatry, 34,* 361–367.

Silsby, H., & Tennant, F. S., Jr. (1974). Short-term, ambulatory detoxification of opiate addicts using methadone. *International Journal of the Addictions, 9*(1), 167–170.

Sorensen, J. L., Hargreaves, W. A., & Weinberg, J. A. (1982). Withdrawal from heroin in three or six weeks: Comparison of methadyl acetate and methadone. *Archives of General Psychiatry, 39,* 167–171.

Stitzer, M., Bigelow, G., & Liebson, I. (1982). Comparison of three out-patient methadone detoxification procedures. In *Problems of drug dependence* (NIDA Monograph No. 41). Rockville, MD: U.S. Department of Health and Human Services.

Strain, E. C., Preston, K. L., Liebson, I. A., & Bigelow, G. E. (1992). Acute effects of buprenorphine, hydromorphone and naloxone in methadone-maintained volunteers. *Journal of Pharmacology and Experimental Therapeutics, 261*(3), 985–993.

Sullivan, J. T., Johnson, R. E., Testa, M. S., Stitzer, M., & Jasinski, D. R. (1994). Development of a method to screen for opiate withdrawal suppressing drugs: Clonidine (C) effects. *Clinical Pharmacology and Therapeutics, 55*(1), 131.

Wilson, B. K., Elms, R. R., & Thomson, C. P. (1974). Low-dosage use of methadone in extended detoxification. *Archives of General Psychiatry, 31,* 233–236.

Wen, H. L., & Ho, W. K. K. (1982). Suppression of withdrawal symptoms by dynorphin in heroin addicts. *European Journal of Pharmacology, 82,* 183–186.

Chapter 6

NALTREXONE AND OPIATE ABUSE

Conor K. Farren, M.B., M.R.C.P.I., M.R.C.Psych.
Stephanie O'Malley, Ph.D.
Bruce Rounsaville, M.D.

This chapter outlines the use of naltrexone in opiate abuse over the past 25 years, examines ways of improving its effectiveness, and looks at the profile of subjects that appear to benefit from it the most. We examine the different ways in which naltrexone has been used in opiate abusers and look at both the advantages and the disadvantages of the programs that have used it. We suggest various methods of improving the success rate of naltrexone in opiate abuse, from patient selection to adjunctive behavioral techniques.

The need for a long-acting narcotic antagonist had been explored as far back as 1948 by Wikler (1948). He suggested that antagonists could extinguish drug-seeking behavior by their ability to block the effect of narcotics if the patient tried to get high, or could extinguish the conditioned withdrawal response occurring in the presence of the stimuli previously associated with the use of drugs. Wikler also suggested that the urge to use opioids might be extinguished if patients lived in the environment that previously had been associated with drug addiction without being able to get high from the narcotics (Wikler, 1948).

Naltrexone, synthesized in 1965 by Blumberg and Dayton (1973), has a number of advantages over other opioid antagonists. It is more potent than naloxone and nalorphine (Martin et al., 1973) and, unlike newer pharmacotherapies like buprenorphine, is devoid of agonist activity. Being a pure antagonist means that naltrexone not only fails to produce opioid effects but also prevents any opioid agonist from binding to the opioid receptor and producing opioid effects. Thus, there is no opioid-induced euphoria, respiratory depression, or pupillary constriction (Martin et al., 1973). Resnick et al. (1974) suggested that naltrexone would be useful for the treatment of individuals who were no longer opioid dependent but who were at significant risk for recidivism, that is, individuals who were recently detoxified from opioids or who were returning to a high-risk environment.

Other advantages include a relatively long half-life and an oral administration route. However, there have been reports of dysphoric reactions in experimental subjects who were given naltrexone (Mendelson et al., 1980), and Hollister et al. (1981) found some adverse mood effects in normal volunteers who were given naltrexone. In general, however, there appears to be a consensus that in normal persons there is no difference in mood effects between naltrexone and placebo (O'Brien et al., 1978), and most large-scale studies on recovering opiate addicts have not found dysphoria or other mood changes to be a problem in the clinical use of naltrexone (Brahen et al., 1984; Greenstein et al., 1984; Tennant et al., 1984; Washton et al., 1984). Those persons who are maintained on naltrexone for months or even years report no mood effects.

Naltrexone as a medication is also very easy to administer and is generally well tolerated. It can be administered as a daily 50-mg dose or as a triweekly regime of 100 mg on Monday, 100 mg on Wednesday, and 150 mg on Friday. It can even be given as 150 mg on Monday and 200 mg on Thursday (Ginzberg, 1986). It has very few contraindications and is very safe in clinical dosages. It has no addictive potential and has no tolerance induced by use over long periods of time. Its ease of induction and its lack of withdrawal make it relatively easy to start and very easy to discontinue (Kleber, 1985). In the presence of naltrexone, heroin self-administration is no longer rewarding, and the behavior is observed to stop (Mello et al., 1980). Naltrexone has also been used to successfully extinguish opioid-conditioned responses in a laboratory setting (O'Brien et al., 1984).

INDUCTION INTO A NALTREXONE PROGRAM

Because naltrexone will precipitate withdrawal in opiate-addicted individuals, much of the research has examined the efficacy of various strategies to induct patients into a naltrexone program. Although gradually reducing doses of methadone for 5–10 days constitutes one approach, this program requires an additional 10 days to elapse after the last dose of methadone before the naltrexone can be started. At the other end of the spectrum, a rapid detoxification from opiates assisted by clonidine can have the patient ready for commencement of naltrexone in as little as 48 hours after being opiate dependent (Kleber & Kosten, 1984). In an outpatient randomized clinical trial comparing clonidine alone to a standard 30-day-dosage tapering of methadone for detoxification, the rate of remaining opioid free for a week was 45% with no difference between the two treatments (Kleber et al., 1985). The choice between these two types of detoxification depends upon the type of opiate agonist that the patient was using, whether it was short or long acting, the motivation of the patient, and the need for speed in returning to work.

While inpatient induction into a naltrexone program is usually more successful than the use of other therapies, initially it is more expensive in the cost of the program and in the cost to the patient, who may have to leave a job and who may have hospital expenses as well. "Street" addicts are usually more willing to enter an inpatient unit than methadone-maintained patients are. It is suggested that while outpatient induction has a lower initial success rate, at the end of 1 month both inpatient and outpatient approaches are left with approximately the same number of clients. "Street" addicts appear to benefit from supports, such as counseling or behavioral techniques, given during the induction period, whereas methadone-maintained patients do not appear to benefit to the same extent. In general, methadone-maintained patients have a high dropout rate when first inducted onto naltrexone (Kleber, 1985).

In early studies where both naltrexone and clonidine were used for induction of naltrexone maintenance, naltrexone was started at 1 mg and gradually increased to 50 mg over a 6-day period (Charney et al., 1982). In later studies, starting with a single first-day dose of 12.5 mg produced only mild withdrawal symptoms when patients were given clonidine (Vining et al., 1988). Furthermore, the duration of withdrawal with this approach was equivalent for the methadone- or the heroin-dependent patients. This equivalence was interesting because withdrawal symptoms after abruptly stopping methadone use ordinarily last nearly twice as long as they do after stopping heroin use (Kleber, 1981).

Administering an antagonist such as naltrexone precipitates withdrawal within minutes for both methadone-maintained and ordinary heroin addicts, and this process of precipitation appears to equalize the duration of subsequent withdrawal symptoms. The amount of clonidine needed to ameliorate these symptoms when naltrexone and clonidine are used together is also lessened by using larger initial doses of naltrexone. When a clonidine and a low-dose naltrexone regime are used, the clonidine doses needed are almost 8 mg of clonidine over a 6-day period with a peak daily dose of 2.9 mg (Charney et al., 1982).

When a higher starting dose of clonidine is used (12.5 mg), clonidine is only needed for 4 days, with a total dose of 1.7 mg and a peak dose of 0.6 on day 1 (Vining et al., 1988). Giving high doses of both clonidine and naltrexone on the first day can reduce the average withdrawal time from 3.3 days to 2.3 days, despite lower clonidine dosage on the second day (Brewer et al., 1988). When clonidine and high-dose naltrexone were used in a day hospital setting, over 90% of patients were started successfully on naltrexone, but only half remained for over 2 weeks (Vining et al., 1988). Alternatively, high-dose naloxone and short-acting intravenous benzodiazepine midazolam has been used in an inpatient setting and has shortened the transition from methadone to naltrexone maintenance in opioid addicts to a period as short as a few hours (Loimer et al., 1991).

NALTREXONE MAINTENANCE

The long-term outcome after induction is critical but essentially depends on the strategies to maintain the patients on naltrexone rather than on the induction process; however, if the patients have a severe withdrawal reaction, they are not likely to be willing to stay on naltrexone. Relapse to illicit opiate use is frequent (usually over 90%) over even a 6- to 12-month period without sustained outpatient treatment (Kosten, 1990).

Success or failure of naltrexone maintenance is determined by the nature and structure of the sustained outpatient treatment program, the patients individual characteristics, and the matching of the program to those characteristics.

The best results with naltrexone treatment have been reported in studies of physicians and other medical professionals. Washton et al. (1984) studied the use of naltrexone in a group of addicted physicians who were working in a variety of specialties and who were addicted to a variety of morphine-based medications that they were self-prescribing. The subjects had a large amount of social disruption secondary to their addiction. All 15 of the subjects completed detoxification and entered an intensive 6-month outpatient program. Seventy-four percent of the subjects completed the program, returned to medical practice, and were opiate free at a 1-year follow-up. Another 13% of the subjects gave up naltrexone but remained opiate free. Ling and Wesson (1984) followed a group of 60 addicted health care professionals who were treated in private physicians' offices for an average of 8 months. Forty-seven subjects, or 78% were rated much "improved" or "moderately improved" on a global scale that rated the degree of improvement in drug abuse, professional activities, and psychosocial adjustment. It was found that subjects in the "much improved" group were older, did not drink. and remained in naltrexone treatment longer than 6 months relative to the less-successful group. Both studies provided comprehensive programs that involved full medical evaluations, detoxification, psychiatric and family evaluations, with provisions for therapy as well as confirmation of naltrexone ingestion. An outpatient treatment program designed to treat addicted health care professionals with naltrexone and cohesive group therapy reported a greater than 60% rate of professional reinstatement during the program, based at Yale University (Roth et al., 1997). The average subject duration on naltrexone was 9 months, and subjects typically remained on the program for a further 11 months before being discharged. Liaison with professional licensing bodies was an intrinsic component of the treatment. All of the above programs involved a group of highly motivated subjects whose careers depended upon successful completion of the prescribed treatment.

Groups of patients with the greatest material and psychological assets tend to do the best in any treatment program, and treatment with naltrexone is no exception. Thus, patients with good educational backgrounds and recent employment, and especially those who are under threat of losing employment unless compliant with treatment, tend to do best. Tennant et al. (1984) studied 160 patients in the setting of suburban community health project clinics. The patients had an average history of opiate use of 10.5 years, and the majority (64%) were employed. Most (71%) were active heroin addicts, and 26% were former addicts maintained on methadone, levo-alpha-acetylmethadol (LAAM), or propoxyphene napsylate. All expressed a desire for abstinence-oriented treatment. Treatment began with a naloxone challenge given after complete detoxification. Patients were then started on a dose of naltrexone that started at 50 mg and was increased to 100 mg on Monday and Wednesday, and to 150 mg on Friday. Patients were given a weekly urine drug screen, needle mark examination, and alcohol breath test. Each patient was assigned a counselor for weekly consultation. Patients remained in treatment for a period of 51 days on average. Twenty-eight percent of the patients dropped out in the first week, and only 17% of the patients remained in treatment for over 90 days. Less than 1% of urine screens and alcohol breath tests showed the presence of abusable drugs or alcohol, and only about 3% of urine screens showed the presence of heroin. In the light of subsequent studies examining the effects of naltrexone on alcohol consumption in alcoholics (O'Malley et al., 1992; Volpicelli et al., 1992), the findings of decreased alcohol consumption by the heroin addicts on naltrexone were interesting.

Another study of predominantly middle-class business executives reported success. Washton et al. (1984) reported treating 114 opiate-addicted business executives within a highly structured abstinence-oriented aftercare program following an inpatient detoxification program that used clonidine. The patients were all addicted for at least 2 years to some form of opiate. Most of the patients were white males, average age was 30 years, and mean incomes were $42,000. All patients successfully completed inpatient detoxification and induction into naltrexone program. This induction phase lasted from 4 to 10 weeks and included group therapy, peer group meetings, family therapy, individual therapy, and educational sessions. The patients continued to take naltrexone during the transition from hospital to home. Sixty-one percent of the patients successfully completed 6 months of naltrexone treatment in the outpatient program with no missed visits or drug-positive urines. An additional 20% of patients discontinued naltrexone before 6 months, but remained in the program with drug-free urines. Of the entire group, 64% were opiate free at the 12- to 18-month follow-ups. It is notable that those who were under stipulated and unequivocal job jeopardy (just under half of patients) did significantly better than those who were not.

When naltrexone is used in other structured settings with a definite incentive for maintenance of abstinence, it can be very successful. Brahen et al. (1984) reported on their study of naltrexone treatment in a work release program. Inmates with a history of opiate addiction had traditionally been excluded from work release programs because of their high likelihood of returning to their former drug habit. In Long Island in 1974, a program was developed to try to decrease the figures for recidivism and relapsed drug use among the prison population. Addicted inmates who previously had been excluded from the work release program were allowed on if they took naltrexone. Once the inmates were examined and approved for the program, they were quickly inducted by taking 150 mg of naltrexone. In this program, the inmates lived outside the prison in transitional housing and obtained work of some sort in the community. Naltrexone was used for approximately 4 months. Urine samples were collected randomly twice per week to monitor the inmates' illicit drug use. The consequences for repeated alcohol or drug use was reincarceration. Inmates also received vocational education, supervision, and regular weekly counseling during this period. After the introduction of naltrexone, the success of former opiate addicts on the work release program was equal to that of non-addicts, with a 25% attrition rate for both groups. Follow-up data suggests that once they had completed their sentences and left the work release program, naltrexone-treated inmates had fewer drug-related arrests than those inmates who did not go on naltrexone.

In the less structured world of "street" addicts, with less incentive to become opiate free, naltrexone has been less successful. In a heterogenous opiate-abusing population based at the Philadelphia Veterans Administration Medical Center, Greenstein et al. (1984) found that one third of subjects were opiate free 6 months after stopping naltrexone. The population of 327 patients averaged 7 years of opiate dependence, ranging from 2 to 20 years. Sixty percent of the subjects were black, and 40% were white. They came from working-class or lower-class backgrounds. Just under half of them were employed, and 80% were veterans. The vast majority had multiple treatment experiences with previous detoxifications, residences in theraputic communities, and varying periods of methadone maintenance.

The authors found that drug-free patients or those well stabilized on low-dose methadone were the most likely to start naltrexone. Those using high-dose methadone or using heroin on top of methadone were less likely to begin naltrexone. Initially, the program used a short period of opiate freedom, less then 5 days, prior to induction into the naltrexone phase. The program was then changed because many patients experienced precipitated withdrawal after receiving a naloxone challenge. The program was changed: the drug-free interval prior to induction was increased to at least 5 days, and there was a more liberal prescription of ancillary medication. Interestingly, the dropout rates were similar for those two induction protocols, with a third of each group failing to complete naltrexone induction. The high initial dropout rate was felt to be due to spur-of-the-moment decisions by some addicts to try naltrexone, leading to early default from the program and to severity of precipitated withdrawal for some addicts. In general, those addicts did poorly who had low motivation and who had ambivalence about naltrexone and about the concept of becoming entirely drug free. Those addicts who successfully remained abstinent seemed to either mature out, convert to religion or communal causes, retire from the drug scene, or have significant changes in their situation or environment.

In an important multicenter double-blind treatment trial, carried out in 17 centers in the United States, treatment outcome for naltrexone was not considered successful (Bradford et al., 1975). This program involved less structure and had less behavioral emphasis than some of the other programs mentioned above. Both naltrexone and placebo groups received routine counseling and supervision. After 6 weeks, only 50% of the patients were still taking naltrexone, just higher than the figure for placebo. By 3 and 6 months, the retention figures were 30% and 20%, respectively. By 9 months, the retention rate had fallen to 10% for both the naltrexone group and the group on placebo.

When naltrexone was introduced to Spain, a pilot program was

instituted that utilized an inpatient induction period of 7 days, combined with a subsequent outpatient regime of maintenance naltrexone
combined with counseling, individual psychotherapy, and family group
psychotherapy together with ancillary treatment such as antidepressants, neuroleptics, or lithium, if indicated (Garcia-Alonzo et al., 1989).
The patients consisted of 113 opiate dependents who had a history of
greater than 18 months and less than 4 years of opiate addiction and
who were not on methadone treatment, and 37 opiate abusers without
dependence. The median retention time for the subjects was 12 weeks,
and 40% of the subjects remained in the study for at least 24 weeks
from the onset of induction into naltrexone treatment. The authors
attributed the success of the program to the use of highly motivated
investigators and to the recruitment of non-methadone-treated patients,
as well as to the benefits of naltrexone itself.

In contrast, when naltrexone was introduced in Israel, and a
double-blind placebo-controlled trial was carried out on a group of 31
postdetoxification opioid addicts for a period of 2 months, the authors
reported that while naltrexone blocked opioid-induced euphoria and
indeed decreased the craving for opium, it did not inhibit drug usage
(Lerner et al., 1992). The program involved both regular urine monitoring and individual and group psychotherapy. When the patients were
followed up for a year, with no pharmacotherapy treatment for the in-
tervening 10 months, 8 of the 15 original naltrexone group patients
remained opioid free, and 6 of the placebo group patients remained
opioid free. The authors found that such factors as higher education
level, steady employment, marriage, completion of military service, and
lesser criminal records were all significant factors in positive outcome,
while pharmacotherapy was not. The authors noted that patients with
a good profile who are motivated and cooperative would probably do
better in any kind of rehabilitation program.

A different style of program was reported by Meyer et al.(1976)
at McLean Hospital in Boston (Altman et al., 1976; Meyer et al., 1976a,
1976b). In these studies, patients had to start as inpatients for a period
of up to 2 months. Following inpatient behavioral extinction experiments, the patients were discharged and were referred to a nearby phar-
macist for completion of therapy. The majority of patients, who were
by and large from a lower socioeconomic class patients and who had
few family ties and no current jobs, did not complete the inpatient stay.
Of those who did, the mean number of pharmacy visits was 59 days.
The authors concluded that naltrexone was of limited use in the rehabilitation of opiate abusers, at least in their particular behavioral-
oriented setting and with their particular profile of patients.

Goldstein (1976) developed the notion of sequential treatment of opiate addiction. He proposed a progression from heroin to metha-done on a daily basis, to LAAM on a three-times-weekly basis, detoxifi-cation to an opiate antagonist such as naltrexone, and then drug-free status. He indicated that patients would probably not achieve perma-nent abstinence immediately and would have to be recycled through this process repeatedly. This interesting idea, which appears pharmaco-logically and practically sound, has not caught on in practice.

Overall the retention rate on naltrexone programs, whatever the actual design, appears to be best for health professionals and individuals of similar high social and economic status, such as business executives (Kleber, 1985). It works best on those who are willing to remain on a program for 6–12 months and who have good family support. From the program's point of view, a high ratio of therapists to patients ap-pears to be essential. Poorest results have been obtained with post-methadone-maintained patients, and in between come other groups such as street addicts going straight from detoxification to naltrexone and former street addicts who have been clean for a time in some sort of hospital or theraputic community or having come out of prison.

Other potential suitable candidates for naltrexone include addicts early in their opiate abuse career or opiate addicts with no previous treatment; individuals who have been clean but who have recently relapsed; individuals currently abstinent but afraid of relapse because of stress; and individuals on a methadone program waiting list. No one has focused on these potential candidates in either a research or a ther-apeutic setting and would appear ideal for naltrexone (Kleber, 1985). Table 6.1 lists the characteristics of the ideal naltrexone patient and can be used to match patients with different programs.

NALTREXONE AND METHADONE

Naltrexone has not caught on as well as might be expected from such a theoretically ideal drug. In considering naltrexone maintenance treat-ment, it should be recognized that naltrexone will not appeal to the majority of opioid-dependent persons. Of "street" heroin addicts who enter treatment, not more than 10–15% show any interest in a drug that "keeps you from getting high" (Greenstein et al., 1984). In contrast, methadone has been found to be a very successful treatment for the majority of "street" heroin users because, among other things, metha-done satisfies heroin users' drug craving. Indeed, the effectiveness of methadone treatment has produced retention rates on methadone maintenance that are the mirror image of those on naltrexone, with 50–90% of patients remaining in treatment for 6 months or more on

TABLE 6.1. Profile of Ideal Naltrexone Program Patient

- Patient is motivated and committed to opiate abstinence.
- Patient is under specific pressure from employer or legal system to complete program.
- Family/spouse is involved directly in therapy.
- Patient is of higher socioeconomic status, is educated, has steady employment, is married, and has no/small criminal record.
- Patient is early in his substance abuse career.
- Patient has been clean and has recently relapsed.
- Patient is properly inducted into the naltrexone program with minimal withdrawal symptoms.
- Patient with concurrent alcohol misuse may derive benefit from naltrexone on alcohol-related outcomes.

methadone (Lowinson et al., 1992). Methadone also provides a mild opiate "high" and does not preclude the use of illicit opiates to boost this effect, unlike naltrexone treatment that produces no opiate high. In addition, the protracted and often severe withdrawal syndrome on abrupt cessation of methadone maintenance serves to enhance retention, whereas there is no withdrawal syndrome associated with naltrexone.

Methadone has another major advantage over naltrexone in that there is no required detoxification phase. Hence, there is no initial discomfort in taking methadone. This aspect of methadone therapy is unlike naltrexone treatment, in which the patient must first detoxify from opiates prior to naltrexone induction.

On the other hand, naltrexone has many potential advantages compared with methadone. First, naltrexone is nonaddicting and, as such, can be used in a variety of settings, such as medical clinics and primary care centers, and it can be safely prescribed without fear of diversion. Second, it can work out to be cheaper than methadone maintenance because of the elimination of the need for daily or near-daily visits. Third and most important, the chances for long-term opiate abstinence are greatly enhanced in the long run on naltrexone since protracted withdrawal has already been handled during the initial phase of naltrexone treatment. In contrast, the periods of detoxification and immediate postdetoxification are the period of most vulnerability for relapse in methadone-maintained patients because of the lengthy withdrawal symptoms and long detoxification. Fourth, addicts are less likely to continue intravenous drug abuse while on naltrexone than on methadone because naltrexone is associated neither with continued partial reinforcement from heroin use nor with potential synergistic effects from cocaine use, all of which reduces the risks for spread of HIV and other needle-borne diseases.

Despite these potential advantages, the immediate pharmacological rewards of using naltrexone are not as great to the patient as the rewards of using methadone. Recruitment problems for naltrexone can also be attributed to rigid protocols, suspicion of "experimental" drugs, community pressure, and the reluctance of those in charge of methadone programs to decrease their census by referral. Patients may also confuse naltrexone with Antabuse and may have to be advised that they will feel neither discomfort nor an opiate high when using opiates on naltrexone.

ALCOHOL AND NALTREXONE

The matter of alcohol consumption and the opiate system is one of intense interest at present. Naltrexone has been shown to be of benefit in the treatment of alcohol dependence in two separate trials and has been shown to increase abstention rates, reduce craving, reduce relapse rates, reduce alcohol-related problems, and reduce numbers of drinking days in alcoholics (O'Malley et al., 1992; Volpecilli et al., 1992). When one examines the rates of alcohol abuse and dependence in patients maintained on the narcotic agonist methadone, there is a high prevalence of alcohol problems that varies between 14% and 74% depending upon the criteria used (Jackson et al., 1983). A more consistent figure of approximately 25% of methadone patients with active or inactive alcohol dependence appears in a number of reports (El-Basel et al., 1993; Jackson et al., 1983; Joseph & Appel, 1985; Stimmel et al., 1983). There is evidence that excessive drinking existed in most of the alcoholics on methadone prior to admission to the methadone program. For example, Green et al. (1978) reported that 12 out of 14 methadone patients with excessive-drinking patterns in a random sample of 96 patients in a New York City methadone clinic had alcohol problems prior to admission to the program. In a prospective study of 214 patients. Kreek (1978, 1981) noted that 20% of the patients were heavy drinkers at the time of their admission to methadone maintenance; and in a study of 193 male heroin addicts conducted in St. Louis, Weller et al. (1980) found that 37% had alcohol problems.

If an opiate antagonist such as naltrexone decreases alcohol consumption in alcoholics, what happens to alcoholic opiate addicts who take opiate agonists such as methadone for long periods of time? Joseph and Appel (1985) surveyed 1,251 patients in a New York methadone program and found that 27% of the patients drank excessively during the 3 months prior to their first period of methadone treatment. About 80% of patients at the low and the excessive levels of alcohol consumption maintained their pretreatment level of daily alcohol consumption. Of patients with moderate pretreatment alcohol consumption, one third remained at their pretreatment level of alcohol consumption, slightly more than one third increased their consumption, and slightly less than one third decreased their consumption. The authors concluded that methadone did not have a substantial systematic effect on patients' level of drinking. Notable increases in the consumption of alcohol are evident, however, after detoxification from methadone, if only to alleviate the discomfort associated with withdrawal and the protracted abstinence syndrome. Stimmel et al. (1983) found that there were no differences in alcoholism remission in a 2½-year prospective study of alcoholic methadone patients randomly assigned to abstinent (Alcoholics Anonymous), controlled-drinking, and control groups. Instead, active alcoholics who participated decreased their consumption of alcohol with time in methadone treatment unrelated to the method of intervention. An earlier study from the same group (Jackson et al., 1983) reported no difference between patients on a methadone maintenance treatment program for 1 year and new admissions to the methadone program in the patients' rates of current alcoholism. Although a number of studies have reported an increase in alcoholism among patients when they are admitted to methadone maintenance programs (Joseph & Appel, 1985; Kaufman, 1982; Liebson et al., 1973; Stimmel et al., 1983), other studies, reporting the heavy consumption of alcohol among patients in methadone programs, have noted that these drinking problems existed prior to the patients' entering the programs (Grabowski, 1979; Green et al., 1978; Kreek, 1978, 1981; Weller et al., 1980).

It has been possible to decrease the alcohol consumption by methadone-maintained patients through the use of disulfiram and a behavior therapy regime (Liebson et al., 1973). In this regime, the patients were only granted access to methadone if they also ingested disulfiram, while the within-subject controls were given disulfiram but were not required to ingest it as a condition of receiving methadone. Although most patients were reluctant to take disulfiram, they preferred this treatment to discharge from the methadone program. There was a noteworthy drop in alcohol consumption in the treatment group that was significant at the .001 level. Unfortunately, there were only six patients in the whole study, and the regime, though it appears successful, has not been adapted as standard treatment of alcoholism in methadone-maintained patients. Treatment studies that have examined abstinence-oriented, controlled-drinking therapies or voluntary disulfiram therapies have not been successful (Bickel et al., 1987).

What is not specifically available at present is information about the amount of alcohol consumption among patients who are opiate dependent and maintained on naltrexone. While the information concerning potential increases in alcohol consumption on methadone programs is contradictory, there is no detailed information to date about the expected decline in alcoholism on naltrexone maintenance. In Ling and Wesson's (1984) study of addicted health professionals, 32 of the 60 subjects were drinkers. Although Ling and Wesson did not report the decrease or increase in alcohol consumption on naltrexone, they did note that the drinkers did significantly worse than the nondrinkers in global outcome scales. This finding probably is a reflection of the greater psychosocial difficulties — and, thus, poorer outcomes — associated with patients who are polysubstance abusers and not single-substance abusers rather than a reflection of the failure of naltrexone to reduce alcohol intake in this group. Tennant et al. (1984) reported a positive breath alcohol test rate of 0.8% in the 1,008 breath tests carried out on 160 patients in their naltrexone-for-opiates program but did not report the alcoholism rate among subjects prior to starting the program. This is, however, an encouraging figure given the opiate-abusing population's prevalence of alcoholism. Anecdotally, naltrexone appears to decrease alcohol consumption and the abuse of other drugs and to decrease craving for all substances of abuse, relative to a methadone-maintained population (Kleber, 1985). In contrast, Greenstein et al. (1984) noted that a few patients increased their alcohol consumption early in their naltrexone treatment.

Thus, the relation between naltrexone and alcohol consumption in an opiate-abusing population has yet to be systematically studied. What may be inferred from the evidence so far — and especially from the trials of naltrexone in pure alcoholics — is that naltrexone may be useful in the treatment of opiate abusers who also have alcohol problems by encouraging not only opiate but also alcohol abstinence.

HOW TO MAKE NALTREXONE MORE USEFUL

We have already described ideal patient characteristics for naltrexone programs. But what can be done for patients on the existing programs to make them more successful? Suggestions come from some early programs. Callahan (1980), in his HALT program, reported that 21% of the patients completed 6 weeks on naltrexone alone compared with 49% of the patients who completed 6 weeks with behavior therapy and naltrexone. The program used such behavioral techniques as contingency contracting and thought stopping. This program reported that time on naltrexone lengthened from an average of 44 days up to 85 days, a significant difference (Callahan, 1976). But, unfortunately, while the behavior therapy group had better program retention and less drug use at 0–7 months, there was no differences evident at 8–14 months or 15–21 months (Callahan, 1980).

Anton et al. (1981) at Yale demonstrated that during the first month of naltrexone therapy addicts in family therapy had a very low drop-out rate (92% retention) that was significant at the .001 level. This was, however, a nonrandomized trial. Although the rate of retention dropped off in this study, it remained higher than the retention rates for Callahan (1980) and his behavior therapy regime, and also higher than that of Resnick et al. (1979). The latter authors used a system of individual counseling, and they randomized 37 addicts to either individual counseling or to no counseling (Resnick et al., 1979). At one month, 77% of the addicts were still in treatment in the counseling group, and only 33% of the addicts were in treatment in the noncounseling group. This was a significant difference. When the addicts were stratified by "street" versus postmethadone status, overall program retention was better for the street addicts with counseling but not for the postmethadone addicts. As time went on, the difference between the counseling and noncounseling groups lessened, with 54% of the addicts opiate free at 3 months in the counseling group and 40% of the addicts opiate free in the noncounseling group. The percentage of patients taking naltrexone also diminished by 3 months, with 27% of the patients taking it in the counseling group and no patients taking it in the noncounseling group. By 6 months, only 2 patients (or 9%) were taking naltrexone, both of whom were in the counseling group.

A study of contingency payment by Grabowski (1979), showed an 89% success rate at both 1 month and 2 months in the paid addicts, while previous addicts who were paid a similar amount of money without a contingency program had only a 60% success rate at 1 month and a 40% success rate at 2 months.

Thus, it can be shown that by judicious assessment of patient characteristics, and by the use of various psychotherapeutic or behavioral interventions, naltrexone can be made more successful and more broadly useful.

In order to address naltrexone's lack of immediate positive pharmacological reinforcement, it is necessary to provide positive incentives for initiation and maintenance of naltrexone. This could take the form of payment of a simple contingent fee, which has helped compliance in several studies (Callahan, 1980; Grabowski, 1979; Meyer et al., 1976b). It might be possible to choose some of the positive incentives relative to the methadone program (e.g., shorter waiting list, more privileges, lower fees). An appropriate choice of incentive, such as the potential loss of licensing or employment, makes a significant impact on the retention in a program (Ling & Wesson, 1984; Washton et al., 1984).

An important weakness for naltrexone is the initial presence of aversive naltrexone side effects or protracted withdrawal symptoms. While this issue can be addressed by the use of inpatient initiation and by pharmacological strategies (Brewer et al., 1988; Charney et al., 1982; Kleber & Kosten, 1984; Loimer et al., 1991; Meyer et al., 1976a; Vining et al., 1988), such psychosocial interventions as the provision of added support, involvement of the addict's social network, and preparedness training could be added.

Another weakness of naltrexone is that there is no pharmacological negative reinforcement for premature dropout. Naltrexone can be discontinued easily, unlike methadone, which can cause an immediate and sometimes severe withdrawal. One way to address this problem would be with contingency contracting, possibly involving family members, in which negative consequences are linked to premature dropout. The importance of establishing a significant theraputic link — whether with individual counseling or with other techniques, such as family therapy — cannot be overstated. It is this link — together with the beneficial effects of naltrexone itself, as well as with the benefits of a positive or negative reinforcement scheme — that ultimately determines the likely outcome. As Ginzburg (1986) said:

> Theraputic use of naltrexone is as an adjunct in the treatment of opiate abusers. Thus while naltrexone has a promising future, it needs to be placed in a context of being a part of the overall treatment plan. Treatment failure cannot be blamed on the failure of naltrexone to block opioids, nor is its treatment success likely to be the consequence of the use of naltrexone alone. (pp. 98–99)

There are other methods that could be employed to increase the use of naltrexone. The first method might involve selecting the patients that fit the profile of those who have best responded to naltrexone and placing them on a naltrexone program, and then referring the other patients to methadone. Another method might involve a program decision to require an initial course of naltrexone treatment prior to acceptance into a methadone program. This method would circumvent the problem of methadone's initial attractiveness vis a vis naltrexone; and even if this method is effective for only a small number of patients, the long-term disadvantages and expense of methadone would be avoided for those patients. Because methadone is sometimes seen as a treatment of indefinite duration, any kind of successful intervention that promoted opiate abstinence would be welcome. The main problem is that each center's entire opiate treatment program would have to be geared to acceptance and promotion of naltrexone, which clearly is not the case at present.

Naltrexone could be offered to a broad range of subjects in the context of a contract that would call for negative contingencies for discontinuation, in order to address the problem that naltrexone is relatively easy to discontinue. This strategy has been successful in very specific and controlled situations: for example, in testing addicted physicians, for whom the alternative would be the loss of their licenses (Brahen et al., 1984; Washton et al., 1984); or business executives, who might lose their jobs if they are noncompliant (Washton et al., 1984); or prisoners, who might be removed form a work release program if they do not take naltrexone (Brahen et al., 1984). This type of contingency contracting might be used in any group that is under legal pressure, such as patients on parole or on probation. Unfortunately, the subjects are as likely not to restart illicit drug use with the expiration of the contract, which is the experience with cocaine abusers (Anker & Crowley, 1982).

An approach that has not yet been tried would be to adapt the community reinforcement approach to naltrexone maintenance. While early attrition from naltrexone programs has been improved by such positive reinforcements as money, this superiority in retention has not endured over time. Higgins et al. (1991, 1994) have reported substantial benefits from this approach in ambulatory cocaine abusers. The community reinforcement approach involves combining cognitively oriented coping-skills training, providing positive behavioral reinforcements for drug-free urines, and involving significant others in the treatment. The authors have demonstrated the approach's superiority over standard treatment and have shown the effectiveness of the individual components, including the involvement of the significant other and the use of a voucher system to reward drug-free urines. Adapting such an approach to naltrexone could deal with the early dropout problems by providing vouchers for taking medication or for giving drug-free urines. The willingness of the patients to endure mild withdrawal symptoms during induction and maintenance may be increased by the appropriate use of a voucher system. A study to evaluate this particular methodology is currently under way at Yale University.

Although naltrexone has not been universally adopted for the treatment of opiate addiction, it remains a powerful tool if used on the appropriately matched patient in the setting of a comprehensive behavioral and psychotherapeutic program. It remains to be seen whether naltrexone's utility in certain settings will be appreciated by the treatment community at large or whether naltrexone will retain its current status of limited use in opiate addiction around the world.

REFERENCES

Altman, J. L., Meyer, R. E., Mirin, S. M., & McNamee, H. B. (1976). Opiate antagonists and the modification of heroin self administration in man: An experimental study. *International Journal of the Addictions, 11*(3), 467.

Anker, A. A., & Crowley, T. J. (1982). Use of contingency contracts in speciality clinics for cocaine abuse. In L. S. Harris (Ed.), *Problems of drug dependence 1981* (NIDA Research Monograph No. 41, pp. 452–459). Washington DC: U.S. Government Printing Office.

Anton, R. F., Hogan, I., Jalai, B., Riordan, C. E., & Kleber, H. D. (1981). Multiple family therapy and naltrexone in the treatment of opiate dependence. *Drug and Alcohol Dependence, 8,* 157–168.

Bickel, W. K., Marion, I., & Lowinson, J. H. (1987). The treatment of alcoholic methadone patients: A review. *Journal of Substance Abuse Treatment, 4*(1), 15–19.

Blumberg, H., & Dayton, H. B. (1973). Naloxone, naltrexone, and related noroxymorphones. *Advances in Biochemistry and Psychopharmacology, 8,* 33–43.

Bradford, H. A., Hurley, F. L., Golondzoeske, O., & Dorrier, C. (1975). Interim report on clinic intake and safety data from 17 NIDA funded naltrexone centers. In D. Julius & P. Renault (Eds.), *Narcotic antagonists: Naltrexone* (NIDA Research Monograph No. 9, pp. 163–171). Washington, DC: U.S. Government Printing Office.

Brahen, H. S., Henderson, R. K., Capone, T., & Kondal, N. (1984). Naltrexone treatment in a jail work release program. *Journal of Clinicial Psychiatry, 45*(9, Sec. 2), 49–52.

Brewer, C., Rezae, H., & Bailey, C. (1988). Opioid withdrawal and naltrexone induction in 48–72 hours with minimal drop out, using a modification of the naltrexone–clonidine technique. *British Journal of Psychiatry, 153,* 340–343.

Callahan, E. J. (1976). Comparison of two naltrexone programs: Naltrexone alone versus naltrexone plus behavior therapy. In D. Julius & P. Renault (Eds.), *Narcotic antagonists: Naltrexone* (NIDA Research Monograph No. 9, pp. 150–157). Washington DC: U.S. Government Printing Office.

Callahan, E. J. (1980). The treatment of heroin addiction: Naltrexone alone with behavior therapy. *American Journal of Drug and Alcohol Abuse, 7,* 795–807.

Charney, D. S., Riordan, C. E., Kleber, H. D., Murburg, M., Braverman, P., Sternberg, D. E., Heninger, G. R., & Redmond, D. E. (1982). Clonidine and naltrexone: A safe, effective and rapid treatment of abrupt withdrawal from methadone therapy. *Archives of General Psychiatry, 39,* 1327–1332.

El-Basel, N., Schilling, R. F., Turnbull, J. E., & Su, K.-H. (1993). Correlates of alcohol use among methadone patients. *Alcoholism: Clinical and Experimental Research, 17*(3), 681–686.

Garcia-Alonzo, F., Gutierrez, M., San, L., Bedate, J., Forteza-Rei, J., Rodriguez-Artalejo, F., Lopez-Allvarez, M., Perez de los Cobos, J. C., & Cami, J. (1989). A multicenter study to introduce naltrexone for opiate dependence in Spain. *Drug and Alcohol Dependence, 23*(2), 117–121.

Ginzburg, H. M. (1986). Naltrexone: Its clinical utility. *Advances in Alcohol and Substance Abuse, 5*(1–2), 83–101.

Goldstein, A. (1976). Heroin addiction: Sequential treatments employing pharmacological supports. *Archives of General Psychiatry, 33,* 353.

Grabowski, J. (1979). Effects of contingent payment on compliance with a naltrexone regime. *American Journal of Drug and Alcohol Abuse, 6*(3), 355–365.

Green, J., Jaffe, J. H., Carlisi, J. A., & Zaks, A. (1978). Alcohol use in the opiate use cycle of the heroin addict. *International Journal of the Addictions, 13*(7), 1021–1033.

Greenstein, R. A., Arndt, I. ., McLellan, A. T., O'Brien, C. P., & Evans, B. (1984). Naltrexone: A clinical perspective. *Journal of Clinical Psychiatry, 45,* 25–28.

Higgins, S. T., Budney, A. J., Bickel, W. K., Foerg, F. E., Donham, R., & Badger, G. J. (1994). Incentives improve outcome in outpatient behavioral treatment of cocaine dependence. *Archives of General Psychiatry, 51*(7), 568–576.

Higgins, S. T., Delaney, D. D., Budney, A. J., Bickel, W. K., Hughes, J. R., Foerg, F., & Fenwick, J. W. (1991). A behavioral approach to achieving initial cocaine abstinence. *American Journal of Psychiatry, 148,* 1218–1224.

Hollister, L. E., Johnson, K., Boukhabya, D., & Gillespie, H. K. (1981). Aversive effects of naltrexone in subjects not dependent upon opiates. *Drug and Alcohol Dependence, 8,* 37–41.

Jackson, G., Cohen, M., Hanbury, R., Korts, D., Sturiano, V., & Stimmel, B. (1983). Alcoholism among narcotic addicts and patients on methadone maintenance. *Journal of Studies on Alcohol, 44*(3), 499–504.

Joseph, H., & Appel, P. (1985). Alcoholism and methadone treatment: Consequences for the patient and program. *American Journal of Drug and Alcohol Abuse, 11*(1–2), 37–53.

Kaufman, E. (1982). The relationship of alcoholism and alcohol abuse to the abuse of other drugs. *American Journal of Drug and Alcohol Abuse, 1,* 1–17.

Kleber, H. D. (1981). Detoxification from narcotics. In J. H. Lowinson & P. Ruiz (Eds.), *Substance abuse: Clinical problems and perspectives* (pp. 317–338). Baltimore: Williams & Wilkins.

Kleber, H. D. (1985). Naltrexone. *Journal of Substance Abuse Treatment, 2,* 117–122.

Kleber, H. D., & Kosten, T. R. (1984). Naltrexone induction: Psychologic and pharmacologic strategies. *Journal of Clinical Psychiatry, 45,* 29.

Kleber, H. D., Riordan, C. E., Rounsaville, B. J., Kosten, T. R., Charney, D., Gaspari, J., Hogan, I., & O'Connor, C. (1985). Clonidine in outpatient detoxification from methadone maintenance. *Archives of General Psychiatry, 42,* 391–398.

Kosten, T. R. (1990). Current pharmacotherapies for opioid dependence. *Psychopharmacology Bulletin, 26*(1), 69–74.

Kreek, M. J. (1978). Medical complications in methadone patients. *Annals of the New Yoek Academy of Sciences, 311,* 110–114.

Kreek, M. J. (1981). Metabolic interactions between opiates and alcohol. *Annals of the New York Academy of Sciences, 362,* 36–49.

Lerner, A., Sigal, M., Bacalu, A., Shiff, R., Burganski, I., & Gelkopf, M. (1992). A naltrexone double blind placebo controlled study in Israel. *Israel Journal of Psychiatry and Related Sciences, 29*(1), 36–43.

Liebson, I., Bigelow, G., & Flamer, R. (1973). Alcoholism among methadone patients: A specific treatment method. *American Journal of Psychiatry, 130*(4), 483–485.

Ling, W., & Wesson, D. R. (1984). Naltrexone treatment for addicted health care professionals: A collaborative private practice experience. *Journal of Clinical Psychiatry, 45*(9, Sec. 2), 46–48.

Loimer, N., Lenz, K., Schmid, R., & Presslich, O. (1991). Technique for greatly shortening the transition from methadone to naltrexone maintenance of patients addicted to opiates. *American Journal of Psychiatry, 148,* 933–935.

Lowinson, J. H., Marion, I. H., Joseph, H., & Dole, V. P. (1992). Methadone maintenance. In J. H. Lowinson, P. Ruiz, R. B. Millman, & J. G. Langrod (Eds.), *Substance abuse: A comprehensive textbook* (pp. 550–561). Baltimore: Williams & Wilkins.

Martin, W. R., Jasinski, D. R., & Mansky, P. A. (1973). Naltrexone, an antagonist for the treatment of heroin dependence: Effects in man. *Archives of General Psychiatry, 28,* 784–791.

Mello, N. K., Mendelson, J. H., Keuhnle, J. C., & Sellers, M. (1980). Operant analysis of human heroin self administration and the effects of naltrexone. *Journal of Pharmacology and Experimental Therapeutics, 216,* 45–54.

Mendelson, J. H., Ellingboe, J., Keuhnle, J. C., & Mello, N. K.(1980). Effects of naltrexone on mood and neuroendocrine function in normal adult males. *Psychoneuroendocrinology, 3,* 231–236.

Meyer, R. E., McNamee, H. B., Mirin, S. M., & Altman, J. L. (1976a). Analysis and modification of opiate reinforcement. *International Journal of the Addictions, 11*(3), 476.

Meyer, R. E., Mirin, S. M., Altman, J., & McNamee, H. B. (1976b). A behavioral paradigm for the evaluation of narcotic antagonists. *Archives of General Psychiatry, 33,* 371.

O'Brien, C. P., Childress, A. R., McLellan, A. T., Ternes, J., & Ehrman, R. N. (1984). Use of naltrexone to extinguish opioid-conditioned responses. *Journal of Clinlical Psychiatry, 45*(9, Sec. 2), 53–56.

O'Brien, C., Greenstein, R., Ternes, J., & Woody, G. (1978). Clinical pharmacology of narcotic antagonists. *Annals of the New York Academy of Sciences, 311,* 232–240.

O'Malley, S. S., Jaffe, A. J., Chang, G., Schottenfeld, R. S., Meyer, R. E., & Rounsaville, B. (1992). Naltrexone and coping skills therapy for alcohol dependence: A controlled study. *Archives of General Psychiatry, 49,* 881–887.

Resnick, J., Volavka, J., Freedman, A., & Thomas, M. (1974). Studies of EN-1638A (naltrexone): A new narcotic antagonist. *American Journal of Psychiatry, 131,* 646–650.

Resnick, R., Schuyten-Resnick, E., & Washton, A. M. (1979). Narcotic antagonists in the treatment of opioid dependence: Review and commentary. *Comprehensive Psychiatry, 20,* 116–125.

Roth, A., Hogan, I., & Farren, C. K. (1997). Naltrexone plus group therapy the treatment of for opiate abusing health care professionals. *Journal of Substance Abuse Treatment, 14,* 1–4.

Stimmel, B., Cohen, M., Sturiano, V., Hanbury, R., Korts, D., & Jackson, G. (1983). Is treatment for alcoholism effective in persons on methadone maintenance? *American Journal of Psychiatry, 140,* 862–866.

Tennant, F. S., Rawson, R. A., Cohen, A. J., & Mann, A. (1984). Clinical experience with naltrexone in suburban opioid addicts. *Journal of Clinical Psychiatry, 45*(9, Sec. 2), 42–45.

Vining, E., Kosten, T. R., & Kleber, H. D. (1988). Clinical utility of rapid clonidine naltrexone detoxification for opioid abusers. *British Journal of Addictions, 83,* 567–575.

Volpecilli, J. R., Alterman, A. I., Hayashida, M., & O'Brien, C. P. (1992). Naltrexone in the treatment of alcohol dependence. *Archives of General Psychiatry, 49,* 886–880.

Washton, A. M., Pottash, A. C., & Gold, M. A. (1984). Naltrexone in addicted business executives and physicians. *Journal of Clinical Psychiatry, 45*(9, Sec. 2), 39–41.

Weller, R. A., Halikas, J. A., & Darvish, H. S. (1980). Alcoholism in black male heroin addicts. *British Journal of Addictions, 75,* 381–388.

Wikler, A. (1948). Recent progress in research on the neurophysiological basis of morphine addiction. *American Journal of Psychiatry, 105,* 329–338.

Chapter 7

COMORBID SUBSTANCE ABUSE IN OPIATE-DEPENDENT PATIENTS

Beatrice Burns, M.S.N., A.P.R.N.

While opioid maintenance is increasingly acceptable as a treatment model for opioid addiction, concerns remain about the use of other illicit drugs in methadone programs (Cushman, 1988; T. A. Kosten et al., 1989; T. R. Kosten et al., 1987). This is not a new or unusual situation, as concurrent drug use has been prevalent in methadone programs since the early history of this form of treatment. One of the major benefits of methadone maintenance treatment is rapid social stabilization with dramatic decrease in intravenous (as well as other routes of) heroin use once an addict is admitted to a program (Ball et al., 1988, 1989; Hall, 1993). Even so, cocaine use may persist or increase in the population that abuses it. Since the 1980s, an added concern with intravenous drug use is the increased risk of transmission of HIV and other infectious diseases in the intravenous drug abuse population, compromising an important goal of methadone treatment (Abdul-Quader et al., 1987; Chaisson et al., 1989; White et al., 1994). The particular subset of treatment refractory individuals who abuse both opioids and cocaine via the intravenous route are increasingly seroconverting to HIV positive. In addition, it has been noted that this population is especially difficult to engage in treatment, since these individuals generally choose to use emergency rooms in crises. When this population does get into treatment, the course is often one of unremitting substance use; or if abstinence is attained, it is generally punctuated by frequent relapse (National Institute on Drug Abuse, 1989; T. R. Kosten et al., 1986; Rosenblum et al., 1991). Treatment compliance is poor in general, and surveys of patients from this population indicate that many patients unsuccessfully cycle through treatment. Outpatient follow-up, in particular, after inpatient rehabilitation or detoxification from alcohol, for example, is remarkably poor (Corty & Ball, 1987; Des Jarlais & Friedman, 1987; Hubbard et al., 1983).

Alcohol abuse has received less recent attention than intravenous drug use—and especially cocaine abuse—but remains a prevalent problem of continued special concern in the methadone maintenance population. This chapter will initially consider the general problem of concurrent drug use but will focus particularly on cocaine and alcohol problems.

HISTORY OF CONCURRENT DRUG USE IN METHADONE TREATMENT PROGRAMS

Since methadone treatment became formalized in the 1960s, concurrent drug use has been a knotty issue for treaters. Initially, alcohol and marijuana were considered "soft drugs" that were not of concern and, compared to the larger problems of heroin use, were even considered an acceptable alternative. Concern developed, however, when studies began reporting widespread alcohol abuse (Joseph & Appel, 1985; Senay et al., 1986) in methadone maintenance populations. Treaters responded with closer scrutiny of treatment outcome and problems that may develop as a result of methadone treatment. Programs emerged that focused on improving treatment models by using goal-oriented psychosocial interventions and clearer counseling methods. Alcohol problems were directly addressed through specific, alcohol-focused counseling and education (Stark, 1989). For example, contingency contracting emerged and was widely explored as a behavioral control in the management of concurrent illicit drug use and alcohol abuse by reinforcing drug-free urines through various methods (Dolan et al., 1985; Stitzer et al., 1980).

Subsequently, cocaine became the focus of attention. The cocaine epidemic of the 1980s illustrated, among other things, the cycling popularity of drug use, along with the growing specter of HIV in the intravenous drug abuse population. Studies of methadone maintenance treatment programs consistently reported diminished intravenous drug abuse in the active treatment populations (Gottheil et al., 1993; White et al., 1994) while increasing intravenous drug abuse grew with length of time out of treatment (Serpelloni et al., 1994).

Concern with cocaine's ascendance in the drug world is reflected in a review of cocaine citations in the *Cumulative Index Medicus* for the years 1973, 1983, and 1993. In 1973 there were 26 articles on cocaine;

none included opioids. In 1983 there were 80 articles; one cited combined use with opioids. In 1993 there were more than 650 citations on cocaine, 9 about cocaine use with methadone and 20 on cocaine in combination with opioids. Thus, it is clear that this problem has persisted; but understanding of the special nature of this comorbidity has lagged behind the productivity in this field in general. These trends are summarized in Figure 7.1.

Further evidence of increased cocaine abuse in methadone treatment is reflected in the volume of published studies of drug use in methadone programs. In a review of methadone publications in the *Cumulative Index Medicus* for 1973, there were 2 articles on "other drug" use in methadone treatment, 1 on alcohol and 1 on cocaine. In 1983, 8 articles identified alcohol (6), mixed drugs (1), and benzodiazepine (1) use in methadone programs; there were no articles on cocaine or combined cocaine/opioids. In 1993, 15 articles cited heroin (3), alcohol (1), benzodiazepines (3), combined cocaine/opioids (1), and cocaine (7) (see Figure 7.1). Thus, by the 1990s publications started to reflect increasing cocaine use in methadone programs, evident in the treatment arena for years.

A CLOSER LOOK AT CURRENT COCAINE USE IN METHADONE PROGRAMS

As reported earlier, many addicts who also abuse other substances decrease substance use shortly after admission to methadone maintenance programs. Rates of substance use continue to decrease with length of time in methadone treatment when patients are medicated with adequate doses (Abdul-Quader et al., 1987; Anglin & McGlothlin, 1984; D'Aunno & Vaughn, 1992; Gottheil et al., 1993; Hubbard et al., 1989; Schottenfeld et al., 1993a; Shaffer & SaSalvia, 1992; Stine et al., 1991).

However, cocaine remains a major drug of abuse. Its prevalence, availability, and decreasing cost make it a drug of choice for the polydrug abuser. T. R. Kosten et al. reported that 74% of opiate addicts who applied for treatment used cocaine in 1980 (T. R. Kosten et al., 1986). Ball et al. reported 47–60% of inner-city methadone patients were using cocaine on admission. A 1990 General Accounting Office study reported that 20–40% of patients in methadone treatment programs used cocaine. The rate of cocaine abuse among methadone-maintained patients has increased considerably in the last 10 years (T. R. Kosten et al., 1989a). For instance, rates of cocaine abuse among

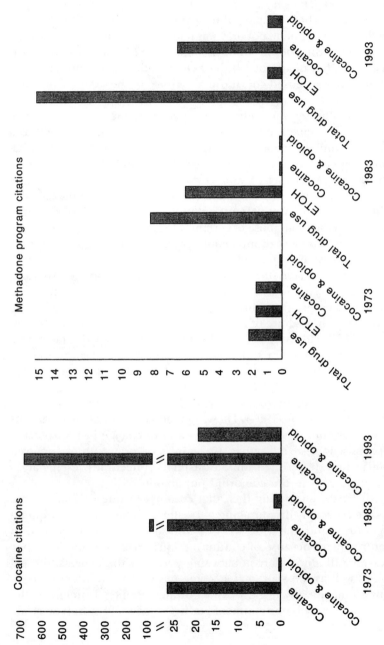

FIGURE 7.1. Rising interest in cocaine use as reflected by published articles in *Cumulative Index Medicus* over three decades: 1973, 1983, and 1993.

those entering treatment averaged 58% in one trial, and rates of cocaine abuse during treatment can be as high as 40% (T. R. Kosten et al., 1988, 1990). Data from the Tristate Ethnographic Project suggest that cocaine has become part of the drug use and social life of clients in methadone treatment: not only was it used by the most deviant clients (80% of those using heroin while in methadone maintenance programs use cocaine), but nearly one fifth of clients otherwise compliant with program rules also used cocaine at least once in the week prior to being interviewed (Strug et al., 1985).

Newly admitted methadone treatment patients, whose substance abuse lifestyles remain intact, are likely to continue their opioid drug use, at least until the medication reaches therapeutic dose. At that point, although opiate use usually decreases, the treatment response of individuals who are using cocaine is not so clear.

The interaction of methadone with cocaine is complex, and a troublesome minority of patients not only fail to respond to treatment but may increase their abuse of certain substances, particularly cocaine, once admitted to methadone maintenance treatment (Condelli et al., 1991; T. R. Kosten et al., 1986, 1987).

Certain characteristics of opioid addicts in methadone programs place them at risk for concurrent cocaine abuse and other social problems. There is often a history of heavy drug use, usually including experience with or abuse of multiple drugs, such as stimulants, depressants, and hallucinogenics (Condelli et al., 1991). Other risk factors include responses to interactions between methadone and cocaine (Stine et al., 1992, 1993), their increased likelihood for psychiatric comorbidity (T. R. Kosten et al., 1987; Woody et al., 1983), and race. African Americans are overrepresented in surveys on cocaine use (Kang & De Leon, 1993, Meandzija et al., 1994). These methadone maintenance patients tend to share needles for cocaine use and to engage in unprotected and promiscuous sexual activity (for money or as a result of impaired judgment and diminished inhibitions). HIV infection presents additional challenges in the comorbid population.

It is hardly surprising then that cocaine-abusing methadone patients are especially discouraging to treaters. These patients frequently do not respond to a wide array of clinical interventions, they drop out of treatment because of continuing illicit drug use, and they may negatively influence their nonabusing peers. In the process, the patients, as well as the staff, may become pessimistic and demoralized, adding to the already negative views of methadone treatment by the public and methadone treatment staffs (Woody, 1983; Sutker et al., 1978).

METHADONE-MAINTAINED HIV PATIENTS WITH COMORBID COCAINE ABUSE

One of the more baffling questions in methadone treatment is how to handle HIV-positive cocaine-abusing patients in order to decrease and eliminate their drug use and retain them in treatment. These HIV-positive opioid/cocaine addicts are targeted and actively recruited by methadone programs to control the spread of HIV, as well as to treat the addicts' illness and addiction (White et al., 1994; Serpelloni et al., 1994). This subset of addicts presents an even more formidable set of social, medical, and legal problems than the non-HIV-infected opioid addict in methadone treatment.

An example of the special problems of this population is illustrated by our clinical experience. The West Haven Veterans Administration Medical Center has a small methadone population of 65 patients. The program offers intensive day treatment that all patients are required to attend Monday through Friday for up to 12 weeks (shorter if working, longer if appropriate). Two weeks of clean urine screens are required before advancing to a less intensive involvement. Most patients enter the program, stop their drug use, engage in treatment, and advance to their preferred level of involvement. A small percentage, however, do not stop their drug use and even with increased clinical attention get discharged for continued illicit drug use, generally cocaine, and for noncompliance with treatment.

During the past 2 years, the West Haven program has discharged 53 patients, 12 of whom were HIV positive. Of the 41 non-HIV discharges, 12 (29%) were for drug use. Eight (20%) of those were discharged because of cocaine or cocaine/opioid use. Of the 12 HIV-positive discharges, 9 (75%) were for drug use, 6 (50%) of which were for cocaine or cocaine/opioid use (see Figure 7.2).

In this sample of drug-abusing treatment failures, there is a remarkable difference in the percentage of HIV (75%) versus non-HIV (29%) patients discharged for continuing drug use. Additionally, 6 (50%) of the HIV-infected patients were discharged for cocaine use, while 8 (20%) of the non-HIV patients were discharged for cocaine use. From this data one could infer that HIV patients on methadone who use cocaine are at risk for discharge and may benefit from a unique approach. (For further exploration of this topic see Chapters 4 and 8).

METHADONE AND ALCOHOL DEPENDENCE

Alcohol has always been the primary "other" substance abused in methadone programs. Alcohol is used to excess by 20–50% of methadone-

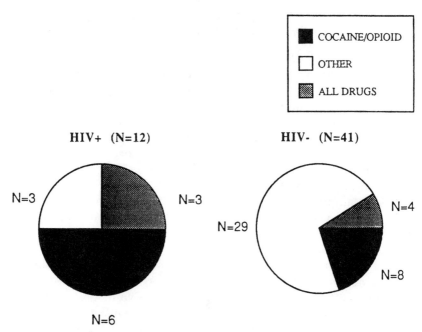

FIGURE 7.2. Reasons for discharge of HIV-positive and HIV-negative patients (*n* = 53) from MMP. Data from West Haven VA Medical Center methadone maintenance program for the years 1992–1994.

maintained patients (Kreek et al., 1978; Kreek, 1981a, 1981b). A study by Anglin et al. (1989) supports the thesis that use of alcohol and narcotics are not independent problems. In that study, which included both white and Mexican American subjects, an inverse relation was seen between the use of alcohol and heroin. Both populations that were studied exhibited decreased alcohol use while using street heroin and increased alcohol use during periods of outpatient drug treatment (methadone maintenance and drug free) and during periods of opiate abstinence. D'Amada (1983) found similar results with an interesting variation: a significant percentage (31%) of alcohol-abstinent methadone patients began to drink alcohol while in methadone treatment, whereas only 12% of drug-free treatment patients relapsed to alcohol.

Physiological and metabolic issues are also important in comorbid opiate and alcohol abuse. Alcohol use with methadone maintenance is likely to cause methadone patients to request more methadone. This may be due to enhanced hepatic metabolism (Kreek et al., 1978; Kreek, 1981a, 1981b), leading to opiate withdrawal, or due to alcohol withdrawal itself, which the patient may identify as opiate withdrawal. Alcohol withdrawal symptoms overlap with, but do not share cross-tolerance with, opiate withdrawal symptoms, adding a new layer of complexity to methadone dosing.

TREATMENT OF COMORBID DRUG AUBSE IN OPIATE-DEPENDENT PATIENTS

Opioid addicts, the majority of whom are not in treatment, often hold a fatalistic view that abstinence is not worth struggling for, since in the past they have failed at treatment, abstinence, and changing their lives in general. Health care workers may also lose hope in treating frequently relapsing patients, which has a significant impact on the treatment of recidivist addicts. Additionally, discouragement may come from limited treatment space, narrow treatment options, and dwindling financial support. Nevertheless, addicts who continue illicit cocaine use have multiple foci for intervention.

The first focus of intervention, extensively studied, is psychosocial treatment. It is generally recognized, as stated previously, that most addicts stop or significantly reduce their use of illicit drugs upon entry into methadone maintenance treatment. When that does not occur and illicit drug use continues, especially cocaine use, routine drug counseling has not proved effective. An intensive psychosocial focus needs to begin on admission, supporting initial efforts to discontinue illicit substance use and to improve life situations.

Especially useful in early treatment are increased contact, involving psychotherapy directed at the stage of recovery that the patient is in, and psychoeducation that provides facts about substance use, along with eliciting patients' feelings and thinking about substance use. Effective in later treatment are contingency management that provides immediate consequences for patients' behavior (generally in the form of loss of take-home medication for a positive urine sample) and relapse prevention that is tailored to drug use. Interventions are individually developed and then presented to the treatment team meetings for consensus and uniform follow-through.

Treatment needs to focus on teaching, supporting, and modifying those behaviors that are known to correlate with positive outcomes. Characteristics of treatment-responsive individuals are stable relationships, absent psychiatric comorbidity, noninvolvement with the legal system, stable housing, participation in valued activity (e.g., work, volunteering, child care), and financial stability, including welfare. Psychosocial stressors, even when severe, do not necessarily precipitate use of illicit substances when these characteristics are present; thus, it is vital to strengthen each of these areas during the course of treatment. A case study illustrates the complexity of the clinical presentation and the need for integrated treatment.

Brief Case Study

Ms. A. is a 37-year-old divorced white woman. She has been on a methadone maintenance program for 4 years. In addition to her heroin diagnosis, she carries diagnoses of cocaine, marijuana, and alcohol dependence as well as borderline personality disorder. She is HIV positive, seroconverting in 1991. She has been depressed since the death of her son in a motor vehicle accident in 1983. From 1988 until admission to methadone maintenance treatment, she had been homeless, with multiple admissions to inpatient psychiatric and substance treatment programs.

Ms. A.'s first year in treatment was remarkable in the number of brief relapses to the use of substances (cocaine, opioids, benzodiazepines, and amphetamines). Each relapse was short, typically characterized by two consecutive urines containing an illicit drug. She was hospitalized on a psychiatric ward twice for depression with suicidal thoughts.

Toward the end of her first year, she began using cocaine regularly and was placed on a cocaine contract; that is, her dose of methadone was increased for each of a series of positive cocaine urines that she gave (see methadone dose below). By the time Ms. A. was at 100 mg/day, her urines were cocaine free. She continued on the high dose of methadone for 2 years and then requested a series of decreases to 80 mg/day.

Ms. A. was frequently in crisis. Her style was to meet each problem in her life by amplifying, embellishing, and overreacting to, or ignoring her problems, thus assuring that any of her responses would eventually become a crisis. Initially, her group contact was typified by gentle confrontation from other, primarily male, patients. This confrontation proved ineffective for changing her "victim" stance and may have even supported it. Her failure to accept responsibility for her actions was met squarely in individual therapy. Psychoeducational groups that included improved self-esteem, assertiveness training, relapse prevention, and the methadone program "adoption" of a child in Appalachia were all components of her team-developed treatment.

By the end of the first year of her focused psychotherapy and increased methadone dose, Ms. A. had stopped relapsing and had started to consider returning to work. She had been a lab technician prior to her involvement with drugs. Around that time, her mother was diagnosed with cancer. Ms. A. had been estranged from her family for years. Her relationship with her parents was highly ambivalent, oscillating between over involvement and distance. Her siblings mistrusted her and did not want her near the family.

Ms. A. was hospitalized again for depression and pneumonia. Her

HIV infection had become symptomatic. The family situation waxed and waned; her two siblings formed a block to prevent her having contact with her increasingly ill mother. Ms. A. had a series of positive drug urines but quickly stopped her drug use. Treatment again focused on her use of drugs, considering the consequences and honing her relapse prevention skills.

Her mother died; and then her father, with whom she was closest, became ill and died. During this period of time, her psychotherapy focused on family and intimate relationships. In addition to her chaotic relationships with her family, Ms. A. was going through a series of relationships with men. Relationships remain a conflictual, highly charged arena for her.

Currently, she has not had a positive drug urine for nearly a year, but continues to have crises, mostly self-generated. Psychosocial, educational and therapeutic contact is generally increased at these times with variable responses.

This brief case study suggests that, in addition to neurobiological mechanisms, psychosocial factors are extremely important in the persistence of comorbid cocaine abuse in methadone-maintained patients. Additionally, pharmacological interventions may prove beneficial. These interventions are discussed below.

OPIOID AGONISTS AS A PHARMACOTHERAPY STRATEGY FOR COCAINE ABUSE

It has been reported that methadone treatment has a complex interaction with cocaine use. Treatment with the opioid agonist methadone did not reduce cocaine-positive urines in heroin-dependent patients (T. R. Kosten et al., 1987, 1989b), but morphine pretreatment suppressed cocaine self-administration in a dose-dependent manner in squirrel monkeys (Stretch, 1977). Clinical and preclinical studies of the effects of opioid antagonists on cocaine self-administration have also yielded conflicting results. There is considerable evidence that opioid antagonists, such as naloxone and naltrexone, do not suppress cocaine self-administration in primates or in rodents (Carroll et al., 1986; Ettenberg et al., 1982; Goldberg et al., 1971; Killian et al., 1978; Woods & Schuster, 1972). In rats, naltrexone pretreatment did not produce a change in cocaine self-administration (Ettenberg et al., 1982) or an increase in cocaine self-administration (Carroll et al., 1986). However, in contrast to these studies of opioid antagonist effects on cocaine self-administration in preclinical models, there is one clinical report that, compared to methadone therapy, naltrexone treatment (100–150 mg, three times per week) of opiate-dependent polydrug abusers significantly reduced cocaine-positive urines (Kosten et al., 1989a).

Since it is not clearly demonstrated whether agonist treatment itself promotes, attenuates, or has no effect on cocaine abuse, this problem has been an ongoing subject of clinical research. Both psychosocial and pharmacological factors may play a role in the interactions between opioid substitution treatment and cocaine abuse. For example, methadone maintenance may facilitate the use of cocaine by (1) freeing up money to buy cocaine — money that would otherwise have been used to buy opiates; (2) providing a high that is not dampened by methadone; or (3) being readily accessible to the addicts on the program (since it is often sold in the proximity of the maintenance programs). Mixing an opioid agonist like methadone with cocaine may prolong or even increase the euphoria of cocaine while also attenuating the dysphoria afterward. There is also the perception that the methadone program is for the treatment of opiate addiction, not cocaine addiction, leading in some cases to less-intense program attention to the problem. This perception may prevent an early intervention in cocaine use that could interrupt a prolonged "run," leading to discharge from methadone maintenance programs.

There is some limited preliminary indication that methadone dose may influence cocaine abuse in methadone-maintained patients. Some studies of cocaine use in methadone programs have indicated that methadone may put some patients at risk for cocaine use (Kosten, 1990); but a study of an increasing-dose contingency protocol (methadone dose was increased in response to positive cocaine toxicology) showed that 8 of 10 patients stopped cocaine use when they reached higher (greater than 100 mg) methadone doses (Stine et al., 1992). This variable effect of methadone (entry into the program may increase cocaine use, but higher methadone doses may decrease such use) could be explained by the behavioral component of the contingency treatment described above. Using a pharmacological model, however, the results could also be explained by the differential effects of low versus high dose on the withdrawal-like symptoms of opiates. One survey demonstrated that opiate-dependent patients do report cocaine-precipitated, opioid, withdrawal-like symptoms (Stine et al., 1991), and a later study in a low-versus-high methadone and buprenorphine maintenance dose confirmed greater symptoms of withdrawal in patients who used cocaine while maintained on the higher doses (Stine & Kosten, 1994). These results remain preliminary, and confirmation of methadone dose effect on cocaine use is needed by a larger, randomized, dose–response study (in progress) of methadone dose and cocaine use. However, these results do call into question any simple concept of the relation between

methadone and cocaine use and also cast further doubt on the practice of decreased methadone dose as a punishment for cocaine use.

The newer opioid agonist pharmacotherapies are now being investigated for possible therapeutic effects on cocaine abuse. Levo-alpha-
acetylmethadol (LAAM), the longer-acting methadone derivative (see
Chapter 12), may avoid quick changes in opioid blood levels that have
been said to potentiate cocaine effects (euphoria, or "high") and to increase abuse liability. This medication is also being studied for its effects on cocaine abuse (Alison Oliveto, personal communication). It has
been suggested that buprenorphine, a partial opioid antagonist with
relatively low opioid agonist activity (T. A. Kosten et al., 1989; T. R. Kosten et al., 1989a; Jacob et al., 1979; Jasinski et al., 1978; Leander, 1983;
Lewis, 1985; Mello & Mendelson, 1980; Mello et al, 1981), may decrease
the "speedball" interaction with cocaine and thereby reduce cocaine
abuse. Pilot studies in our program documented cocaine use in 3%
of the urines from 41 patients treated on buprenorphine, compared
to 24% of the urines from 61 patients on methadone maintenance, and
in 12 patients switched from methadone to buprenorphine, the rate
of cocaine-positive urines declined from 20% to 2% (T. A. Kosten et
al., 1989; T. R. Kosten et al., 1989a). While three larger, controlled, clinical trials have shown no efficacy of buprenorphine over methadone
in reducing cocaine abuse, T. R. Kosten and associates have found a
dose-related reduction in cocaine use with buprenorphine (Fudala et
al., 1990; T. R. Kosten et al., 1993; Schottenfeld et al., 1993b). Thus, a
relatively high buprenorphine dose (e.g., 16 mg/day) may be more effective (similar to the methadone dose hypothesis above) (see also Chapter 13). Clinical trials to test this hypothesis are also in progress (T. R.
Kosten, personal communication).

ADDITIONAL PHARMACOTHERAPIES
FOR COCAINE ABUSERS ON METHADONE

A long list of medications have been tested in clinical trials on cocaine
abusers. In addition to the tricyclic antidepressants (TCAs) and serotonin reuptake inhibitors (SRIs), bromocriptine, trazadone, lithium, and
methylphenidate have been used. Various classes of pharmacotherapies continue to be tested, including (but not exclusively) stimulants
(mazindol), anticonvulsants (carbamazepine), and a widely used medication for treating alcoholism (Antabuse). Antidepressants, opioid
blockers, and opioid agonist–antagonists have been the most extensively
tested medications.

Desipramine hydrochloride (DMI) has probably been the most

studied TCA for cocaine abuse. Clinical trials of DMI with cocaine-abusing methadone-maintained patients have been equivocal. Those mixed results may be due to high dropout rates, time-limited trials, diagnostically complex patients, poor subject recruitment, and, especially with methadone, the overlap effects of clinical therapies. T. R. Kosten (1989) has postulated that methadone patients tend to be more resistant to pharmacotherapies than cocaine abusers who are not dependent on opioids. One mitigating factor, however, is that methadone patients are more compliant in clinical cocaine treatment trials since medications can be dispensed with methadone. In a medication trial of amantadine, desipramine. and placebo, T. R. Kosten et al. (1992), using a cocaine-abusing methadone population, reported that cocaine use initially decreased at 4 weeks with DMI and became nonsignificant at 8 weeks. Arndt et al. (1992) reported in their study of 59 cocaine-abusing patients in a methadone program that, aside from improved psychiatric status in the DMI group, there were no other differences from the placebo group, including use of cocaine. In fact, improvement in patients' statuses was considered to be the result of enhanced attention and strict program policy adherence. Since methadone programs are required to provide clinical treatment along with the medication, it has been difficult to determine which effects are attributed to which treatment.

The major working hypothesis guiding pharmacotherapy trials has been that cocaine use leads to dopamine depletion, thus causing depression-like symptoms commonly observed in the cocaine-abstinent state. Rao et al. (1995) also report that pharmacotherapies for the treatment of cocaine have focused on the phases of cocaine withdrawal, acute versus chronic. Because dopamine hypoactivity may occur during the acute phase and dopamine depletion may occur in the chronic phase, there has been testing of such medications as the dopamine agonists amantadine, bromocriptine, and others in all phases. Bupropion has shown some promise (Margolin et al., 1991) for decreasing cocaine use as well as for improving mood, thus decreasing craving because of dysphoria; however a recent multisite trial showed no efficacy of bupropion over placebo (Margolin et al., 1995). Amantadine trials have been equally disappointing. In a random assignment of different amantadine doses to two groups, Handelsman et al. (1995) recently reported that amantadine was no more effective than placebo in reducing cocaine use and craving.

A more recent biological hypothesis exphasizes the role of serotonin in cocaine abuse. Although serotonergic medications (specific serotonin reuptake inhibitors, or SSRIs) have fewer side effects, they have many of the same clinical problems of the TCAs and dopaminergic medications when used for treatment of cocaine abuse in that their efficacy has not been clearly demonstrated. Additionally, serotonergic research is in its early stages, and the effects of drugs on the serotonin system are yet to be unraveled. Some data indicate that enhancing the serotonin (5-hydroxytryptamine [5-HT]) system appears to play a role in decreasing the self-administration of drugs, possibly by altering some of the reinforcing aspects of the substance (Sellers et al., 1991). This behavior change may be one of many possible effects of serotonin. Batki et al. (1991) used fluoxetine and group therapy in a trial with cocaine-abusing methadone patients. They reported a decrease in quantitative cocaine urine and money spent on cocaine. However, since the medication was combined with group therapy, effects may be attributed to overlapping interventions. Currently novel pharmacotherapeutic approaches to cocaine treatment are being explored in general and this research will in turn lead to novel approaches to cocaine treatment in methadone programs.

In conclusion, the role of medications in the treatment of methadone-maintained patients with comorbid cocaine abuse is unclear. However, researchers have identified three distinct groups of patients, who may benefit from pharmacotherapy: heavily abusing addicts who may experience neurochemical alterations; patients with psychiatric comorbidity, expecially depression; and those who are medically compromised with serious illnesses such as HIV (T. R. Kosten, 1989). Integrating medications into the psychosocial treatment plan is also necessary for maximizing effectiveness. The treatment team should understand the reasons for and possible effects of medications in order to heighten the team's awareness and involvement in this aspect of treatment.

TREATMENT OF ALCOHOL ABUSE AND DEPENDENCE

Careful assessment of patients for alcohol problems on admission to methadone treatment is vital to the patients' success in the program. Differentiating between alcohol-dependent problem drinkers and non-dependent drinking patients is a fundamental step in the process (Chatham et al., 1995). In a study of alcoholic methadone patients to determine the relation between blood alcohol levels (BALs), admission Michigan Alcohol Screening Test (MAST) scores, clinic absenteeism, and depression (measured by the Beck Depression Inventory, or BDI), Bickel and Amass (1993) found significant positive correlations between mean BAL and MAST, mean BAL and clinic absenteeism, and MAST and BDI. An important finding of this study was that the MAST predicted mean BAL. This could be a potentially useful tool for assisting in identifying alcohol-dependent patients on admission to methadone programs.

Most drinking severity is positively related to urine screens containing illicit drugs (Hunt et al., 1986; Roszell et al., 1986). Generally, staff are inclined to respond to a positive drug urine by addressing the drugs in use, interestingly, this study finding may indicate the need for an alcohol intervention as well. Clearly this body of literature indicates a number of ways to assess the presence of an alcohol problem. Developing treatment plans that address alcohol issues must begin in the early stages of treatment in order to assure a higher likelihood of treatment success. However, whenever an indication of alcohol abuse arises, early or later, it must be dealt with immediately and directly in order to prevent a worsening of the clinical condition.

Herd (1993) found that, of four publicly funded treatment programs, methadone programs reported the lowest rates of heavy drinking and alcohol problems. Factors that predicted heavy drinking and drunkenness were context and reasons for combining drug and alcohol use. Thus, methadone programs may provide built-in protection since the setting promotes drug- and alcohol-free behavior; and as reported earlier, drug use decreases with the length of time spent in a methadone treatment program.

Most programs consistently screen (with Breathalyzer; with BAL rarely) for the presence of alcohol and are watchful for clinical indications of abuse. Once alcohol abuse or dependence is established, there are several options available: self-help (Alcoholics Anonymous or other), special within-program alcohol groups, in- or outpatient rehabilitation programs, or pharmacotherapies.

Methadone programs are frequently responding to the use of both alcohol and cocaine with specifically designed treatments, often using groups. These treatments may incorporate creative use of contingency contracting, family and couples treatment, and peer confrontation and support.

Pharmacotherapies can also be a benefit to alcohol treatment with opiate-maintained individuals. Disulfiram (Antabuse) has been useful in alcoholic opiate addicts. Up to 25% of patients in methadone programs have been reported to have drinking problems. These problems are often successfully managed by behavioral means, including Breathalyzer testing, withholding methadone for a positive Breathalyzer reading, increasing specialized therapy for alcohol, or attending Alcoholics Anonymous. In a subgroup of patients who are refractory to these methods, disulfiram may be indicated. Liebson et al. (1973), in a successful study, found that the rewarding effects of methadone complemented the use of disulfiram. Another large Veterans Administration collaborative study (Ling et al., 1983), however, found that patients tended to test themselves with alcohol to determine whether they were receiving placebo. These investigators also found no disulfiram–placebo differences in the methadone-maintained patients, but the drinking problems in both groups showed improvement. This improvement was attributed to the structure imposed by the disulfiram study. The investigators concluded that willingness to accept disulfiram was a significant factor in the beneficial effects observed and that there was no evidence of adverse interaction between methadone and disulfiram. When psychosocial treatment and disulfiram are not effective, some patients may respond to naltrexone maintenance (instead of opioid agonist substitution) for the combination of opiate and alcohol dependence. Naltrexone treatment is discussed in detail in Chapter 6 in this volume.

SUMMARY

Treating the opioid addict who abuses other substances, especially alcohol and cocaine, remains a clinical challenge in the mid-1990s. To the credit of the substance treatment field, many creative approaches have been tried, some with varying success. Nevertheless, it continues to be crucial for those of us in the research and clinical arenas to develop unique treatments to engage this treatment-refractory population.

Matching patients to treatment appears to be the most successful model for engaging and treating addicts. Within that model, creative thinking and unusual approaches must be encouraged. The particularly recondite subpopulation of cocaine/opioid addicts, who are more and more frequently also HIV positive, would benefit from continuing efforts to engage them in a combination of psychopharmacological and psychosocial therapies.

REFERENCES

Abdul-Quader, A. S., Friedman, A. S., DesJarlais, D., Marmor, D., Maslansky, R., & Bartelme, S. (1987). Methadone maintenance and behavior by intravenous drug users that can transmit HIV. *Contemporary Drug Problems, 14*, 425–434.

Anglin, M. D., Almog, I. J., Fisher, D. G., & Peters, K. R. (1989). Alcohol use by heroin addicts: Evidence for an inverse relationship. A study of methadone maintenance and drug-free treatment samples. *American Journal of Drug and Alcohol Abuse, 15*(2), 191–207.

Anglin, M. D., & McGlothlin, W. H. (1984). Outcome of narcotic addict treatment in California. In F. Tims & J Ludford (Eds,), *Drug abuse treatment evaluation: Strategies, progress and prospects* (NIDA Research Monograph No. 51, pp. 106–128). Washington, DC: National Institute on Drug Abuse.

Arndt, I. O., Dorozynsky, L., Woody, G. E., McLellan, A. T., & O'Brien, C. P. (1992). Desipramine treatment of cocaine dependence in methadone-maintained patients. *Archives of General Psychiatry, 49,* 888–893.

Ashery, R. S., Carlson, R. G., Falck, R. S., & Siegal, H. A. (1995). Injection drug users, crack cocaine users, and human services utilizaion: An exploratory study. *Social Work, 40*(1), 75–82.

Ball, J. C., Myers, P. C., & Friedman, S. R. (1988). Reducing the risk of AIDS through methadone maintenance treatment. *Journal of Health and Social Behavior, 29,* 214–226.

Ball, J. C., Ross, A., & Jaffe, J. H. (1989). Cocaine and heroin use by methadone maintenance patients. In L. S. Harris (Ed.), *Problems of drug dependence: Proceedings of the Committee on Problems of Drug Dependence* (NIDA Research Monograph No. 95, p. 328). Rockville, MD: National Institute on Drug Abuse.

Batki, S. L., Manfredi, L. B., Sorensen, J. L., Jacob, P., Dumontet, R., & Jones, R. T. (1991). *Fluoxetine for cocaine abuse in methadone patients: Preliminary findings* (NIDA Research Monograph No. 105, pp. 516–517). Rockville, MD: National Institute on Drug Abuse.

Bickel, W. K., & Amass, L. (1993). The relationship of mean daily blood alcohol levels to admission MAST, clinic absenteeism and depression in alcoholic methadone patients. *Drug and Alcohol Dependence, 32*(2), 113–118.

Carroll, M. E., Lac, S. T., Walker, M. J., Kragh, R., & Newman, T. (1986). Effects of naltrexone on intravenous cocaine self-administration in rats during food satiation and deprivation. *Journal of Pharmacology and Experimental Therapeutics, 238,* 1–7.

Chaisson, R. E., Bacchetti, P., Osmond, D., Brodie, B., Sande, M. A., & Moss, A. R. (1989). Cocaine use and HIV infection in intravenous drug users in San Francisco. *Journal of the American Medical Association, 261,* 561–565.

Chatham, L. R., Rowan-Szal, G. A., Joe, G. W., Brown, B. S., & Simpson, D. D. (1995). Heavy drinking in a population of methadone-maintained clients. *Journal of Studies on Alcohol, 56*(4), 417–422.

Condelli, W. S., Fairbanks, J. A., Dennis, M. L., & Rachal, J. V. (1991). Cocaine use by clients in methadone programs: Significance, scope and behavioral interventions. *Journal of Substance Abuse Treatment, 8,* 203–212.

Corty, E., & Ball, J. C. (1987). Admissions to methadone maintenance: Comparisons between programs and implications for treatment. *Journal of Substance Abuse Treatment, 4,* 181–187.

Cushman, P. (1988). Cocaine use in a population of drug abusers on methadone. *Hospital and Community Psychiatry, 39,* 1205–1207.

Daly, J. M., & Salloway, S. (1994). Dopamine receptors in the human. *Psychiatric Times,* pp. 25–32.

D'Amanda, C. D. (1983). *Program policies and procedures associated with treatment outcome* (NIDA Treatment Research Monograph No. 83-1281). Rockville, MD: National Institute on Drug Abuse.

D'Aunno, T., & Vaughn, T. E. (1992). Variations in methadone treatment practices. *Journal of the American Medical Association, 267*(2), 253–258.

Des Jarlais, D. C. & Friedman, S. R. (1987). HIV infection among intravenous drug users: Epidemiology and risk reduction [editorial review]. *AIDS, 1*(2), 67–76.

Des Jarlais, D. C., Friedman, S. R., & Hopkins, W. (1985). Risk reduction for the acquired immunodeficiency syndrome among intravenous drug users. *Annals of Internal Medicine, 103,* 755–759.

Dolan, M. P., Black, J. L., Penk, W. E., Robinowitz, R., & DeFord, H. A. (1985). Contracting for treatment termination to reduce illicit drug use among methadone maintenance treatment failures. *Journal of Consulting and Clinical Psychology, 53*(4), 549–551.

Dole, V. P., & Nyswander, M. E. (1968). Methadone maintenance and its implication for theories of narcotic addiction. In A. Wilker (Ed.), *The addictive state* (pp, 359–366). Baltimore: Williams & Wilkins.

Ettenberg, A., Pettit, H. O., Bloom, F. E., & Koob, G. F. (1982). Heroin and cocaine intravenous self-administration in rats: Mediation by separate neural systems. *Psychopharmacology* (Berlin), *78,* 204–209.

Fudala, P. J., Johnson, R. E., & Jaffe, J. H. (1991). *Outpatient comparison of buprenorphine and methadone maintenance: II. Effects on cocaine usage, retention time in study and missed clinic visits* (NIDA Research Monograph No. 105, pp. 587–588). Rockville, MD: National Institute on Drug Abuse.

Gawin, F. H., Kleber, H. D., Byck, R., Rounsaville, B. J., Kosten, T. R., Jatlow, P., & Morgan, C. (1987). Desipramine facilitation of initial cocaine abstinence. *Archives of General Psychiatry, 46,* 117–121.

General Accounting Office, United States (1990). *Methadone maintenance: Some treatment programs are not effective. Greater federal oversight needed* (Publication No. GAO/HRD-90-104) Washington, DC: U.S. Government Printing Office.

Goldberg, S. R., Woods, J. H., & Schuster, C. R. (1971). Nalorphine-induced changes in morphine self-administration in rhesus monkeys. *Journal of Pharmacology and Experimental Therapeutics, 176,* 464–471.

Gottheil, E., Sterling, R. C., & Weinstein, S. P. (1993). Diminished illicit drug use as a consequence of long-term methadone maintenance. *Journal of Addictive Disease, 12*(4), 45–57.

Gronbladh, L., Ohlund, L. S., & Gunne, L. M. (1990). Mortality in heroin addiction: impact of methadone treatment. *Acta Psychiatrica Scandinavica, 82,* 223–227.

Hall, W. (1993). Perfectionism in the therapeutic appraisal of methadone maintenance [Editorial]. *Addiction, 88,* 1181–1182.

Handelsman, L., Limpitlaw, L., Williams, D., Schmeidler, J., Paris, P., & Stimmel, B. (1995). Amantadine does not reduce cocaine use or craving in cocaine-dependent methadone maintenance patients. *Drug and Alcohol Dependence, 39*(3), 173–180.

Herd, D. (1993). Correlates of heavy drinking and alcohol related problems among men and women in drug treatment programs. *Drug and Alcohol Dependence, 32*(1), 23–35.

Hubbard, R. L., Allison, M., Bray, R. M., Craddock, S. G., Rachol, J. V., & Ginzburg, H. M. (1983). An overview of client characteristics, treatment services and treatment outcomes for outpatient methadone clinics in the treatment outcome prospective study (TOPS). In J. R. Cooper, F. Altman, B. S. Brown, & D. Czechowicz (Eds.), *Research on the treatment of narcotic addiction: State of the art* (pp. 714–647). Rockville, MD: National Institute on Drug Abuse.

Hubbard, R. L., Marsden, M. E., Rachal, J. V., Hardwod, H. J., Cavanaugh, E. R., & Ginzburg, H. M. (1989). *Drug abuse treatment: A national study of effectiveness.* Chapel Hill: University of North Carolina Press.

Hunt, D. E., Strug, D. L., Goldsmith, D. S., Lipton, D. S., Robertson, K., & Truitt, L. (1986). Alcohol use and abuse: Heavy drinking among methadone clients. *American Journal of Drug and Alcohol Abuse, 12*(1–2), 147–164.

Jacob, J. J. C., Michaud, G. M., & Tremblay, E. C. (1979). Mixed agonist–antagonist opiates and physical dependence. *British Journal of Clinical Pharmacology, 7,* 291S–296S.

Jaffe, J. H. (1992). Opiates: Clinical aspects. In J. Lowinson, P. Ruiz & R. Millman (Eds.), *Substance abuse: A comprehensive textbook* (pp. 186–194). Baltimore: Williams & Wilkins.

Jasinski, D. R., Pevnick, J. S., & Griffith, J. D. (1978). Human pharmacology and abuse potential of the analgesic buprenorphine. *Archives of General Psychiatry, 35,* 501–516.

Joseph, H., & Appel, P. (1985). Alcoholism and methadone treatment. *American Journal of Drug and Alcohol Abuse, 11,* 37–53.

Judson, B. A., Goldstein, A., & Inturrisi, C. E. (1983). Methadyl acetate (LAAM) in the treatment of heroin addicts: A double-blind comparison of gradual and abrupt detoxification. *Archives of General Psychiatry, 40,* 834–840.

Kang, S. Y., & De Leon, G. (1993). Criminal involvement of cocaine users enrolled in a methadone treatment program. *Addiction, 88*(3), 395–404.

Killian, A. K., Bonese, K., & Schuster, C. R. (1978). The effects of naloxone on behavior maintained by cocaine and heroin injections in the rhesus monkey. *Drug and Alcohol Dependence, 3,* 243–251.

Koob, G. F., & Bloom, F. E. (1988). Cellular and molecular mechanisms of drug dependency. *Science, 242*(4879), 715–723.

Kosten, T. A. (1990). Cocaine attenuates the severity of naloxone-precipitated opioid withdrawal. *Life Sciiences, 47,* 1617–1623.

Kosten, T. A., Jacobsen, L. S., & Kosten, T. R. (1989). Severity of precipitated opiate withdrawal predicts drug dependence by DSM-III-R criteria. *Amerian Journal of Drug and Alcohol Abuse, 15,* 237–250.

Kosten, T. R. (1989). Pharmacotherapeutic interventions for cocaine abuse: Matching patients to treatments. *Journal of Nervous and Mental Disease, 177,* 379–389.

Kosten, T. R., Kleber, H. D., & Morgan, C. (1989a). Role of opioid antagonists in treating intravenous cocaine abuse. *Life Sciences, 44,* 887–892.

Kosten, T. R., Kleber, H. D., & Morgan, C. (1989b). Treatment of cocaine abuse with buprenorphine. *Biological Psychiatry, 26,* 537–639.

Kosten, T. R., Morgan, C., Falcione, J., & Schottenfeld, R. S. (1992). Pharmacotherapy for cocaine-abusing methadone-maintained patients using amantadine or desipramine. *Archives of General Psychiatry, 49,* 894–898.

Kosten, T. R., Rounsaville, B. J., & Foley, S. H. (1990). Inpatient versus outpatient cocaine abuse treatments. In L. S. Harris (Ed.), *Proceedings of the Com-*

mittee on Problems of Drug Dependence (NIDA Research Monograph No. 95, pp. 312–313). Rockville, MD: National Institute on Drug Abuse.

Kosten, T. R., Rounsaville, B. J., Gawin, F. H., & Kleber, H. D. (1986). Cocaine abuse among opioid addicts: Demographic and diagnostic characteristics. *American Journal of Drug and Alcohol Abuse, 12,* 1–16.

Kosten, T. R., Rounsaville, B. J., & Kleber, H. D. (1987). A 2.5-year follow-up of cocaine use among treated opioid addicts: Have our treatments helped? *Archives of General Psychiatry, 44,* 281–284.

Kosten, T. R., Rounsaville, B. J., & Kleber, H. D. (1988). Antecedents and consequences of cocaine abuse among opioid addicts: A 2.5 year follow-up. *Journal of Nervous and Mental Disease, 176,* 176–181.

Kosten, T. R., Schottenfeld, R., Ziedonis, D., et al. (1993). Buprenorphine versus methadone maintenance for opioid dependence. *Journal of Nervous and Mental Disease, 181*(6), 358–364.

Kozel, N., & Adams, E. (1986). Epidemiology of drug abuse: an overview. *Science, 234,* 970–974.

Kreek, M. J. (1981a). Metabolic interactions between opiates and alcohol. *Annals of the New York Academy of Sciences, 362,* 36–49.

Kreek, M. J. (1981b). Medical management of methadone-maintained patients. In J. H. Lowinson & P. Ruis (Eds.), *Substance abuse: Clinical problems and perspectives* (pp. 660–673). Baltimore: Williams & Wilkins.

Kreek, M. J., Oratz, M., & Rothschild, M. A. (1978). Hepatic extraction of long- and short-acting narcotics in the isolated perfused rabbit liver. *Gastroenterology, 75,* 88–94.

Kreek, M. J., Schoeller, D., Wong, W., & Klein, P. (1981). Identification of cirrhosis by the 13C-aminopyrine breath test (ABT) in methadone maintained patients. *Gastroenterology, 80,* 1338.

Leander, J. D. (1983). Opioid agonist and antagonist behavioral effects of buprenorphine. *British Journal of Pharmacology, 78,* 607–615.

Lewis, J. W. (1985). Buprenorphine. *Drug and Alcohol Dependence, 14,* 363–372.

Liebson, I., Bigelow, G., & Flamer, R. (1973). Alcoholism among methadone patients: A specific treatment method. *American Journal of Psychiatry, 130,* 483–485.

Ling, W., Klett, J., & Gillis, R. D. (1978). A cooperative clinical study of methadyl acetate. *Archives of General Psychiatry, 35,* 345–353.

Ling, W., Weiss, D. G., & Charuvastra, C. V. (1983). Use of disulfiram for alcoholics in methadone maintenance programs. *Archives of General Psychiatry, 40,* 851–854.

Lipton, D. S., & Maranda, M. J. M. (1983). Detoxification from heroin dependency: An overview of methods and effectiveness. In B. Stimmel (Ed.), *Evaluation of drug treatment programs.* New York: Haworth Press.

Magura, S., Siddiqi, Q., Freeman, R. C., & Lipton, D. S. (1991). Changes in cocaine use after entry to methadone treatment. *Journal of Addictive Diseases, 10*(4), 31–45.

Margolin, A., Kosten, T. R., Avants, S. K., Wilkins, J., Ling, W., Beckson, M., Arndt, I. O., Carnish, J., Ascher, J. A., Li, S. H., & Bridge, P. (1995). A multicenter trial of bupropion for cocaine dependence in methadone-maintained patients. *Drug and Alcohol Dependence, 40,* 125–131.

Margolin, A., Kosten, T., Petrakis, I., Avants, S. K., & Kosten, T. (1991). *An open pilot study of bupropion and psychotherapy for the treatment of cocaine abuse in methadone-maintained patients* (NIDA Research Monograph No. 105, pp. 367–368). Rockville, MD: National Institute on Drug Abuse.

Meandzija, B., O'Connor, P. G., Fitzgerald, B., Rounsaville, B. J., & Kosten, T. R. (1994). HIV infection and cocaine use in methadone maintained and untreated intravenous drug users. *Drug and Alcohol Dependence, 36*(2), 109–113.

Mello, N. K., & Mendelson, J. H. (1980). Buprenorphine suppresses heroin use by heroin addicts. *Science, 207,* 657–659.

Mello, N. K., Mendelson, J. H., & Kuehnle, J. C. (1981). Buprenorphine effects of human heroin self-administration: An operant analysis. *Journal of Pharmacology and Experimental Therapeutics, 223,* 30–39.

National Institute on Drug Abuse (1989). *Drug abuse warning network: Emergency room cocaine mentions (C-89-01).* Rockville, MD: Author.

Novick, D. M., Khan, I., & Kreek, M. J. (1986). Acquired immunodeficiency syndrome and infection with hepatitis viruses in individuals abusing drugs by injection. *Bulletin of Narcotics, 38*(1–2), 15–25.

Rao, S., Ziedonis, D., & Kosten, T. (1995). The pharmacotherapy of cocaine dependence. *Psychiatry Annals, 25*(6), 363–368.

Rosenblum, A., Magura, S., & Joseph, H. (1991). Ambivalence toward methadone treatment among intravenous drug users. *Journal of Psychoactive Drugs, 23*(1), 21–27.

Roszell, D. K., Calsyn, D. A., & Chaney, E. F. (1986). Alcohol use and psychopathology in opioid addicts on methadone maintenance. *American Journal of Drug and Alcohol Abuse, 12*(3), 269–278.

Segal, D. L., & Schuster, C. R. (1995). Buprenorphine: what interests the National Institute on Drug Abuse? In A. Cowan & J. W. Lewis (Eds.), *Buprenorphine: Combatting drug abuse with a unique opioid* (pp. 309–320). Wiley-Liss.

Senay, E. C., Mahta, C., Dorus, W., Soberu, K., & Baumgardner, M. (1986). Comprehensive treatment for heroin addcits: A pilot study. *Journal of Psychoactive Drugs, 18,* 107–115.

Schottenfeld, R. S., O'Malley, S., Abdul-Salaam, K., & O'Connor, P. G. (1993a). Decline in intravenous drug use among treatment-seeking opiate users. *Journal of Substance Abuse Treatment, 10,* 5–10.

Schottenfeld, R. S., Pakes, J., Ziedonis, D., & Kosten, T. R. (1993b). Buprenorphine: Dose related effects on cocaine and opiate use in cocaine abusing opiate dependent humans. *Biological Psychiatry, 34,* 66–74.

Sellers, E. M., Higgins, G. A., Tomkins, D. M., Romach, M. K., & Toneatto, T. (1991). Opportunities for treatment of psychoactive substance use disorders with serotonergic medications. *Journal of Clinical Psychiatry, 52*(12), 49–54.

Serpelloni, G., Carrieri, M. P., Rezza, G., Morganti, S., Gomma, M., & Binki, N. (1994). Methadone treatment as a determinant of HIV risk reduction among injecting drug users: A nested case-control study. *AIDS Care, 6*(2), 215–220.

Shaffer, H. J., & SaSalvia, T. A. (1992). Patterns of substance use among methadone maintenance patients. *Journal of Substance Abuse Treatment, 9,* 143–147.

Stark, M. J. (1989). A psychoeducational approach to methadone maintenance treatment. *Journal of Substance Abuse Treatment, 6,* 169–181.

Stine, S. M. (1992). Cocaine abuse within methadone programs. In T. Kosten & H. E. Kleber (Eds.), *Clinician's guide to cocaine addiction: Theory, research and treatment* (pp. 359–373). New York: Guilford Press.

Stine, S. M., Burns, B., & Kosten, T. (1991). Methadone dose for cocaine abuse. *Amerian Journal of Psychiatry, 148*(9), 1268.

Stine, S. M., Freeman, M., Burns, B., Charney, D. S., & Kosten, T. R. (1992). The effect of methadone dose on cocaine abuse in a methadone program. *American Journal on Addictions, 1,* 294–303.

Stine, S. M., & Kosten, T. R. (1994). Reduction of opiate withdrawal-like symptoms by cocaine abuse during methadone and buprenorphine maintenance. *American Journal of Drug and Alcohol Abuse, 20*(4), 445–458.

Stine, S. M., Satel, S., & Kosten, T. R. (1993). Cocaine precipitation of patient-identified opiate withdrawal. *American Journal on Addictions, 2*(3), 255–258.

Stitzer, M. L., Bigelow, G. E., & Liebson, I. (1980). Reducing drug use among methadone maintenance clients: Contingent reinforcement for morphine-free urines. *Addictive Behaviors, 5,* 333–340.

Strain, E. C., Stitzer, M. L., Liebson, I. A., & Bigelow, G. E. (1994). Comparison of buprenorphine and methadone in the treatment of opioid dependence. *American Journal of Psychiatry, 151*(7), 1025–1030.

Stretch, R. (1977). Discrete-trial control of cocaine self-injection behavior in squirrel monkeys: Effects of morphine, naloxone, and chlorpromazine. *Canadian Journal of Physiology and Pharmacology, 55*(4), 778–790.

Strug, D. L., Hunt, D. E., Goldsmith, D. S., et al. (1985). Patterns of cocaine use among methadone clients. *International Journal of the Addictions, 20,* 1163–1175.

Sutker, P. B., Allain, A. N., Smith, C. J., & Cohen, G. H. (1978). Addicts' descriptions of therapeutic community, multimodality and methadone maintenance treatment clients and staff. *Journal of Consulting and Clinical Psychology, 46,* 508–517.

White, J. M., Dyer, K. R., Ali, R. L., Gaughwin, M. D., & Cormack, S. (1994). Injecting behavior and risky needle use amongst methadone maintenance clients. *Drug and Alcohol Dependence, 34,* 113–119.

Wise, R. A. (1988). The neurobiology of craving: Implications for the understanding and treatment of addiction [Review]. *Journal of Abnormal Psychology, 97*(2), 118–132.

Woods, J. H., & Schuster, C. R. (1972). Opiates as reinforcing stimuli. In T. Thompson & R. Pickens (Eds.), *Stimulus properties of drugs* (pp. 163–173). New York: Appleton-Century-Crofts.

Woody, G. E. (1983). *Treatment characteristics associated with outcome* (Treatment Research Monograph No. 83-1281). Rockville, MD: National Institute on Drug Abuse.

Woody, G. E., Luborsky, L., McLellan, A. T., O'Brien, C. P., Bek, A. T., Blaine, J., Herman, I., & Hole, A. (1983). Psychotherapy for opiate addicts: Does it help? *Archives of General Psychiatry, 40,* 639–645.

Zahniser, N. R., Peris, J., Dwskin, L. P., Curella, P., Yaruda, R. P., O'Keefe, L., & Boyson, S. J. (1988). *Sensitization to cocaine in the nigrostriatal dopamine system* (NIDA Research Monograph No. 88). Rockville, MD: National Institute on Drug Abuse.

Section B

ANCILLARY SERVICES
AND SPECIAL POPULATIONS

Chapter 8

MATCHING METHADONE-MAINTAINED PATIENTS TO PSYCHOSOCIAL TREATMENTS

S. Kelly Avants, Ph.D.
Robert Ohlin, Psy.D.
Arthur Margolin, Ph.D.

There is wide variability in the type and intensity of psychosocial interventions provided to individuals enrolled in methadone maintenance programs (MMPs). At one extreme are programs that distribute methadone and offer only the minimal additional services required by U.S. Food and Drug Administration (FDA) standards; at the other extreme are programs that provide intensive services, such as those provided in day hospitals. In this chapter we will describe some of the ancillary psychosocial services that are, or could potentially be, offered to methadone-maintained patients; and we will discuss efforts under way to identify strategies for matching patients to the most appropriate and cost-beneficial treatment intensity.

ARE ANCILLARY PSYCHOSOCIAL INTERVENTIONS NECESSARY?

Although methadone maintenance was based on a disease model of addiction, social rehabilitation has always been one of its primary goals (Dole & Nyswander, 1965). In its original formulation, Phase I of methadone maintenance treatment was a 6-week inpatient stay during which the patient was stabilized on methadone, a medical and psychiatric work-up was performed, and individualized treatment plans were developed, which included preparation for high school equivalency examinations, job placement studies, and a review of family and housing problems. A focus on psychosocial rehabilitation continued on an outpatient basis in Phase II of treatment, during which time the emphasis was on employment, housing, education, and reconciliation with family members. Patients remained in the second phase until they reached Phase III, at which time the ex-addict was described as having become "a socially normal, self-supporting person" (Dole & Nyswander, 1965, p. 82).

Since this original formulation of methadone maintenance in the mid-1960s, there have been major changes in the type of medical and psychosocial problems that MMPs must face. The most urgent of these problems is the HIV epidemic. Intravenous drug users now constitute the second largest group of HIV-infected individuals in the country, with HIV-seroprevalence rates of approximately 50% (Des Jarlais, Friedman & Casriel, 1990). Furthermore, 71% of the heterosexual AIDS cases reported in 1990 were believed to be the result of sexual contact with an intravenous drug user (Lewis & Watters, 1991). Although methadone maintenance has the potential to reduce the spread of HIV through the reduction of intravenous opiate use and needle sharing (Ball & Ross, 1991; Novick et al., 1986; Senay, 1985), MMPs are still faced with an escalating medical and psychosocial service burden. There is a pressing need for medical services for patients already infected, especially since methadone patients are less likely to receive medical attention unless these services are offered on site (Umbricht-Schneiter et al., 1992). There is also a need for behavioral interventions targeting high-risk behaviors among MMP patients, such as unsafe sexual practices or the intravenous use of other drugs (e.g., cocaine).

Cocaine use, now endemic in many inner cities, constitutes another of the serious problems faced by MMPs (Condelli et al., 1991). Cocaine use not only undermines a fundamental goal of methadone treatment—the cessation of all illicit drug use, which is the basis for medical and psychosocial rehabilitation (Ball & Ross, 1991)—but adds to the spread of HIV. Cocaine use during methadone treatment has been found to be related to poor treatment retention (Joe et al., 1991a) and to poor treatment outcome (Ball & Ross, 1991). Cocaine use appears to have become a part of the social life of many MMP patients, not only the most "deviant" patients but also a significant proportion of patients who are otherwise compliant with program rules (Strug et al., 1985). The following are several factors that may contribute to cocaine use in MMPs (Avants et al., 1994a; Strug et al., 1985): (1) the lack of effective pharmacological treatments for cocaine abuse (Meyer, 1992); (2) the appeal of cocaine as a new "high;" (3) the use of cocaine (a) to self-medicate the sedating and other side effects of higher doses of methadone or (b) in combination with methadone, to diminish some of the unpleasant effects of cocaine, such as the "crash" and cocaine-induced paranoia; (4) the availability of money, previously spent on heroin, to buy cocaine; (5) the abundance of conditioned drug cues and the availability of cocaine in the inner-city neighborhoods where MMPs are frequently located; and (6) the social networks created when drug-addicted patients congregate in an MMP, thus maintaining the drug subculture.

Exacerbating the difficulties posed by the HIV epidemic and the abuse of cocaine in MMPs are characteristics of inner-city patients who are most at risk. Patients drawn from inner-city areas frequently have few resources, are often unemployed and undereducated, and may have additional psychiatric or medical problems. African Americans may be especially at risk. They are more likely than whites to drop out of methadone treatment prematurely (Joe et al., 1991a), to use cocaine at time of entry into methadone treatment (Kosten et al., 1986), and to increase their cocaine use while in treatment (Kosten et al., 1987). They are also disproportionately represented among HIV-positive patients (Meandzija et al., 1995); and HIV-positive status, in turn, is associated with high unemployment rates and increased illicit substance use.

Psychiatric disorders, especially depression, are also prevalent at high rates in opiate users who enter treatment (Kosten & Rounsaville, 1986). More than 50% of inner-city methadone patients are estimated to have a lifetime diagnosis of depression at admission (Ball & Ross, 1991; Kosten & Rounsaville, 1986); and depression is a predictor of poor outcome, especially in the domain of continued or increased illicit drug use (Kosten et al., 1986). In addition, patients with high levels of psychiatric disturbance are most likely to engage in high-risk behaviors, such as needle sharing (Metzger et al., 1991).

Personality disorders are also prevalent in patients who enter methadone treatment. Antisocial personality disorder is the most frequently diagnosed of these disorders. Between 45 and 55% of opiate-dependent patients who enter methadone treatment meet criteria for antisocial personality disorder (Kosten & Rounsaville, 1986; Gill et al., 1992). This disorder is associated with unemployment (Chambers et al., 1972), with increased incidence of cocaine abuse, and with additional psychosocial problems (Kosten et al., 1986). Patients with antisocial personality disorder typically respond very poorly to treatment (Leal et al., 1994; Woody et al., 1985) and are more likely to engage in high-risk behaviors (Gill et al., 1992).

These are indeed challenging times for MMPs. With an increase in the need for medical and psychosocial interventions has come a decrease in funding for these services (Lowinson et al., 1992). As the number of MMPs increased throughout the 1970s, high-volume low-cost treatment settings, providing few interventions other than the administration of methadone, became increasingly prevalent (Weddington, 1990). In the mid-1980s, federal funding was cut still further for community-based drug treatment programs (Meyer, 1992); and in the 1990s, MMPs may be faced with further constraints posed by managed care.

The need for services, however, is clear. In a study of 590 methadone patients who were entering treatment at 21 clinics, approximately half were in need of medical services; one third were in need of financial, employment, and educational assistance; one fifth were in need of family and legal services, and one third were in need of mental health services (Joe et al., 1991b). Although methadone programs provide as many services as their budgets and staffing will allow, the medical and psychosocial needs of most patients are not met during the course of treatment (Ball & Ross, 1991; Joe et al., 1991b).

The spread of HIV among drug-addicted populations, the prevalence of cocaine abuse and psychiatric disorders in MMPs, and the general degradation of inner-city living conditions suggests that the question is not, whether ancillary psychosocial and medical services are necessary in MMPs, but what type and intensity of services are appropriate, and what is the most cost-effective way to provide these services? In the sections that follow, we will attempt to address these questions. First, we will describe various psychosocial interventions that have been used in MMPs or that have the potential to be adapted for use with methadone patients. Grouped under the heading "Low-Intensity Interventions" are treatments that range from the minimal FDA requirements to case management and counseling, behavioral contingency management programs, and individual and group psychotherapy. Grouped under the heading "High-Intensity Interventions" are day hospitals and the community reinforcement approach.

LOW-INTENSITY PSYCHOSOCIAL INTERVENTIONS

Minimal FDA Requirements

FDA regulations (Federal Register, 1994) state that rehabilitative services play an important role in the treatment of opioid dependence and recommend that MMPs have access to a comprehensive range of medical and rehabilitative services. However, the regulations do not mandate specific rehabilitative services, nor the frequency with which services should be offered. General requirements include (1) the provision of vocational rehabilitation, education, and employment services to patients who desire and are ready to participate in job training programs or to gain employment; (2) the provision of prenatal care to pregnant patients; and (3) the provision of counseling on prevention and transmission of HIV disease. If services are not available on site, the MMP is required to make the appropriate referral for these services to community agencies. All MMP patients are assigned a primary counselor; although a counselor–patient ratio of 1:50 is recommended, this ratio is no longer mandated. During the first year of treatment, treatment plans should be developed and reviewed every 90 days, and eight random urine screens are required. Thus, an MMP that is functioning at the minimal level set by FDA regulations needs to medically supervise methadone dispensing, conduct random urine toxicology screens and periodic treatment plans, and provide referrals to community agencies for medical and psychosocial services. Interim methadone maintenance (Yancovitz et al., 1991), now available for patients for up to 120 days while they await comprehensive methadone treatment, requires even less intensive intervention; random urine screens are required, but no primary counselor assignment needs to be made and no treatment plans are required to be developed.

Case Management and Counseling

A study of six MMPs conducted by Ball and Ross (1991) found that the psychosocial services that are typically provided consist of methadone dispensing as well as urine monitoring, case management, and twice-monthly face-to-face individual counseling sessions focusing on program compliance and rehabilitation. Counselors in that study had an average caseload of 41 patients; and in addition to providing twice-monthly counseling, the counselors offered "as needed" brief contacts with patients and made referrals to community agencies. Less than 3% of patients received on-site family or vocational counseling, less than 6% attended educational classes, less than 10% received psychotherapy, and less than 25% received group therapy.

Is this level of intervention sufficient? The addition of counseling in and of itself may not suffice for all patients. Studies have shown that methadone patients who receive minimal counseling show no significant change in HIV-risk behaviors (Childress et al., 1991; Hartgers et al., 1992). Ball and Ross (1991) found that the rate of continued intravenous drug use varied considerably depending upon the program.

Programs with an effective director, with quality counseling services, and with an orientation toward maintenance and rehabilitation had the lowest rates of intravenous drug use. Psychosocial interventions that can be provided to methadone patients in addition to case management and counseling range from those interventions that require minimal staff involvement and formal training to those that require extensive time and expertise, as will be discussed below.

Behavioral Interventions

A number of behavioral treatment approaches have shown promise in MMPs. Perhaps the most widely used behavioral approaches to increase compliance with MMP treatment goals come under the umbrella of contingency management, which can be accomplished with minimal additional burden on existing staff. Positive contingency programs provide patients with rewards that are contingent upon drug abstinence; negative contingency programs are based on a withholding of rewards that is contingent upon drug use. The most systematically studied positive contingencies used in MMPs are the provision of take-home privileges and monetary rewards that are contingent upon the submission of negative urine screens (Iguchi et al., 1988; Magura et al., 1988; Milby et al., 1978; Stitzer & Bigelow, 1984; Stitzer et al., 1979, 1992). Voucher systems (Higgins et al., 1993), by which patients receive vouchers that can be exchanged for goods and services that are contingent upon documented abstinence, have also recently been introduced into some methadone programs. Negative contingencies that have been investigated include a reduction of the methadone dose and ultimate detoxification that is contingent upon the submission of positive urine screens (Dolan et al., 1985; McCarthy & Borders, 1985; Nolimal & Crowley, 1990; Saxon et al., 1993; Stitzer et al., 1986). An increase in the methadone dose that is contingent upon drug use has also been investigated (Kirby et al., 1991; Rhoades et al., 1990) and in one study has been shown to be more effective in reducing cocaine use than a reduction of the methadone dose (Stine et al., 1992).

Another behavioral intervention—cue exposure therapy—is based on a conditioning model of addiction that views conditioned cues in the drug user's environment as having an important role in sustaining drug-using behavior (Margolin & Avants, 1992). Support for this model is provided by research that has found that the majority of drug-dependent subjects who are exposed to drug cues in the laboratory respond with physiological reactivity and increased craving (Avants et al., 1993; Childress et al., 1988). An alternative explanatory model for cue reactivity posits that a response to cues is a function of self-efficacy and drug expectancies (Marlatt & Gordon, 1985). Some evidence for this social-learning perspective was provided by a study that compared cue responders and nonresponders (Avants et al., 1995). In that study, it was found that the nonresponders perceived their drug of choice as less positively and negatively reinforcing than the cue responders did and that the nonresponders reported greater self-efficacy in certain high-risk situations. Cue exposure interventions are being investigated in a number of treatment settings. Originally, these interventions consisted of the basic extinction paradigm wherein the patient is repeatedly exposed to the conditioned stimuli (e.g., drug paraphernalia) in the absence of an unconditioned response (e.g., effect of the drug) with the goal of extinguishing the conditioned craving and thus reducing drug use. However, extinction paradigms today now include teaching coping skills during cue exposure with the goal not only of extinguishing the conditioned response but also of increasing the patient's self-efficacy in the presence of cues (Childress et al., 1991).

Individual Psychotherapy

In view of the high rate of psychopathology (particularly depression, anxiety disorders, and antisocial personality disorder) in opiate users who enter MMPs (Rounsaville et al., 1982), individual psychotherapy has also been suggested as an adjunct to methadone maintenance (Woody et al., 1990). However, few MMPs actually provide psychotherapeutic services (Ball & Ross, 1991). The few studies that have investigated the efficacy of psychotherapy as an adjunct to methadone treatment have provided mixed results. Rounsaville and his colleagues (1983) compared counseling alone to counseling and interpersonal psychotherapy and found no significant differences in various psychological measures: both groups improved in several of these measures; however, neither group improved in measures of illicit drug use. In contrast, Woody and his colleagues (1983) compared counseling alone to counseling and supportive expressive therapy and to counseling and cognitive behavioral therapy and found that all patients improved but that those who received additional psychotherapy had better outcomes than those who received only counseling.

Group Psychotherapy

Surprisingly few MMPs provide group therapy on a regular basis, and little is known about the content of the therapy groups that are provided. One manual-guided group approach used in our own MMP is an adaptation of the coping skills training program developed for alcoholics by Monti and his colleagues (1989). Each group session begins with a 30-minute open-forum discussion and is followed by a 60-minute, structured, coping skills group that covers such topics as relapse prevention, vocational training, stress management, health issues, leisure activities, and problem solving. Each session ends by providing patients with a list of people who can give them, or of places where they can receive, additional information and services relating to the topic covered during a group session. Preliminary analysis of efficacy data suggests that this group approach shows promise for the reduction of illicit substance abuse during the first 3 months of methadone treatment. A combination of twice-weekly individual therapy and twice-weekly group therapy that uses a cognitive–behavioral approach is also reported as showing promise for reducing illicit substance abuse in methadone patients (Magura et al., 1992). For those patients who have achieved stability in treatment—and who might otherwise receive few, if any, additional services—a clinically guided self-help group approach has been recommended that focuses on fostering responsibility and on assisting the patient's reintegration into the drug-free community (Nurco et al., 1991).

HIGH-INTENSITY PSYCHOSOCIAL INTERVENTIONS

When ancillary psychosocial services are provided in sufficient intensity, and by qualified providers, those services may have a significant effect. Evidence for this effect is suggested by a study that investigated three intensities of ancillary psychosocial treatment for methadone-maintained patients (McLellan et al., 1993). Patients who were randomly assigned to receive the minimal services possible under FDA standards fared poorly as far as continued drug use and psychological functioning were concerned, with many patients having to transfer to more-intensive services prior to completion of the study. Patients who were randomly assigned to receive more frequent counseling in addition to their methadone had better outcomes. Patients in this condition received weekly counseling, during which they received help with various problems common to recovering patients. Patients who had access to more-intensive psychosocial services, such as on-site medical/psychiatric care, family therapy, and employment counseling, had the best outcomes. In the section that follows, we describe two high-intensity interventions: a day treatment program, which provides numerous services on site, and the community reinforcement approach, in which a significant other, rather than the program staff, plays a key role in the patient's recovery.

Intensive Day Treatment

Day treatment programs (DTPs) have shown promise for the treatment of alcohol and cocaine dependence in non-MMP settings (Alfs & McLellan, 1992; Alterman et al., 1992). When compared to an even higher-intensity treatment such as inpatient stay, DTPs have been shown to have comparable results, at lower cost, both for the treatment of alcoholism (McCrady et al., 1986) and for the treatment of cocaine dependence (Alterman, 1991).

The DTP provided at our own MMP, modeled on a DTP begun in 1990 at the West Haven Veterans Administration MMP, is based on the premise that the typical inner-city opiate addict who has newly entered an MMP has had little exposure to, or has derived few rewards from, a drug-free lifestyle, having been extensively socialized in the norms and precepts of the drug subculture. As a result, extensive resocialization is necessary at many levels if the patient is to achieve and maintain the MMP's goal of rehabilitation. Our DTP's approach to the goal of resocialization is to create a community in which patients—through interaction with staff, rehabilitated peers, and other patients, begin to internalize more constructive and adaptive norms and values (cf. Catalano & Hawkins, 1985; Platt & Metzger, 1987). Patients participate on two levels. At one level, patients attend instructional modules in which specific skills are taught. At another level, patients participate in meetings and activities designed to increase their sense of being active members of a functional community and are given first hand experience of the attendant responsibilities inherent in sustaining this relationship to other individuals. Upon entry into our MMP, all unemployed patients attend the DTP for 5 hours per day, for 5 days per week, for 12 weeks. Modules that compose the DTP were drawn from a number of sources and encompass diverse approaches to treatment but in general cover five basic areas: (1) physical and emotional health, (2) substance abuse treatment, (3) community development, (4) development of alternative reinforcers, and (5) basic daily living skills. A description of the modules in each of these five areas follows.

1. *Physical and emotional health.* The objective of the modules in this area is to promote physical and mental health through didactic and experiential groups. Modules include (a) three-times-weekly physical activity, (b) stress management and relaxation training, (c) a health and hygiene class taught by nursing staff, and (d) twice-weekly psychotherapy group.

2. *Substance abuse treatment.* The modules in this area focus specifically on abstinence from illicit drug use. Modules include (a) a relapse

prevention group in which patients are taught cognitive behavioral relapse prevention techniques (Carroll et al., 1991; Marlatt & Gordon, 1985), (b) a 12-step group (modified from Nowinski et al., 1992), (c) a Narcotics Anonymous group, and (d) a "concern status" group attended by patients identified by the community as having difficulty following community rules for abstinence and attendance.

3. *Community development.* The objective of the modules in this area is to encourage a sense of community on several levels. Modules in this area include (a) a peer group in which patients, without staff in attendance, interact with "peer guides" (other MMP patients who have been in the program longer, have done well in treatment, and act as positive role models), (b) a community meeting in which all staff members and patients are in attendance to discuss issues of concern to the entire DTP community, (c) a current events group in which patients discuss how local events reported in the newspaper affect them, their families, and the community, and (d) a community speakers group in which members of the larger community describe and provide referrals to community resources.

4. *Development of alternative reinforcers.* The objective of the modules in this area is to provide patients with the opportunity to identify non-drug-related positive reinforcers (cf. Vuchinich & Tucker, 1988) by exposing patients to various leisure time activities, hobbies, and modes of artistic expression within an interactive non-drug-using context. The modules include (a) a leisure group in which patients discuss and participate in non-drug-related pleasurable activities, (b) an art therapy group in which patients express themselves through sketching and painting, (c) a music group in which patients learn to listen to music in a non-drug-related atmosphere, and (d) a focus games group in which patients are taught and practice games of skills.

5. *Basic daily living skills.* The objective of this general area is to prepare the patient for daily living by providing the following modules: (a) a prevocational training group in which job-seeking skills are taught and referrals are provided for on-site vocational training, GED classes, and counseling regarding continued education; (b) a money management group that teaches the basics of budgets, banking, and saving while also addressing the issue of money as a drug cue; and (c) an educational film group that shows videos depicting various aspects of functioning productively within one's family, community, and society.

THE COMMUNITY REINFORCEMENT APPROACH

The community reinforcement approach (CRA) was developed in 1973 for the treatment of alcoholism. Several studies have suggested that CRA may be more effective that traditional therapies for the treatment of alcoholism (Sisson & Azrin, 1989). CRA was recently adapted for the treatment of cocaine dependence at the University of Vermont by Higgins and his colleagues (Higgins et al., 1993, 1994a, 1994b) who have tested it with reported success, and more recently CRA has been suggested for the treatment of illicit substance use in opioid-dependent patients who are being maintained on buprenorphine (Schottenfeld, personal communication).

The basic components of CRA are as follows: (1) pharmacotherapy that targets the substance of abuse (e.g., Antabuse or, potentially, buprenorphine or methadone), (2) vocational training that specifically targets the acquisition of employment that promotes abstinence, (3) reciprocity marriage counseling that teaches the patient and his or her partner more positive communication skills, (4) social skills training that emphasizes problem solving and drug refusal skills and that encourages active involvement in recreational and leisure activities, (5) relapse prevention counseling that identifies antecedents and consequences of drug/alcohol use, and (6) a contingency management system as adapted by Higgins et al. (1994b), involving both the patient and the patient's significant other, in which abstinence is reinforced with pleasant activities and with vouchers for the purchase of goods and services (the program is 6 months in duration).

Similar to the DTP described previously, CRA is based on the premise that the relative value of drug use decreases as the psychosocial environment becomes more positively reinforcing; thus, the focus of both treatments is to help the patient develop a social support network and social environment that is supportive of abstinence. Although there are similarities between the DTP described earlier and CRA, there are several important differences. The primary difference is the active involvement of a non-substance-using significant other in CRA programs. When a patient enters a CRA program, he or she selects a significant other who will be responsible for monitoring the patient's progress in treatment. This person is a spouse, family member, friend, or lover who is willing to play an active role in the therapy. The significant other is informed of the results of urine screens and implements the behavioral contingencies. The involvement of a significant other in treatment has been found to be a robust predictor of abstinence initiation and maintenance (Higgins et al., 1994b; Sisson & Azrin, 1989).

The involvement of a significant other and the focus on off-site sources of reinforcement in CRA programs points to a basic difference in the philosophy of the two approaches. A premise underlying our own DTP is that our inner-city patients have little access to the benefits of a drug-free lifestyle and have few non-drug-using friends or family members to support their abstinence. Therefore, if resocialization is to occur, on-site access must be provided by staff and rehabilitated peers in an intensive daily program. In contrast, CRA assumes that an off-site drug-free lifestyle is available to the patient and that such a lifestyle can be accessed with the help of the significant other, with guidance from the MMP counselor. The feasibility of implementing CRA with unemployed inner-city methadone patients who are just entering treatment, of course, remains to be tested. However, one promising approach is to integrate the two programs such that an intensive day hospital is provided for unemployed patients during the first 3 months of methadone treatment, followed by CRA during the subsequent 6 months. As patients stabilize and are reintegrated into a non-drug-using lifestyle, they could then begin to participate in less intensive aftercare programs (Nurco et al., 1991; Weddington, 1990).

WHICH LEVEL OF PSYCHOSOCIAL TREATMENT FOR WHICH METHADONE PATIENT?

Given the findings in the addiction — and, more generally, in the psychotherapy — literature that a wide range of patient characteristics may affect treatment outcome and that no single treatment is optimal for all patients (Marlatt, 1988; Tims & Holland, 1984), there has been a movement in substance abuse treatment outcome research toward identifying patient characteristics that may ultimately help match patients with the optimal treatment (Carroll & Rounsaville, 1993; Woody & O'Brien, 1991). However, to date, only a few studies have focused on matching MMP patients to treatments. McLellan and his colleagues (1983) investigated hypothesized matching and mismatching of drug- and alcohol-dependent patients to different treatment modalities (including methadone maintenance) on the basis of psychiatric severity, employment, substance abuse severity, family relations, and legal status and found that patients matched to treatment had better outcomes than mismatched patients had immediately after treatment and at a 6-month follow-up. Another study (Woody et al., 1990) provided three different treatments (counseling, counseling and supportive expressive therapy, and counseling and cognitive behavioral therapy) to methadone-maintained patients and found that the addition of psychotherapy was particularly helpful for patients who had the highest level of psychiatric impairment, as well as for patients with a diagnosis of antisocial personality disorder, if they were also depressed. A third study (Mclellan et al., 1984) found that patients with high levels of psychiatric disturbance benefited more from MMP treatment compared to a therapeutic community treatment, perhaps because the confrontational nature of encounter group therapy practiced in the therapeutic community was a cause of distress for patients who were more psychiatrically impaired.

In an attempt to further examine patient–treatment matching in methadone-maintained patients, our clinical research team at Yale is conducting a study investigating the differential efficacy of two intensities of psychosocial interventions at two sites: a small Veterans Administration site and a large community-based inner-city site. The low-intensity intervention is the 90-minute, manual-guided, weekly, group intervention, described earlier in this chapter, that provides skills training and ongoing referrals to additional services (Avants, 1993). The high-intensity group is the day treatment program described in the previous section on high-intensity treatments. The goals of the study are fourfold: (1) to determine whether an intensive day hospital modeled on a Veterans Administration program will generalize to a community-based inner-city MMP, (2) to determine whether it is possible to identify subgroups of MMP patients that differentially benefit from the two intensities of treatment, and (3) to determine which intensity of treatment is most cost effective and cost beneficial overall and for each subgroup.

Studies that expressly adopt a matching perspective go beyond an examination of the "main effects" of treatment and emphasize the interaction of patient characteristics with type of treatment. In order to investigate which treatment intervention is most efficacious for different subpopulations of MMP patients, several patient–treatment matching strategies may have to be considered. Our strategy was to specify five putative matching variables, to balance the groups on these variables, using urn randomization (Wei, 1978), and to conduct retrospective analyses to determine patient–treatment interactions. A higher level of specificity would be to formulate a priori predictions about which patient subtypes would benefit from which treatment. At this time, there is a paucity of data in the literature to guide formulation of such predictions. There is also little data to construct an even higher level of research design specificity—an assignment of patients on a priori grounds to either matched or mismatched conditions. At this stage in our knowledge, such an approach weakens our ability to identify patient characteristics that may interact with treatment outcome because only a small number of matching characteristics could be chosen as a basis for assignment into matched or mismatched conditions. The patient characteristics selected as matching variables for our ongoing study are race, sex, antisocial personality disorder, depression, and cocaine dependence.

HOW MUCH WILL IT COST,
AND CAN WE AS A SOCIETY AFFORD IT?

Studies investigating the cost-effectiveness of MMPs have provided mixed results (Anglin et al., 1989; Hubbard et al., 1989; McGlothlin & Anglin, 1981) and have not attempted to determine the cost effectiveness of the psychosocial interventions provided by the MMP. Cost effectiveness analysis, of course, does not attempt to evaluate all of the benefits of a program but simply determines which program produces a single desired outcome at the lowest cost. Although cost effectiveness analyses are often used to direct government funding, they may not be wholly appropriate in the evaluation of an MMP that can—and perhaps should—be measured, not by a single outcome, but by numerous desired outcomes, such as the reduced spread of HIV, increased employment, improved psychiatric status, and reduced crime (Sindelar, 1993).

Another approach for evaluating MMPs is the use of cost–benefit analysis (Sindelar & Manning, 1994), which, in its simplest interpretation, is an analytic method designed to consider and quantify, where possible and appropriate, all of the costs and benefits, not just one desirable outcome, associated with a specific program. There is a small but growing literature on the extent to which the costs of MMPs are offset by gains to society in the form of social costs averted (e.g., reduced crime or slower spread of HIV). Two cost–benefit simulations (Maidlow & Berman, 1972; Rufener et al., 1977) have suggested that MMPs are beneficial (cf. Apsler & Harding, 1991). However, little is known about whether one type of psychosocial intervention provided by an MMP is more beneficial than another—and if so, for whom. Different intensities of psychosocial interventions in MMPs may produce different amounts of averted social cost. More-intensive psychosocial interventions provided by qualified staff may cost more per patient but could produce a higher level of averted social costs and lower levels of recidivism. Moreover, certain patients may need less-intensive treatment to produce the same level of averted social costs, thus saving scarce resources for individuals who require more-intensive care.

The economists working on the ongoing study plan to conduct a comprehensive cost–benefit analysis in addition to cost effectiveness analyses (see Sindelar, 1993 for a complete description of the procedures to be employed). The cost effectiveness analyses will provide specific data, for example, on the cost of a single outcome (e.g., the cost of a drug-free day) for each intensity of psychosocial intervention and for each patient subgroup. Cost–benefit tables will then be constructed (Weisbrod et al., 1980) using recommended methods for quantifying costs and benefits (e.g., Anglin et al., 1989; Ball et al., 1981; Hunt et al., 1986; McGlothlin & Anglin, 1981). Dollar values will be placed on costs and benefits, where appropriate, using extant literature to guide in the valuing of the more complex outcomes. In addition, since many of the potential benefits are nonpecuniary (e.g., reduced spread of HIV, better family functioning, reduced crime, increased self-esteem, better parenting), some benefits will need to be quantified without assigning a dollar value.

The goal of these analyses is to aid in our understanding of whether and to what extent the costs of the different intensities of MMP psychosocial services are offset by averted costs to society. For example, it has been reported (Kreek, 1992) that drug-free residential community programs ranged in cost from $12,000 to $30,000 per year, and a private or institution-based drug-free program ranged from $400 to over $1,000 per day. Furthermore, cost to society in crimes committed by addicts in their attempt to procure drugs was estimated to be from $50,000 to $200,000 per addict per year, and the cost of incarcerating an addict for crimes committed ranged from $25,000 to $80,000 per year. The cost to manage an AIDS patient ranged from $50,000 to $200,000. Kreek (1992) compared these costs to the $1,800–$2,500 per capita annual funding for an average methadone patient. It remains an open question whether, and to what extent, any increase in cost necessitated by the provision of more-intensive psychosocial services in MMPs would be offset by increased earnings of patients, less crime committed against individuals, and fewer legal, medical, and social costs to society.

CONCLUSIONS

Until research results are available that could guide MMPs in matching patients to the appropriate and most effective and beneficial intensity of ancillary psychosocial treatment as far as the cost of that treatment is concerned, one commonsense approach with the potential to make the best use of scarce resources is an elaboration of the original three-phase model of methadone maintenance. This "revisited" model would provide intensive psychosocial services early in treatment to those patients who clearly lack the psychosocial skills and resources necessary for successful rehabilitation (e.g., the unemployed, psychiatrically impaired, medically compromised, polysubstance abuser, as well as patients who lack abstinent social support). Unlike Phase I of the original model, however, which provided these services on an inpatient basis, services would be provided on an outpatient basis, preferably onsite, but perhaps by necessity through referrals to outside agencies. It is therefore essential that at this phase resources be allocated to conduct follow-ups to ensure that services are received as recommended. Once some degree of stabilization is attained (e.g., after 6–12 weeks), less-intensive interventions (e.g., counseling, contingency management, group therapy, and family involvement through CRA) can be provided, based on the individual patient's needs and the resources of the MMP. In Phase III, when, in the words of Dole and Nyswander (1965), the patient becomes "a socially normal, self-supporting person," there could be aftercare programs, such as those recommended by Nurco and his colleagues (1991) and Weddington 1990), that require little staff involvement and that encourage patient self-reliance.

ACKNOWLEDGMENTS

Portions of this chapter have been published previously in Avants et al. (1994a). Copyright 1994 by Haight Ashbury Publications. Reprinted by permission. Research supported by the National Institute on Drug Abuse (Grant Nos. R01-DA08754 [SKA] and K21-DA00277 [SKA]).

REFERENCES

Alfs, D. S., & McLellan, T. A. (1992). A day hospital program for dual diagnosis patients in a VA medical center. *Hospital and Community Psychiatry, 43,* 241–244.

Alterman, A. I. (1991). Day hospital versus inpatient cocaine dependence rehabilitation: An interim report. In L. S. Harris (Ed.), *Problems of drug dependence* (NIDA Research Monograph No. 105, pp. 363–364). Rockville, MD: National Institute on Drug Abuse.

Alterman, A. I., Droba, M., & McLellan, A. T. (1992). Response to day hospital treatment by patients with cocaine and alcohol dependence. *Hospital and Community Psychiatry, 43,* 930–932.

Anglin, M. D., Speckart, G. R., Booth, M. W., & Ryan, T. M. (1989). Consequences and costs of shutting off methadone. *Addictive Behaviors, 14,* 307–326.

Apsler, R., & Harding, W. M. (1991). Cost-effectiveness analysis of drug abuse treatment: Current status and recommendations for future research. In L. S. Harris (Ed.), *Problems of drug dependence* (NIDA Drug Abuse Services Research Monograph No. 1, pp. 58–81). Rockville, MD: National Institute on Drug Abuse.

Avants, S. K. (1993). *Project Methadone Match weekly group treatment manual: Ancillary psychosocial group therapy for methadone-maintained patients.* Unpublished treatment manual.

Avants, S. K., Margolin, A., & Kosten, T. R. (1994a). Cocaine abuse in methadone maintenance programs: Integrating pharmacotherapy with psychosocial interventions. *Journal of Psychoactive Drugs, 26,* 137–146.

Avants, S. K., Margolin, A., Kosten, T. R., & Cooney, N. L. (1995). Differences
between responders and non-responders to cocaine cues in the laboratory. *Addictive Behaviors, 20,* 215–224.

Avants, S. K., Margolin, A., Kosten, T. R., & Singer, J. L. (1993). Changes concurrent with initiation of abstinence from cocaine abuse. *Journal of Substance Abuse Treatment, 10,* 577–583.

Avants, S. K., Ohlin, R., Floyd, K. R., & Badger, E. (1994b). *Project Methadone
Match day treatment program manual: Intensive psychosocial intervention for
methadone-maintained patients.* Unpublished treatment manual.

Ball, C. J., Rosen, L., Flueck, J. A., & Nurco, D. (1981). The criminality of heroin
addicts when addicted and when off opiates. In J. A. Inciardi (Ed.), *The
drug–crime connection* (pp. 39–65). Beverly Hills, CA: Sage.

Ball, C. J., & Ross, A. (1991). *The effectiveness of methadone maintenance treatment.*
New York: Springer-Verlag.

Ball, C. J., Shaffer, J. W., & Nurco, D. N. (1983). The day-to-day criminal activity
of heroin addicts in Baltimore: A study in the continuity of offense rates.
Drug and Alcohol Dependence, 12, 119–142.

Carroll, K. M., & Rounsaville, B. J. (1993). Implications of recent research on
psychotherapy for drug abuse. In G. Edwards, J. Strang, & J. H. Jaffe (Eds.),
Drugs, alcohol, and tobacco: Making the science and policy connections (pp. 211–221).
Oxford: Oxford University Press.

Carroll, K. M., Rounsaville, B. J., & Keller, D. S. (1991). Relapse prevention strategies for the treatment of cocaine abuse. *American Journal of Drug and Alcohol Abuse, 17,* 249–265.

Catalano, R. F., & Hawkins, J. D. (1985). Project skills: Preliminary results from
a theoretically based aftercare experiment. In R. S. Ashery (Ed.), *Progress
in the development of cost effective treatment for drug abuse* (NIDA Research Monograph No. 58, pp. 157–181). Rockville, MD: National Institute on Drug
Abuse.

Chambers, C. D., Taylor, W. J. R., & Moffett, A. D. (1972). The incidence of
cocaine abuse among methadone maintenance patients. *International Journal of the Addictions, 7,* 427–441.

Childress, A. R., Hole, A. V., & DePhilippis, D. (1991). *The Coping with Craving
Program.* Philadelphia: Addiction Research Center, University of Pennsyl-
vania School of Medicine, and Philadelphia Veterans Administration Medical Center.

Childress, A. R., McLellan, A. T., Ehrman, R., & O'Brien, C. P. (1988). Classical
conditioned responses in opioid and cocaine dependence: A role in
relapse? In B. A. Ray (Ed.), *Learning factors in substance abuse* (NIDA Research
Monograph No. 84, pp. 25–43). Washington, DC: U.S. Government Printing Office.

Childress, A. R., McLellan, A. T., Woody, G. E., & O'Brien, C. P. (1991). *Are there
minimum conditions necessary for methadone maintenance to reduce intravenous
drug use and AIDS risk behaviors?* In L. S.. Harris (Ed.), *Problems of drug depen-*

dence (NIDA Research Monographs No. 106, pp. 167–177). Rockville, MD: National Institute on Drug Abuse.

Condelli, W. S., Fairbank, J. A., Dennis, M. L., & Rachal, J. V. (1992). Cocaine use by clients in methadone programs: Significance, scope, and behavioral interventions. *Journal of Substance Abuse Treatment, 8,* 203–212.

Des Jarlais, D. C., Friedman, S. R., & Casriel, C. (1990). Target groups for preventing AIDS among intravenous drug users: The "hard" data studies. *Journal of Consulting and Clinical Psychology, 58,* 50–56.

Dolan, M. P., Black, J. L., Penk, W. E., Robinowitz, R., & DeFord, H. A. (1985). Contracting for treatment termination to reduce illicit drug use among methadone maintenance treatment failures. *Journal of Consulting and Clinical Psychology, 53,* 549–551.

Dole, V. P., & Nyswander, M. E. (1965). A medical treatment for diacetylmorphine (heroin) addiction: Treatment with methadone hydrochloride. *Journal of the American Medical Association, 193,* 645–650.

Federal Register (1994). *Food and Drug Administration, regulations on drug used for the treatment of narcotic addicts* (21 CFR ch. 1, pp. 123–145). Washington, DC: U.S. Government Printing Office.

Gill, K., Nolimal, D., & Crowley, T. J. (1992). Antisocial personality disorder, HIV risk behavior and retention in methadone maintenance therapy. *International Journal of the Addictions, 26*(1), 1–22.

Hartgers, C., Van-den-Hoek, A., Krijnen, P., & Coutinho, R. A. (1992). HIV prevalence and risk behavior among injecting drug users who participate in "low-threshold" methadone programs in Amsterdam. *American Journal of Public Health, 82,* 547–551.

Higgins, S. T., Budney, A. J., & Bickel, W. K. (1994a). Applying behavioral concepts and principles to the treatment of cocaine dependence. *Drug and Alcohol Dependence, 34,* 87–97.

Higgins, S. T., Budney, A. J., Bickel, W. K., Foerg, F. E., Donham, R., & Badger, G. J. (1994b). Incentives improve outcome in outpatient behavioral treatment of cocaine dependence. *Archives of General Psychiatry, 51,* 568–575.

Higgins, S. T., Budney, A. J., Bickel, W. K., Hughes, J. R., Foerg, B. A., & Badger, G. J. (1993). Achieving cocaine abstinence with a behavioral approach. *American Journal of Psychiatry, 150*(5), 763–769.

Hubbard, R. L., Marsden, M. E., Rachal, J. V., Harwood, H. J., Cavanaugh, E. R., & Ginzburg, H. M. (1989). *Drug abuse treatment: A national study of effectiveness.* Chapel Hill: University of North Carolina Press.

Hunt, D., Spunt, B., Lipton, D., Goldsmith, D., & Strug, D. (1986). The costly bonus: Cocaine related crime among methadone treatment clients. *Advances in Alcohol and Substance Abuse, 6*(2), 107–122.

Iguchi, M. Y., Stitzer, M. L., Bigelow, G. E., & Liebson, I. A. (1988). Contingency management in methadone maintenance: Effects of reinforcing and aversive consequences on illicit polydrug use. *Drug and Alcohol Dependence, 22,* 1–7.

Joe, G. W., Simpson, D. D., & Hubbard, R. L. (1991a). Treatment predictors of tenure in methadone maintenance. *Journal of Substance Abuse, 3,* 73–84.

Joe, G. W., Simpson, D. D., & Hubbard, R. L. (1991b). Unmet serviced needs in methadone maintenance. *International Journal of the Addictions, 26*(1), 1–22.

Kirby, K. C., Stitzer, M. L., & Brockish, M. (1991). Contingency management aftercare for polydrug abuse in methadone maintenance patients. In L. S. Harris (Ed.), *Problems of drug dependence* (NIDA Research Monograph No. 119, p. 474). Rockville, MD: National Institute on Drug Abuse.

Kosten, T. R., Gawin, F. H., Rounsaville, B. J., & Kleber, H. D. (1986). Cocaine abuse among opioid addicts: Demographic and diagnostic factors in treatment. *American Journal of Drug and Alcohol Abuse, 12,* 1–16.

Kosten, T. R., & Rounsaville, B. J. (1986). Psychopathology in opioid addicts. *Psychiatric Clinics of North America, 9,* 515–532.

Kosten, T. R., Rounsaville, B. J., & Kleber, H. D. (1986). A 2.5 year follow-up of depression, life crises, and treatment effects on abstinence among opioid addicts. *Archives of General Psychiatry, 43,* 733–738.

Kosten, T. R., Rounsaville, B. J., & Kleber, H. D. (1987). A 2.5 year follow-up of cocaine use among treated opioid addicts. *Archives of General Psychiatry, 44,* 281–284.

Kosten, T. R., Rounsaville, B. J., & Kleber, H. D. (1988). Antecedents and consequences of cocaine abuse among opioid addicts: A 2.5 year follow-up. *Journal of Nervous and Mental Disease, 176,* 176–181.

Kreek, M. J. (1992). The addict as a patient. In J. H. Lowinson, P. Ruiz, R. B. Millman, & J. G. Langrod (Eds.), *Substance abuse: A comprehensive textbook* (pp. 997–1009). Baltimore: Williams & Wilkins.

Leal, J., Ziedonis, D., & Kosten, T. R. (1994). Antisocial personality disorder as a prognostic factor for pharmacotherapy of cocaine dependence. *Drug and Alcohol Dependence, 35,* 31–35.

Lewis, D. K., & Watters, J. K. (1991). Sexual risk behavior among heterosexual intravenous drug users: Ethnic and gender variations. *AIDS, 5,* 77–83.

Lowinson, J. H., Marion, I. J., Joseph, H., & Dole, V. P. (1992). Methadone Maintenance. In J. H. Lowinson, P. Ruiz, R. B. Millman & J. G. Langrod (Eds.), *Substance abuse. A comprehensive textbook* (pp. 550–561), Baltimore: Williams & Wilkins.

Magura, S., Casriel, C., Goldsmith, D. S., Strug, D. L., & Lipton, D. S. (1988). Contingency contracting with polydrug-abusing methadone patients. *Addictive Behavior, 13,* 113–118.

Magura, S., Rosenblum, A., Lovejoy, M., Handelsman, L., Foote, J. & Stimmel, B. (1992). Cocaine-using methadone patients show declines in cocaine use and dysphoria during cognitive-behavioral treatment. In L. S. Harris (Ed.), *Problems of drugy dependence* (NIDA Research Monograph No. 132, p. 316). Rockville, MD: National Institute on Drug Abuse.

Maidlow, S. T., & Berman, H. (1972). The economics of heroin treatment. *American Journal of Public Health, 62,* 1397–1406.

Margolin, A., & Avants, S. K. (1992). Cue reactivity and cocaine addiction. In T. R. Kosten & H. D. Kleber (Eds.), *Clinician's guide to cocaine addiction* (pp. 109–127). New York: Guilford Press.

Marlatt, G. A. (1988). Matching clients to treatment: Treatment models and stages of change. In D. M. Donovan & G. A. Marlatt (Eds.), *Assessment of addictive behaviors* (pp. 474–483). New York: Guilford Press.

Marlatt, G. A., & Gordon, J. R. (Eds.). (1985). *Relapse prevention: Maintenance strategies in the treatment of addictive behaviors.* New York: Guilford Press.

McCarthy, J. J., & Borders, O. T. (1985). Limit setting on drug abuse in methadone maintenance patients. *American Journal of Psychiatry, 142,* 1419–1423.

McCrady, B., Longabaugh, R., Fink, E., Stout, R., Beattie, M., & Ruggieri-Authelet, A. (1986). Cost effectiveness of alcoholism treatment in partial hospital versus inpatient settings after brief inpatient treatment: 12-month outcomes. *Journal of Consulting and Clinical Psychology, 54,* 708–713.

McGlothlin, W. H., & Anglin, M. D. (1981). Shutting off methadone: Costs and benefits. *Archives of General Psychiatry, 38,* 885–892.

McLellan, A. T., Arndt, I. O., Metzger, D. S., Woody, G. E., & O'Brien, C. P. (1993). The effects of psychosocial services in substance abuse treatment. *Journal of the American Medical Association, 269,* 1953–1959.

McLellan, A. T., Childress, A. R., Griffith, J., & Woody, G. E. (1984). The psychiatrically severe drug abuse patient: Methadone maintenance or therapeutic community. *American Journal of Drug and Alcohol Abuse, 10*(1), 77–95.

McLellan, A. T., Woody, G. E., Luborsky, L., O'Brien, C. P., & Druley, K. A. (1983). Increased effectiveness of substance abuse treatment: A prospective study of patient–treatment "matching." *Journal of Nervous and Mental Disease, 171,* 597–605.

Meandzija, B., Pakes, J., O'Connor, P., Fitzgerald, B., Rounsaville, B., & Kosten, T.R. (1995). HIV status, demographics, and substance use in a methadone maintenance program. In L. S. Harris (Ed.), *Problems of drug dependence* (NIDA Research Monographs No. 153, p. 63). Rockville, MD: National Institute on Drug Abuse.

Metzger, D., Woody, G., DePhilippis, D., McLellan, A. T., O'Brien, C. P., & Platt, J. J. (1991). Risk factors for needle sharing among methadone treated patients. *American Journal of Psychiatry, 148,* 636–640.

Meyer, R. F. (1992). New pharmacotherapies for cocaine dependence . . . revisited. *Archives of General Psychiatry, 49,* 900–904.

Milby, J. B., Garrett, C., English, C., Fritschi, O., & Clarke, C. (1978). Take-home methadone: Contingency effects on drug-seeking and productivity of narcotic addicts. *Addictive Behaviors, 3,* 215–220.

Monti, P. M., Abrams, D. B., Kadden, R. M., & Cooney, N. L. (1989). *Treating alcohol dependence.* New York: The Guilford Press.

Nolimal, D., & Crowley, T. J. (1990). Difficulties in a clinical application of methadone-dose contingency contracting. *Journal of Substance Abuse Treatment, 7,* 219–224.

Novick, D. M., Kreek, M. J., & Des Jarlais, D. C. (1986). Abstract of clinical research findings: Therapeutic and historical aspects. In L. S. Harris (Ed.), *Problems of drug dependence, 1985* (NIDA Research Monograph No. 67, pp. 318–30). Washington, DC: U.S. Government Printing Office.

Nowinski, J., Baker, S., & Carroll, K. M. (1992). *Twelve-step facilitation therapy manual: A clinical research guide for therapists treating individuals with alcohol abuse and dependence* (NIAAA Project MATCH Monograph No. 1, DHHS Publication No. ADM 92-1893). Rockville, MD: National Institute on Alcohol Abuse and Alcoholism.

Nurco, D. N., Stephenson, P. E., & Hanlon, T. E. (1991). Aftercare/relapse prevention and the self-help movement. *International Journal of the Addictions, 25,* 1179–1200.

Platt, J. J., & Metzger, D. S. (1987). Cognitive interpersonal problem-solving skills and the maintenance of treatment success in heroin addicts. *Psychology of Addictive Behaviors, 1,* 5-13.

Rhoades, H., Ronith, E., Kirby, K., et al. (1990). Joint action of methadone dose and take home dose frequency in treatment compliance. In L. S. Harris (Ed.), *Problems of drug dependence* (NIDA Research Monograph No. 160, p. 453). Rockville, MD: National Institute on Drug Abuse.

Rounsaville, B. J., Glazer, W., Wilber, C. H., Weissman, M. M., & Kleber, H. D. (1983). Short-term interpersonal psychotherapy in methadone-maintained opiate addicts. *Archives of General Psychiatry, 40,* 629-636.

Rounsaville, B. J., Weissman, M. M., Crits-Christoph, K., Wilber, C., & Kleber, H. (1982). Diagnosis and symptoms of depression in opiate addicts: Course and relationship to treatment outcome. *Archives of General Psychiatry 39,* 151-156.

Rufener, B. L., Rachal, J. V., & Cruze, A. M. (1977). *Management effectiveness measures for NIDA drug abuse treatment programs: Vol. 1. Cost benefit analysis* (DHEW Publication No. ADM 77-423). Rockville, MD: National Institute on Drug Abuse.

Saxon, A. J., Calsyn, D. A., Kivlahan, D. R., & Roszell, D. K. (1993). Outcome of contingency contracting for illicit drug use in a methadone maintenance program. *Drug and Alcohol Dependence, 31,* 205-214.

Senay, E. C. (1985). Methadone maintenance treatment. *International Journal of the Addictions, 20,* 803-821.

Sindelar, J. L. (1993). *A blueprint for cost–benefit analyses of methadone maintenance programs.* Unpublished manuscript.

Sindelar, J. L., & Manning, W. G. (1994, July). *Cost–benefit and cost-effectiveness analysis: Issues in the evaluation of the treatment of illicit drug abuse.* Paper presented at a Milbank Memorial Fund and National Institute on Drug Abuse jointly sponsored conference, Arlington, VA.

Sisson, R. W., & Azrin, N. H. (1989). The community reinforcement approach. In R. K. Hester & W. R. Miller (Eds.), *Handbook of alcoholism treatment approaches: Effective alternatives* (pp. 242-258). New York: Pergamon Press.

Stine, S. M., Freeman, M., Burns, B., Charney, D. S., & Kosten, T. R. (1992). Effect of methadone dose on cocaine abuse in a methadone program. *American Journal of the Addictions, 1*(4), 294-303.

Stitzer, M. L., & Bigelow, G. E. (1984). Contingent methadone take-home privileges: Effects on compliance with fee payment schedules. *Drug and Alcohol Dependence, 13,* 395-399.

Stitzer, M. L., Bickel, W. K., Bigelow, G. E., & Liebson, I. A. (1986). Effects of methadone dose contingencies on urinalysis test results of poly-abusing methadone-maintenance patients. *Drug and Alcohol Dependence, 18,* 341-348.

Stitzer, M. L., Bigelow, G., & Liebson, I. (1979). Reducing drug use among methadone maintenance clients: Contingent reinforcement for morphine-free urines. *Addictive Behaviors, 5,* 333-340.

Stitzer, M. L., Iguchi, M. Y., & Felch, L. J. (1992). Contingent take-home incentive: Effects on drug use of methadone maintenance patients. *Journal of Consulting and Clinical Psychology, 60,* 927-934.

Strug, D. L., Hunt, D. E., Goldsmith, D. S., Lipton, D. S., & Spunt, B. (1985).

Patterns of cocaine use among methadone clients. *International Journal of the Addictions, 20,* 1163–1175.

Tims, F. M., & Holland, S. (1984). A treatment evaluation agenda: Discussion and recommendations. In L. S. Harris (Ed.), *Problems of drug dependence* (NIDA Research Monograph No. 51, pp. 167–174). Rockville, MD: National Institute on Drug Abuse.

Umbricht-Schneiter, A., Ginn, D. H., Pabst, K. M., & Bigelow, G. E. (1992). Providing medical care to methadone clinic patients: A controlled study of referral versus on-site care. In L. S. Harris (Ed.), *Problems of drug dependence* (NIDA Research Monograph No. 132, p. 305). Rockville, MD: National Institute on Drug Abuse.

Vuchinich, R. E., & Tucker, J. A. (1988). Contributions from behavioral theories of choice to an analysis of alcohol abuse. *Journal of Abnormal Psychology, 97*(2), 181–195.

Weddington, W. W. (1990). Towards a rehabilitation of methadone maintenance: Integration of relapse prevention and aftercare. *International Journal of the Addictions, 25,* 1201–1224.

Wei, L. J. (1978). An application of an urn model to the design of sequential controlled clinical trials. *Journal of the American Statistical Association, 73,* 559–563.

Weisbrod, B. A., Test, M. A., & Stein, L. I. (1980). Alternatives to mental hospital treatment: Economic cost–benefit analysis. *Archives of General Psychiatry, 37,* 400–405.

Woody, G. E., Mclellan, A. T., Luborsky, L., & O'Brien, C. P. (1985). Sociopathy and psychotherapy outcome. *Archives of General Psychiatry, 42,* 1081–1086.

Woody, G. E., McLellan, A. T., Luborsky, L., & O'Brien, C. P. (1990). Psychotherapy and counseling for methadone-maintained opiate addicts: Results of research studies. In L. S. Harris (Ed.), *Problems of drug dependence* (NIDA Research Monograph No. 104, pp. 9–23). Rockville, MD: National Institute on Drug Abuse.

Woody, G. E., Luborsky, L., McLellan, A. T., O'Brien, C. P., Beck, A. T., Blaine, J., Herman, I., & Hole, A. (1983). Psychotherapy for opiate addicts: Does it help? *Archives of General Psychiatry, 40,* 639–645.

Woody, G. E., & O'Brien, C. P. (1991). Update on methadone maintenance. In N. S. Miller (Ed.), *Comprehensive handbook of drug and alcohol addiction* (pp. 1113–1125). New York: Marcel Dekker.

Yancovitz, S. R., Des Jarlais, D. C., Peskoe Peyser, N., Drew, E., Friedmann, P., Trigg, H., & Robinson, J. W. (1991). A randomized trial of an interim methadone maintenance clinic. *American Journal of Public Health, 81,* 1185–1191.

Chapter 9

ACUPUNCTURE FOR COCAINE ABUSE: RESEARCH FINDINGS, METHODOLOGICAL ISSUES, AND PATIENT–TREATMENT MATCHING

Arthur Margolin, Ph.D.
S. Kelly Avants, Ph.D.

Acupuncture—the insertion of needles in specific points in the body—has been used in China for at least 2,000 years for treating a variety of disorders. The use of acupuncture for the treatment of drug addiction was discovered serendipitously in 1972 by Wen, a Hong Kong neurosurgeon, while conducting a series of studies on the analgesic properties of acupuncture. Heroin addicts who volunteered to be subjects reported that their opiate withdrawal symptoms were lessened on the days when they received the acupuncture treatments. Wen undertook a series of uncontrolled studies on the use of acupuncture for the treatment of opiate addiction and reported good results (Wen & Cheung, 1973; Wen, 1979). Over the past 20 years, numerous studies have been undertaken to investigate the use of acupuncture for treatment of addictions, including opiates (e.g., Clark, 1990), tobacco (e.g., Clavel & Benhamou, 1985; Low, 1977), and alcohol (e.g., Bullock et al., 1989) (for literature reviews. see Brewington et al., 1994; Vincent & Richardson, 1987; Whitehead, 1978). Some of these studies, particularly for alcohol and opiate dependence, have reported a beneficial effect of acupuncture.

The mechanism by which acupuncture constitutes a treatment for addiction is essentially unknown. Knowledge regarding mechanisms underlying acupuncture's effects has resulted almost exclusively from investigations on acupuncture-induced analgesia, which has been hypothesized to be linked to the release of endogenous opioids (for a review see Pomeranz, 1991). Evidence for this hypothesis stems from studies suggesting that acupuncture's analgesic effects are blocked by naloxone (e.g., Mayer et al., 1977) and that acupuncture analgesia is enhanced by enzyme blockers that protect endogenous peptides from degradation (Cheng & Pomeranz, 1980). Cross-tolerance between acupuncture analgesia and morphine has also been reported (Han et al., 1981). (Cross-tolerance between acupuncture and methadone may not occur because acupuncture analgesia has been hypothesized to be dynorphin mediated [Han & Xie, 1984], whereas methadone binds poorly to kappa receptors, the main target of dynorphin.) Traditional Chinese theories of acupuncture (Kaptchuk, 1983), involving the rectification of chi deficiency, or excess, in various "organ" systems, have not been investigated within a Western biomedical framework.

Whatever evidence there is for the mechanisms that underlie acupuncture's effects has primarily been deduced from studies on body acupuncture, not auricular acupuncture, which is the type of acupuncture typically provided in drug treatment facilities. Auricular acupuncture is a nontraditional form of acupuncture discovered by a French physician, Paul Nogier, in the 1940s (Nogier, 1983). Theories concerning auricular acupuncture's mechanism include modulation of neural circuits in the midbrain affected by drugs of abuse (Katims et al., 1992) and stimulation of the vagus nerve in the auricle (Sytinski & Galebsakaya, 1979; Ulett, 1992). Little empirical evidence is available for either of these theories, however.

ACUPUNCTURE FOR THE TREATMENT OF COCAINE DEPENDENCE: RESEARCH FINDINGS

Auricular acupuncture specifically for the treatment of cocaine addiction has been employed for the last decade at Lincoln Hospital's Substance Abuse Division in the Bronx, New York, where over 8,000 cocaine-abusing outpatients have received acupuncture treatments, with approximately 250 patients treated daily (Smith & Khan, 1988). Clinical reports on the psychological and behavioral effects of auricular acupuncture in cocaine-dependent patients suggest that it induces a state of relaxation and promotes homeostasis while relieving withdrawal symptoms and reducing cocaine craving (Smith & Khan, 1988). It has been reported that as many as 40% of patients dependent on cocaine submit a series of negative urine samples after several weeks of treat-ment (Smith & Khan, 1988; Smith, 1988). Despite the increasing popularity of acupuncture for the treatment of cocaine dependence, with approximately 200 clinics nationwide, including over 20 metha-done clinics, offering auricular acupuncture for the treatment of ad-diction (Smith, 1991), it has been evaluated in relatively few studies. Over the past 4 years, our research team at Yale has been focusing on investigating acupuncture for the treatment of cocaine addiction in methadone-maintained patients. Cocaine abuse is widespread among methadone-maintained patients (Condelli et al., 1991) and constitutes a primary route for the transmission of HIV in this patient population (Battjes & Pickens, 1988). Pharmacological treatments for cocaine ad-diction in methadone-maintained patients have not, to date, proved effective. In this chapter we will discuss acupuncture research conducted in both opiate- and non-opiate-dependent cocaine-abusing populations.

In an uncontrolled study conducted at our unit (Margolin et al., 1993a), 32 cocaine-dependent methadone-maintained patients received an 8-week course of daily auricular acupuncture in sites used for the treatment of cocaine dependence at Lincoln Hospital. Fifty percent of patients who entered the study completed the 8-week treatment; 88% of those who completed the study attained abstinence (defined as providing cocaine-free urine samples for the last 2 weeks of the study), yielding an overall abstinence rate for the "intention to treat" sample of 44%. Post hoc comparisons to historical controls that used phar-macotherapy revealed that a higher percentage of patients who received acupuncture initiated abstinence by study completion (44%) compared to subjects who received amantadine (15%) or placebo (13%); the differ-ence between acupuncture (44%) and desipramine (26%) was not statistically significant.

To date, there have been four controlled studies to investigate the efficacy of acupuncture for the treatment of cocaine abuse, three of the studies employing a needle-insertion control. In a study conduct-ed at Lincoln Hospital in the Bronx, New York (Lipton et al., 1992), 150 cocaine-dependent subjects were randomly assigned to receive acupuncture either at points specific for addiction or at points not typi-cally used for the treatment of addiction. Acupuncture was available 6 days per week for up to 1 month. Subjects were encouraged to at-tend 10 consecutive treatment sessions during the month but could dis-continue treatment and return to treatment at any time during the study period. Urine samples were taken at each treatment session. Although this study design reflected the clinical context of the Lincoln Hospital Substance Abuse Treatment Clinic where patients are encouraged to make use of acupuncture treatments whenever they choose, interpretation of the findings was somewhat difficult. Results showed that, on the average, subjects received nine treatments; 30 subjects (15 in each group) completing 2 or more weeks of treatment. A positive finding was reported for acupuncture insofar as subjects who received acupuncture in addiction-specific sites, and who remained in treatment for over 2 weeks, had significantly lower levels of benzoylecgonine in urine screens compared to the needle-insertion control group. However, both groups reported a reduction in cocaine use, and there was no overall difference between the groups in percentage of urines negative for cocaine.

In a randomized clinical trial of acupuncture as an adjunctive treatment for illicit drug use in methadone-maintained patients conducted in Seattle, Washington (Jackson et al., 1994), 60 methadone-maintained patients were randomly assigned to either addiction-specific acupuncture or a needle-insertion control. The needle-insertion control condition was needle insertion into sites close to (i.e., within 2–3 mm) of addiction-specific sites. Collapsed across type of needle insertion, positive outcomes were reported on a number of measures, including cocaine use. Outcomes also compared favorably to a historical control. Methadone patients receiving needle insertion submitted significantly fewer cocaine-positive urines than the no-acupuncture historical control group in 15 of the 26 weeks of treatment. Outcomes, however, did not significantly differ by type of needle insertion.

In a 6-week, randomized clinical trial of acupuncture for cocaine dependence in methadone patients conducted in New Haven, Connecticut (Avants et al., 1995), 40 cocaine-dependent methadone-maintained patients were randomly assigned to receive daily acupuncture in three auricular sites and one body site (LI-4) or in control needle-insertion sites — hypothetically "inactive" sites within 2–3 mm of the four active sites. Treatment retention (75%) was better than in our previous, uncontrolled, acupuncture study (50% retention; Margolin et al., 1993a) and was comparable to retention in pharmacotherapy trials at our unit (Kosten et al., 1992). Overall, there was a positive response to treatment according to a variety of drug-related and psychosocial measures. Cocaine use decreased significantly for patients in both needle-insertion groups. Moreover, when compared to historical pharmacotherapy controls, rates of abstinence initiation in the 6th week were better for both needle-insertion groups than for groups treated with desipramine, amantadine, or placebo (addiction specific acupuncture = 35%; control needle insertion = 20%; amantadine = 0%; desipramine = 17%; placebo = 4%). At a 6-month follow-up, 64% of the subjects who had initiated abstinence during the study were still abstinent, as verified by urine toxicology screens. Despite these otherwise promising results, the only statistically significant difference found between the two types of needle puncture was on subjective ratings of cocaine craving: subjects receiving addiction-specific acupuncture reported significantly less craving during the 6-week study than did subjects receiving control needle insertion.

In a randomized clinical trial of acupuncture conducted in Dade County, Florida (Konefal et al., 1994), the addition of a 16-week program of addiction-specific acupuncture was evaluated and compared to existing drug treatment modalities. Primarily court-referred subjects ($n = 568$) were randomly assigned to one of three groups: (1) standard treatment, (2) standard treatment and frequent urine testing, or (3) acupuncture and standard treatment and frequent urine monitoring. Cocaine-abusing subjects who received acupuncture submitted significantly fewer cocaine-positive urines (21.8%) than did subjects who received standard treatment and frequent urine monitoring (28.3%).

As outlined above, although acupuncture has shown promise when compared to alternative drug treatment modalities, it has not consistently been shown to be more effective than a needle-insertion control. In the next section, we discuss some of the methodological issues that one should consider when conducting research to evaluate the efficacy of acupuncture.

METHODOLOGICAL CONSIDERATIONS FOR CLINICAL TRIALS OF ACUPUNCTURE

Acupuncture arose within a non-Western medical tradition, whose conceptual framework is far removed from the biochemical and scientific foundations of Western medicine. It is a procedure rather than a chemical substance and is thus not easily assimilated into the randomized, placebo-controlled, model of clinical trials. Designing methodologically sound and valid studies for the controlled evaluation of acupuncture is therefore a complex task that poses numerous methodological challenges (McLellan et al., 1993; ter Riet et al., 1990). Primary among the issues to be resolved is the selection of a suitable control condition.

The Needle-Insertion Control

By analogy with the placebo in pharmacotherapy trials, needle insertion into inactive or "sham" points in the ear has been suggested as the appropriate control. However, this is a highly controversial issue both from Eastern and Western theoretical perspectives. Traditional Chinese medicine does not include the concept of a "placebo"; nor does the organismic model that underlies acupuncture theory embody a concept of a systematically "inert" treatment (Wiseman & Ellis, 1985). From a

Western biomedical perspective, Ulett (1992) has argued that auricular acupuncture's effects are due to stimulation of the vagus nerve, which innervates the ear concha—a corollary of this view is that needles placed *anywhere* in the concha, regardless of their alignment with points claimed by acupuncture theory to be ailment specific, should produce the same effects. The task of identifying a suitable control for auricular acupuncture is therefore highly complex. There are many variables that can be considered when inserting a needle into the skin (cf. Liao et al., 1994): for example, depth and angle of needle insertion, needle manipulation, site of insertion, sensations elicited, influence of diffuse noxious inhibitory control mechanisms (Le Bars et al., 1979), patient belief system concerning acupuncture (Vincent, 1990), and patient/treatment–provider relationship.

A commonly used needle-insertion control in addiction research (Bullock et al., 1989) is the placement of needles in the same region as, and relatively close to (i.e., within 2–3 mm), the active sites (i.e., sites used for the treatment of addiction). Using a galvanometer, control sites register as points of relatively high electrical resistance. Because the active and control sites are close together, this control condition has the advantage of making it difficult for subjects who are treated in a group setting to determine which needle insertion condition other subjects were assigned to. However, recent studies that have investigated the usefulness of this procedure as a needle-insertion control suggest that this "proximate needling" may not be the most appropriate control condition.

Our own investigations of the properties of proximate needle-insertion control have concentrated on two key questions: (1) Do active and proximate control sites differ in the intensity of aversive sensations produced (e.g., pain), which could differentially influence dropout rate in the two groups, and (2) Does needle insertion into the proposed active and proximate control sites produce acute or long-term effects so similar that they both constitute "active" treatments.

We addressed the issue of possible aversiveness of needle insertion into proximate control sites by conducting a single-blind study that compared the effects of needle insertion into active and control sites in a nonclinical sample (i.e., staff members and acupuncture students) (Margolin et al., 1993b). In that study, subjects simultaneously received needle placement in active sites in one ear and in control sites, located 2–3 mm from the active sites, in the other ear. We found that the "active" treatment, not the proximate needle-insertion control procedure, was rated as more painful, although neither was considered particularly painful. There were no other differences between the two conditions, and the ability of subjects to guess which ear received which type of needle insertion did not rise above the level of chance. At the time, the results of this study suggested to us that needle insertion close to, and within the same region as, "active" sites might be a suitable control in a randomized clinical trial insofar as such insertion would not be expected to differentially influence treatment dropout or to produce diffuse noxious inhibitory control. However, we soon realized that this study did not address the possibility that the insertion of needles into these control sites could constitute an "active" treatment when given to a clinical sample and therefore that such a condition might not be an appropriate control.

Even though insertion of needles into proximate control sites would not be hypothesized to produce a therapeutic effect based on existent ear maps (O'Conner & Bensky, 1981) or galvanometer readings, little research has been done to validate the suppositions underlying this hypothesis. Therefore, it is certainly possible, and, according to some investigators, even probable (e.g., Liao et al., 1994; Ulett, 1992), that sites proximate to active sites are themselves active. Our research team thus embarked on a second study (Avants et al., 1995) that had the following goals: (1) to derive means and standard deviations that could be used to estimate an effect size for the difference between addiction-specific and proximate needle insertion treatments; (2) to identify acute effects of the two types of needle insertion by having patients complete pre- and postsession ratings (the first two goals would conjointly shed light on the relative "inertness" of the control points); and (3) to determine if we could replicate the findings from our first, uncontrolled, clinical trial of addiction-specific acupuncture for the treatment of cocaine dependence in methadone-maintained patients (Margolin et al., 1993a). Forty patients were randomized to addiction-specific or proximate needle insertion and received daily treatment for 6 weeks. As stated earlier in this chapter, results showed an overall reduction in cocaine use for both groups; however, the difference between the groups, although favoring the addiction-specific treatment group (effect size = 0.28) was not statistically significant. Subjects rated each type of needle insertion as equally credible and perceived no significant differences in the acute effects of the two types of needle insertion. Based on findings from this study, we calculated that 196 patients per group would be necessary for studies that employed this proximate needle-insertion control condition to have adequate power to detect a treatment effect for addiction-specific acupuncture (i.e., power set at 0.80, alpha at 0.05). This is a much larger sample than is typically used in acupuncture studies in the addictions, and may be indicative of a fairly active needle-insertion condition. Jackson et al. (1994), who also used a proximate needle-insertion control, reported positive outcomes for methadone-maintained patients in both needle-insertion groups. Similarly, Lipton et al. (1994), whose control consisted of "nonspecific needling"—acupuncture in auricular sites not typically used for the treatment of addiction—speculated that these "nonspecific" control points may also have been too active to constitute a suitable control.

Since it appeared that a suitable needle-insertion control had yet to be identified, we conducted a third study to assess several different potential controls (Margolin et al., 1995). We employed a within-subjects design study to evaluate the acute effects of four sets of needle-insertion conditions: (1) sites commonly employed for the treatment of cocaine addiction ("addiction specific") and (2) three putative controls, namely, (a) "proximate control," or needle insertion into points within 2–3 mm of addiction specific points; (b) "nonspecific control," or needle insertion into active sites outside of the concha, not indicated for the treatment of cocaine addiction (e.g., "knee," "sciatic," "elbow," "shoulder"); (c) "helix control," or needle insertion into regions on the ear helix. Ten methadone-maintained patients received each of these four treatments on 4 successive days. After each treatment session, subjects completed acute effects ratings that cover a range of possible local and systemic effects of needle insertion. At the end of the last session, subjects rated overall preferences and ranked the four treatments from most to least preferred. We hypothesized that a suitable needle-insertion control would possess two primary characteristics: (1) relatively low subjective ratings of acute systemic effects and (2) relatively low ratings of subject preference. We found that needle insertion into proximate control sites actually had the *highest* systemic effect ratings and was rated second most preferred, after "addiction specific," by a majority of our patients. This relatively high level of activity in the proximate sites may be one reason that clinical trials that utilize this control have failed to find a difference between the active and control groups (cf. Liao et al., 1994). Needle insertion into nonspecific sites also appeared to be a fairly active treatment. The type of needle insertion with the *lowest* overall mean ratings of systemic effects was needling of the helix sites. The helix points were also ranked as least preferred by the majority of patients; in addition, subjects tended to have the least confidence in needling of these sites as a treatment for addiction. Based on these results, we selected needling of the helix sites as the needle-insertion control condition to be employed in our ongoing large-scale randomized clinical trial of acupuncture for the treatment of cocaine dependence in methadone-maintained patients.

A Relaxation Control Condition

Although the physiological mechanisms underlying auricular acupuncture's presumed effects are not understood, it has been proposed, based on clinical reports, that acupuncture induces a state of relaxation that has the effect of reducing craving for cocaine (Smith & Khan, 1988). Hence, it is possible that acupuncture's direct or indirect effects are entirely nonspecific for drug addiction and are based solely on a patient's relaxing for a period of time in a quiet environment. This raises a critical issue of choosing credible comparison and control groups in acupuncture studies. Ideally, a comparison/control group should lack the specific "active ingredients" of the treatment under study while retaining the treatment's nonspecific elements. Some key, nonspecific elements include (1) presentation of a credible rationale for treatment; (3) provision of a comparable patient–therapist relationship and attention; and (3) involvement of a comparable level of desirability or, conversely, patient burden.

Our research team at Yale is currently conducting a randomized clinical trial that compares needle insertion into "active" sites with two control groups, namely, needle insertion into helix sites, as described above, and a relaxation control. These two control conditions retain the nonspecific elements of addiction-specific acupuncture and, in addition, address two different, clinically relevant, questions. The needle-insertion control condition includes all elements of the experimental acupuncture condition with the exception that the points chosen are, presumably, non-addiction specific. Hence, including this comparison group addresses the issue of whether the needling of specific regions of the ear is a crucial, active ingredient in auricular acupuncture. However, it does not, by itself, address the issue of whether other elements of auricular needle insertion are, by themselves, effective. (Thus, e.g., a finding that needle insertion into either addiction-specific or control sites is comparably effective will not rule out the possibility that efficacy is related to nonspecific treatment elements that are unrelated to needle insertion.) Relaxation training provides most of the nonspecific elements of our acupuncture procedure without insertion of needles and thus is promising as a comparison/control condition. Relaxation training includes none of the active elements specific to acupuncture (i.e., needle insertion) but most of the nonspecific elements (i.e., credible rationale, similar time demands, relaxation enhancing conditions). Unlike other control procedures that have been suggested, such as sham TENS (transelectrical nerve stimulation), relaxation training can also be considered an existing treatment modality since it has been employed with varying degrees of success as a treatment for drug addiction (e.g., Chaney & Roswell, 1983; Gelderloos et al., 1991; Klajner et al., 1984). For these reasons, relaxation training serves both as a treatment comparison group and as a control condition. Overall, our two control/comparison conditions should provide different degrees of "dismantling" of the active acupuncture condition.

Other Methodological Considerations: Blinding

Another important issue to consider when conducting efficacy research on acupuncture is whether the study should be single- or double-blind. Double-blind, placebo-controlled designs constitute the "gold standard" for clinical trials. There are several reasons, however, why it may not be practicable to conduct double-blind trials of acupuncture (cf. Vincent & Richardson, 1986).

First, in order for an acupuncture study to be double-blind, the acupuncturist would, of necessity, be inexperienced in delivering acupuncture treatments, since he or she would have to be unaware of the hypothesized "active" or "nonactive" treatment for addiction. This ignorance would contravene one of the criteria enumerated by ter Riet et al. (1990) for sound acupuncture research design, namely, that the acupuncturist administering the treatment be of "good quality" (i.e., experienced and proficient). Although we know of no study that compares treatment effectiveness of acupuncture delivered by inexperienced and experienced acupuncturists, it is possible that acupuncture treatments provided by inexperienced acupuncturists are not as effective as those provided by experienced acupuncturists. Our own observations suggest that treatments delivered by relatively inexperienced acupuncturists may be more painful than treatments delivered by experienced acupuncturists. This difference could be problematic because painful treatments could potentially threaten the study design by increasing dropout rate overall or differentially between groups or by eliciting noxious inhibitory control phenomena in the control group.

Second, unlike conditions in a pharmacotherapy study, in which the active medication and placebo are matched in appearance so that they cannot be differentiated by treatment providers, by other staff members, or by patients receiving the treatment, in clinical trials of acupuncture the control and active treatments are perceptibly different to the treatment provider. The discrimination of treatments by treatment providers, which is not present in double-blind pharmacotherapy trials, provides a basis for preferential treatment of patients according to group.

Third, it would be difficult to rule out the possiblity that acupuncturists delivering the treatments did not detect any differences in treatment effects between the groups. Because the treatments are discriminably different, this discrimation could potentially threaten the blind and again could lead to preferential treatment of patients in one of the groups. It would also be difficult to verify that the acupuncturist had not read any literature, over the course of a multiyear trial, that identified the sites commonly used for the treatment of cocaine addiction. We therefore advocate (1) a single-blind approach, with close monitoring of the acupuncturist for length and quality of the acupuncturist–patient interaction, and (2) posttreatment assessments by patients of acupuncturist skill and interpersonal style.

THE ACUPUNCTURE RESEARCH PROTOCOL AT YALE'S SUBSTANCE ABUSE CENTER

In this section, we provide the research protocol that is currently being followed at our own unit.

Addiction-Specific Acupuncture Condition

Based on the auricular acupuncture treatment protocol for cocaine addiction developed by Michael Smith, M.D., at Lincoln Hospital, needles are inserted into the ear bilaterally at four regions: (1) "sympathetic," located in the deltoid fossa at the junction of the infra-antihelix crus and the medial border of the helix; (2) "lung," located in the center of the cavum concha; (3) "liver," located in the posterior to upper portion of the helix crus; (4) "shen men," located in the inferior corner of the bifurcating point of the antihelix. Needles are inserted into points within these regions that are tender when probed, a commonly accepted characteristic of "active" sites among acupuncture practitioners. Needles are inserted such that they are perpendicular to the surface of the ear and enter the cartilage to a depth of between 1 and 2 mm.

Helix Needle-Insertion Control Condition

Control needle-insertion sites are located in the helix of the ear. Four needles, of the same type and size employed for the active treatment, are inserted subcutaneously at an oblique angle such that they do not penetrate the cartilage. The following regions of the helix are needled:

1. This region is located on the helix from the high point of the helix to just above the superior border of Darwin's tubercle, on the anterior–posterior dividing line border of the auricle.
2. This region is located on the helix at the level of Darwin's tubercle, from just below the superior border of the tubercle to just above the inferior border of the tubercle, on the anterior–posterior dividing line border of the auricle.
3. This region is located from just below the inferior border of Darwin's tubercle to the tail of the helix, on the anterior–posterior dividing line border of the auricle.

One needle is inserted into region 1, another needle in region 2, and two needles in region 3. Needling of the "liver yang" points located near these regions is to be avoided.

In both needle-insertion conditions, needles are left in place for 40–45 minutes. The acupuncture needles (Seirin Co., Ltd.) are 0.20 mm wide and 15 mm long. They are stainless steel, disposable needles, sterilized with ethylene oxide gas, and individually packaged in sterile containers that will be opened by the acupuncturist immediately before insertion (see the guidelines for clean needle technique promulgated by the National Commission for the Certification of Acupuncturists, 1989). Each acupuncture session adheres to the following format:

- Subjects are treated in small groups at the same time of day after receiving their daily methadone dose (groups are composed of subjects who receive the same type of needle puncture).
- Subject is seated in a comfortable, reclining chair and completes daily presession assessment package.
  - Subject cleans both ears with a pad saturated with 70% isopropyl alcohol.
  - Acupuncturist inspects ear area and cleans further with alcohol if needed.
- Acupuncturist inserts four needles into each ear, and subject sits quietly with needles in place for 40 minutes.
- Acupuncturist removes needles and disposes of them in a sharps box.
- Acupuncturist presses on ears with sterile cotton ball.
- Acupuncturist examines subjects' ears for signs of bleeding.
- Subject completes daily postsession assessment package.

Relaxation Control Condition

The relaxation control condition consists of having subjects watch and listen to prerecorded commercially produced videotapes depicting relaxation exercises, such as progressive muscle relaxation, meditation, and guided imagery. All patients receive an introduction to these techniques in an introductory session. All relaxation groups are of the same duration and are conducted at the same time each day as for the needle insertion groups.

MATCHING PATIENTS TO TREATMENT: FOR WHOM IS ACUPUNCTURE EFFECTIVE?

Although clinical research that investigates acupuncture in the addictions is in many respects still in a formative stage, it is nevertheless worthwhile to consider what characterizes an "acupuncture responder." Substance abusers are an extremely heterogeneous group. Thus, even if controlled clinical trials find acupuncture to be generally effective for the treatment of cocaine dependence, it is unlikely that it will be the treatment of choice for all cocaine-addicted patients. Although relatively large samples are necessary to formally test patient–treatment matching hypotheses, results of preliminary studies, as well as clinical experience, can guide future research concerning which patient subgroups to target and which patient characteristics to select for purposes of stratification prior to randomization. We present below some preliminary patient–treatment matching data gleaned from our recent clinical trial (Avants et al., 1995).

Sex

Initiation of cocaine abstinence by study completion did not differ by sex, as it did in our previous, uncontrolled study (Margolin et al., 1992); however, at the 6-month follow-up, 45% of females were abstinent from cocaine compared to 23% of males. In addition, significantly less cocaine craving was reported by those women who received addiction-specific acupuncture (mean = 0.77 on 0–4 point scale) relative to those who received the control needle insertion (mean = 2.90). No such difference between types of acupuncture was found for men.

HIV Status

Forty-seven percent of the patients who completed the 6-week study were HIV-positive. Fifty percent of these HIV-positive treatment completers initiated cocaine abstinence compared to 25% of HIV-negative treatment completers. At the 6-month follow-up, 46% of the HIV-positive patients who had completed treatment were still abstinent compared to 20% of the HIV-negative patients. HIV-positive patients may also have responded differentially to type of needle puncture: HIV-positive patients who received addiction-specific acupuncture reported significantly less cocaine craving (mean = 0.99) than did HIV-positive patients who received control needle insertion (mean = 2.33). This difference was not found for HIV-negative patients.

Severity of Drug Dependence

The percentage of urines that were positive for cocaine during the course of the 6-week study was significantly lower (60%) for patients with low addiction severity index (ASI) scores than for patients with high ASI scores (88%). In addition, patients with low ASI scores may have responded better to addiction-specific acupuncture than to the control needle puncture, insofar as low-severity patients who received addiction-specific acupuncture reported significantly less cocaine craving during the course of the study (mean = 0.77 vs. mean = 1.98) and were more likely to initiate abstinence by study completion (60% vs. 14%) than low-severity patients who received control needle insertion. Patients with high ASI drug severity scores did not respond differentially to addiction-specific and control needle insertion; the percentage of cocaine-positive urines was more than 80% for both types of needle insertion, and mean craving scores were greater than 1.5 for both groups.

Depressed Patients

Beck depression scores were dichotomized by median split (median score = 20). Although "depressed" patients were found to be less likely to initiate abstinence by study completion (24%) than "nondepressed" patients were (54%), the depressed patients did tend to respond better overall to the addiction-specific acupuncture than they did to the needle-insertion control condition; that is, depressed patients who received addiction-specific acupuncture submitted fewer cocaine-positive urines (60%) than depressed patients who received control needle insertion (85%), and they reported less cocaine craving (mean = 0.87) than did depressed patients who received control needle insertion (mean = 2.68). No such differences in response to type of acupuncture were found for the "nondepressed" subgroup.

Route of Cocaine Administration

During the course of the study, intravenous cocaine users submitted significantly fewer cocaine-positive urines (65%) than cocaine smokers did (87%). At the completion of the 6-week study, 47% of in-travenous cocaine users had initiated abstinence compared to 30% of smokers and 20% of snorters. Although this difference was not statisti-cally significant, at follow-up the difference between intravenous users and smokers was even more marked, with 50% of intravenous users and only 11% of smokers abstinent from cocaine (20% of snorters were still abstinent at follow-up).

Although preliminary, these post hoc analyses suggest that certain subgroups of cocaine-abusing patients may respond better than others to acupuncture. Sex, severity of addiction, and comorbid depression have all been found to be useful predictors of treatment outcome in pharmacotherapy and psychotherapy trials (Kosten et al., 1993; Luthar et al., 1993; McLellan et al., 1983a, 1983b; Ziedonis & Kosten, 1991) and therefore are not unique predictors of acupuncture responders. HIV status and route of cocaine administration may be more specific to acupuncture. It is our clinical impression that motivation to receive acupuncture is different for HIV-positive substance abusers relative to HIV-negative patients in that the former may seek out acupuncture not only for its effect on their cocaine abuse but also for its potential ef-fect on other medical problems (e.g., relief of pain). For intravenous drug users, regardless of their HIV status, a treatment that involves needle insertion may be appealing. Given the potential for a strong placebo response to needle puncture by intravenous drug users, it may be particularly difficult to detect a treatment effect for addiction-specific needle puncture relative to control needle puncture in a sample of primarily intravenous drug users.

We concur with ter Reit et al. (1990) in their recommendations of sample homogeneity and stratification prior to randomization. Select-ing a relatively homogeneous sample, although reducing generaliza-bility, may increase the power of the study to investigate acupuncture's effectiveness. For example, a future trial could target HIV-positive pa-tients only, stratified by such variables as sex, addiction severity, depres-sion, and route of administration, using "urn" randomization procedures (Wei, 1978), in order to ensure sufficient power to inves-tigate patient–treatment matching hypotheses, and then could evalu-ate acupuncture on outcomes that are relevant specifically to HIV-positive substance abusers, which would include, but need not be limited to, cocaine abuse.

CLINICAL CONTEXT FOR THE PROVISION OF ACUPUNCTURE

Cocaine-abusing methadone patients have numerous psychosocial problems that acupuncture alone cannot be expected to ameliorate.

Even if acupuncture is found to be a useful tool for helping individuals attain cocaine abstinence—and, therefore, for increasing the individual's readiness for rehabilitation—acupuncture treatments by themselves cannot be expected to improve the individual's vocational, interpersonal, and intrapersonal skills, all of which need to be addressed for successful rehabilitation. Pharmacotherapies have been described as creating a "window of recovery"—as providing relief from the self-depredations of continual cocaine abuse, offering the opportunity to begin the process of rehabilitation (Gawin et al., 1989). Acupuncture treatments may be viewed similarly. For this reason, acupuncture is optimally provided in a clinical context whose resources support the "work of recovery" beyond initiation of abstinence, or, lacking on-site services, whose resources provide appropriate referrals to community resources.

REFERENCES

Avants, S. K., Margolin, A., Chang, P., Kosten, T. R., & Birch, S. (1995). Acupuncture for the treatment of cocaine addiction: Investigation of a needle puncture control. *Journal of Substance Abuse Treatment, 12*(3), 195–205.

Condelli, W. S., Fairbank, J. A., Dennis, M. L., & Rachal, J. V. (1991). Cocaine use by clients in methadone programs: Significance, scope, and behavioral interventions. *Journal of Substance Abuse Treatment, 8*(4), 203–212.

Brewington, V., Lipton, D., & Smith, M. (1994). Acupuncture as a detoxification treatment: A analysis of controlled research. *Journal of Substance Abuse Treatment, 11*(4), 289–307.

Bullock, M., Culliton, P., & Olander, R. T. (1989). Controlled trial of acupuncture for severe recidivist alcoholism. *Lancet, i*(8652), 1435–1439.

Chaney, E. F., & Roswell, D. K. (1983). A cognitive behavioral analysis of relaxation training in drug abusers. *Drug and Alcohol Dependence, 12,* 201–207.

Cheng, R., & Pomeranz, B. (1980). A combined treatment with D-amino acids and electroacupuncture produces a greater analgesia than either treatment alone: Naloxone reverses these effects. *Pain, 8,* 231–236.

Clark, W. (1990). *Trial of acupuncture detoxification (TRIAD).* Final Report to California State Legislature.

Clavel, F., & Benhamou, S. (1985). Helping people to stop smoking: Randomized comparison of groups being treated with acupuncture and nicotine gum with control group. *British Medical Journal, 291,* 1538–1539.

Battjes, R. J., & Pickens, R. W. (1988). *Needle sharing among intravenous drug abusers: National and international perspectives* (NIDA Research Monograph No. 80). Rockville, MD: National Institute on Drug Abuse.

Gawin, F. H., Kleber, H. D., Byck, R., Rounsaville, B. J., Kosten, T. R., Jatlow, P. I., & Morgan, C. (1989). Desipramine facilitation of initial cocaine abstinence. *Archives of General Psychiatry, 46,* 117–121.

Gelderloos, P., Walton, K. G., Orme-Johnson, D. W., & Alexander, C. N. (1991). Effectiveness of the Transcendental Meditation program in preventing and treating substance misuse: A review. *International Journal of the Addictions, 26*, 293–325.

Han, J., Li, S., & Tang, J. (1981). Tolerance to electroacupuncture and its cross tolerance to morphine. *Neuropharmacology, 20*, 593–596.

Han, J. S., & Xie, G. X. (1984). Dynorphin: Important mediator for electro-acupuncture analgesia in the spinal cord of the rabbit. *Pain, 18*, 367–377.

Jackson, R., Wells, E. A., Diaz, O. R., Staton, V., & Saxon, A. J. (1994). *Acupuncture as an adjunct to services provided at methadone treatment facilities.* Paper presented at the 56th annual meeting of the College on Problems of Drug Dependence, Palm Beach, FL.

Kaptchuk, T. J. (1983). *The web that has no weaver.* New York: Congdon & Weed.

Katims, J. J., Ng, L. K. Y., & Lowinson, J. (1992). Acupuncture and transcutaneous electrical nerve stimulation: Afferent nerve stimulation (ANS) in the treatment of addiction. In J. H. Lowinson, P. Ruiz, & R. B. Millman (Eds.), *Substance abuse: A comprehensive textbook* (pp. 574–583). Baltimore: Williams & Wilkins.

Klajner, F., Hartman, L. M., & Sobell, M. B. (1984). Treatment of substance abuse by relaxation training: A review of its rationale, efficacy, and mechanisms. *Addictive Behaviors, 9*, 41–55.

Konefal, J., Duncan, R., & Clemence, C. (1994). The impact of the addition of an acupuncture treatment program to an existing Metro-Dade County outpatient substance abuse treatment facility. *Journal of Addictive Diseases, 13*(3), 71–99.

Kosten, T. A., Gawin, F. H., Kosten, T. R., & Rounsaville, B. J. (1993). Gender differences in cocaine use and treatment response. *Journal of Substance Abuse Treatment, 10*, 1–4.

Kosten, T. R., Morgan, C. M., Falcioni, J., & Schottenfeld, R. S. (1992). Pharmacotherapy for cocaine-abusing methadone maintained patients using amantadine or desipramine. *Archives of General Psychiatry, 49*, 894–899.

Le Bars, D., Dickenson, A. H., & Besson, J. M. (1979). Diffuse noxious inhibitory controls (DNIC): Effects on dorsal horn convergent neurones in the rat. *Pain, 6*, 283–304.

Liao, S. J., Lee, M. H. M., & Ng, L. K. Y. (1994). *Principles and practice of contemporary acupuncture.* New York: Marcel Dekker.

Lipton, D., Brewington, V., & Smith, M. O. (1992). *Acupuncture and crack addicts: A single blind placebo test of efficacy.* Manuscript submitted for publication.

Low, S. (1977). Acupuncture and nicotine withdrawal. *Medical Journal of Australia, 2*, 687.

Luthar, S. S., Glick, M., Zigler, E., & Rounsaville, B. J. (1993). Social competence among cocaine abusers: Moderating effects of co-morbid diagnoses and gender. *American Journal of Drug and Alcohol Abuse, 19*(3), 283–298.

Margolin, A., Avants, S. K., Chang, P., Birch, S., & Kosten, T. R. (1995). A single-blind investigation of four auricular needle puncture configurations. *American Journal of Chinese Medicine, 23*(2), 105–114.

Margolin, A., Avants, S. K., Chang, P., & Kosten, T. R. (1993a). Auricular acupuncture for the treatment of cocaine dependence in methadone-maintained patients. *American Journal of Addictions, 2*(3), 194–200.

Margolin, A., Chang, P., Avants, S. K., & Kosten, T. R. (1993b). Effects of sham and real auricular needling: Implications for trials of acupuncture for cocaine addiction. *American Journal of Chinese Medicine, 21,* 103–111.

Mayer, D. J., Price, D. D., & Raffii, A. (1977). Antagonism of acupuncture analgesia in man by the narcotic antagonist naloxone. *Brain Research, 121,* 368–372.

McLellan, A. T., Grossman, D. S., Blain, J. D., & Haverkos, H.W. (1993). Acupuncture treatment for drug abuse: A technical review. *Journal of Substance Abuse Treatment, 10,* 569–576.

McLellan, A. T., Luborsky, L., Woody, G. E., et al. (1983a). Predicting response to drug and alcohol treatments: Role of psychiatric severity. *Archives of General Psychiatry, 40,* 620–625.

McLellan, A. T., Woody, G. E., Luborsky, L., O'Brien, C. P., & Druley, K. A. (1983b). Increased effectiveness of substance abuse treatment: A prospective study of patient–treatment "matching." *Journal of Nervous and Mental Disease, 171,* 597–605.

National Commission for the Certification of Acupuncturists. (1989). *Clean needle technique for acupuncturists.* Washington, DC: Author.

Nogier, P. F. M. (1983). *From auriculotherapy to auriculomedicine.* Paris: Maisonneuve.

O'Connor, J., & Bensky, D. (1981). *Acupuncture: A comprehensive text.* Seattle, WA: Eastland Press.

Pomeranz, B. (1991). Scientific basis of acupuncture. In G. Stux & B. Pomeranz (Eds.), *Acupuncture: Textbook and atlas* (2nd ed., pp. 4–55). Berlin: Springer-Verlag.

Smith, M. O. (1988). Acupuncture treatment for crack: Clinical survey of 1,500 patients treated. *American Journal of Acupuncture, 16*(3), 241–247.

Smith, M. (1991, December). *NADA Newsletter.*

Smith, M. O., & Khan, I. (1988). An acupuncture programme for the treatment of drug-addicted persons. *Bulletin of Narcotics, 40*(1), 35–41.

Sytinski, I., & Galebsakaya, L. (1979). Physiologo-biochemical bases of drug dependence treatment by acupuncture. *Addictive Behaviors, 4,* 97–120.

ter Riet G., Kleijnen, J., & Knipschild, P. (1990). A meta-analysis of studies into the effect of acupuncture on addiction. *British Journal of General Practice, 40,* 379–382.

Ulett, G. A. (1992). *Beyond yin and yang.* St. Louis: Warren H. Green.

Vincent, C. (1990). Credibility assessments in trials of acupuncture. *Complementary Medical Research, 4,* 8–11.

Vincent, C. A., & Richardson, P. H. (1986). The evaluation of therapeutic acupuncture: Concepts and methods. *Pain, 24,* 1–13.

Vincent, C. A., & Richardson, P. H. (1987). Acupuncture for some common disorders: A review of evaluative research. *Journal of the Royal College of General Practitioners, 37,* 77–81.

Wei, L. J. (1978). An application of an urn model to the design of sequential controlled clinical trials. *Journal of the American Statistical Association, 73,* 559–563.

Wen, H. L. (1979). Acupuncture and electrical stimulation (AES) outpatient detoxification. *Modern Medicine in Asia, 11,* 23–24.

Wen, H. L., & Cheung, S. Y. C. (1973). Treatment of drug addiction by acupuncture and electrical stimulation. *Asian Journal of Medicine, 9,* 138–141.

Whitehead, P. C. (1978). Acupuncture in the treatment of addiction: A review and analysis. *International Journal of the Addictions, 13,* 1–16.

Wiseman, N., & Ellis, A. (1985). *Fundamentals of Chinese medicine.* Brookline, MA: Paradigm Publications.

Ziedonis, D. M., & Kosten, T. R. (1991). Depression as a prognostic factor for pharmacological treatment of cocaine dependence. *Psychopharmacology Bulletin, 27,* 337–343.

Chapter 10

WOMEN AND OPIATE DEPENDENCE

Grace Chang, M.D., M.P.H.

The true extent of opiate abuse and dependence by women is not known. While most estimates suggest that women compose about one quarter of America's addicts, most opiate abuse by the estimated 300,000 women is untreated (Davis, 1994). Powerful social forces, fueled by ignorance, stereotypes, and a traditional emphasis on male addiction, are formidable obstacles to the identification and treatment of women who abuse opiates and incur serious health risks.

In keeping with the focus of this book on novel treatment approaches to opiate addiction, this chapter will synthesize current research on the special treatment needs of opiate-dependent women and perhaps will serve to stimulate further treatment advances. Novel pharmacological approaches will be discussed since the safety of these approaches for women has yet to be definitively established.

ESTABLISHING BASELINE NEEDS FOR PSYCHOSOCIAL TREATMENTS: DISTINCTIVE CHARACTERISTICS OF OPIATE-DEPENDENT WOMEN

Studies of opiate-dependent women suggest gender-specific difficulties. Opiate-dependent women have higher rates of unemployment, depression, and anxiety disorders and have more severe medical problems than men do (Kosten et al., 1985). Because women become opiate dependent more quickly, their dependency histories are compressed and allow less time for identification, intervention, and treatment (Anglin et al., 1987). Opiate-dependent women are more likely to think of themselves as socially deviant, and more likely to be regarded as such by others, than their male counterparts are—and, consequently, have poorer self-images (Johnson, 1987; Sutker, 1981).

There is increasing awareness that female substance abusers have an increased incidence of bulimia when compared to the general population. In comparison to 4% of college females, the prevalence rate of bulimia among female drug abusers is 20%. In a study of 22 women who were undergoing treatment for opiate abuse, 5 had a concomitant eating disorder (Katzman et al., 1991).

Some investigators have sought to identify the etiological basis of drug addiction in women. Risk factors that have been identified include disproportionate rates of substance abuse in the family of origin, sexual abuse before the age of 16, and other family dysfunction, such as conflict, lack of cohesion and expression, and unresolved control issues (Hagan, 1988). Many of these risk factors are associated with the occurrence of child abuse and may further stress the already fragile social system of the female opiate addict (Regan et al., 1984).

Finally, available evidence indicates that the problems of female addiction typically involve heroin-oriented relationships (Ettore, 1992; Gerstein et al., 1979). Unfortunately, substance use in the social networks has been demonstrated to have a substantial negative impact on treatment outcome (Goehl et al., 1993; Hawkins & Fraser, 1987).

TREATMENT SERVICES FOR WOMEN OPIATE USERS

In the past, treatment services for opiate users have typically reflected research results focused on males, have served mostly males, and have been delivered by males. However, in the mid-1970s, with increased awareness of women's needs, treatment programs were designed to be more responsive by including more female staff, limiting services to women, or taking child-care responsibilities into account (Marsh & Simpson, 1986). Different types of programs attracted different types of women, although more women were likely to be retained in methadone maintenance programs than in therapeutic communities, which have been generally perceived to be less suitable for the female drug abuser (De Leon & Jainchill, 1981–1982; Moise et al., 1981).

Still, not all women opiate abusers either initiate or remain in treatment, and it is unclear whether existing services are completely responsive to women's needs. In a study that focused on the detoxification, methadone maintenance, and residential treatment experiences of 208 women opiate users in New York City, a substantial number of respondents reported that they had access to a female counselor and comprehensive counseling, including employment, health, and social issues. However, availability of services oriented to the special needs of women was not affected by the numbers of women drug users in the treatment programs, and, in fact, female-only drug treatment programs were not perceived by female respondents to be especially sensitive to their needs (Hanke & Faupel, 1993).

These results are complemented by those reported in a longitudinal study of changes in alcohol- and other drug-related problems; this study compared 80 subjects from a residential specialist women's service and 80 subjects from two traditional mixed-treatment inpatient services in Australia (Copeland et al., 1993). While both the specialist women's service and the mixed-treatment programs were based on the traditional disease model of addiction and the 12-step philosophy, the specialist women's service employed only female staff and offered residential child care. A 6-month follow-up after treatment revealed no significant differences in any treatment outcome between the two treatment groups, and the researchers concluded that simple provision of women-only treatment and child care without substantive changes in treatment content does not improve outcome. However, the specialist women's service did attract significantly more lesbian women, women with children, women with histories of childhood sexual abuse, and women with positive maternal histories of substance dependence, all of whom may have been more difficult to reach otherwise.

Thus, it appears that while all female staff and child care are well received by female opiate abusers, additional changes in treatment are indicated. Systematic research on which specific changes are needed to render treatment more sensitive to women has been proposed (Copeland et al., 1993).

TREATMENT FOR PREGNANT OPIATE-DEPENDENT WOMEN

The potential medical and social costs of opiate dependence during pregnancy are great. Pregnant opiate-dependent women experience a sixfold increase in maternal obstetric complications and significant increases in neonatal complications (Dattel, 1990). Pregnancy complications include low birth weight, toxemia, third trimester bleeding, malpresentation, puerperal morbidity, fetal distress, and meconium. Neonatal complications include narcotic withdrawal, postnatal growth deficiency, microcephaly, neurobehavioral problems, and a 74-fold increase in sudden infant death syndrome (SIDS) (Dattel, 1990).

Treatment of pregnant opiate abusers has most frequently utilized

methadone maintenance. Benefits conferred by methadone maintenance include removing the addicted woman from a drug-seeking environment, eliminating the need for illicit behavior to support a drug
habit, and preventing the fluctuations in maternal heroin level (Finnegan, 1991.)

Yet, the promise of methadone maintenance has not been consistently supported in the literature. For example, the results of a retrospective case–control study comparing methadone-maintained pregnant
subjects with untreated women showed that both groups used illicit substances at high rates and gave birth to infants of similar weights, even
though the treated women had more prenatal care (Edelin et al., 1988).
On the other hand, a comprehensive care program for pregnant opiate-
dependent women that included methadone maintenance and medical,
counseling, and development services reported improved pregnancy
outcome, but no control group was available for comparison (Suffet &
Brotman, 1984). Information from a nonrandomized pilot study of
an enhanced methadone maintenance program for pregnant addicts
(Chang et al., 1992) and a randomized clinical trial that compared the
two programs (Carroll et al., 1995) confirm improved neonatal outcomes
from the enhanced programs without affecting maternal drug use. Subjects in the enhanced programs had three times as many prenatal visits
as control subjects did, and delivered heavier infants. The enhanced programs offered weekly prenatal care by a nurse/midwife, weekly relapse
prevention groups, positive contingency awards for abstinence (subjects
could earn $15.00 weekly for three negative urine toxicology screens),
and provision of therapeutic child care during treatment visits in addition to daily methadone medication. Standard treatment consisted of
daily methadone medication, weekly group counseling, and thrice-
weekly toxicology screening. Positive contingency awards did not appear to have any effect on outcome; nevertheless, the weekly relapse
prevention group, weekly prenatal care, and therapeutic child care were
well received by participants. The generalizability of these findings is
limited by the small sample size of the studies, a common limitation in
this field of research when randomized trials are attempted.

While it is commonly held that the pregnant heroin addict is
difficult to detoxify and that maternal abstinence may cause fetal withdrawal in utero with a high risk of morbidity and mortality (Finnegan,
1991; Zweben & Payte, 1990), the controversial treatment option of opiate detoxification of the pregnant addict has been raised (Finkelstein,
1993). Highly motivated women who have extensive social supports or
who may be entering long-term residential care postdetoxification may
be candidates for this approach, which has not been widely examined
in the research literature (Finkelstein, 1993).

The issues surrounding methadone maintenance during pregnancy notwithstanding, investigators in the United Kingdom have attempted to attract drug-dependent women into treatment through the use of a pregnancy liaison and outreach service as part of a community drug team (Dawe et al., 1992). This service was directed toward women who either did not receive prenatal or substance abuse treatment or did not disclose their drug use to obstetric caregivers. The liaison service coordinated treatment planning that involved drug treatment and prenatal care offered at a clinic or general practitioner's office. The women were encouraged to work through a hierarchy of drug treatment, beginning with cessation of illicit substance use, methadone replacement, and methadone reduction to abstinence or low-dose maintenance. As a result of the Community Drug Team/Liaison Service, 45 women sought help over a 30-month period and represented a substantial increase in the number of opiate-addicted women who were previously served in the same time period. Thirty-four women began methadone detoxification and 10 were hospitalized for treatment of drug abuse. About a quarter of the deliveries were premature, and a third of the infants were below the tenth percentile in birth weight; no information on the degree of maternal abstinence from illicit substances was given.

The pregnant opiate-dependent woman confronts a multitude of social, medical, and, perhaps, interpersonal problems that would defy any one treatment approach. It appears that what is indicated is to increase outreach, in order to improve the rate of treatment and to coordinate services, and to augment standard treatment approaches with services designed to address the special needs of the pregnant addict. Treatment research findings will be invaluable for the advancement of program design; but in order to increase the generalizability of investigations, pooled data from multiple sites and appropriate use of control groups will be necessary.

TREATMENT FOR HIV-POSITIVE OPIATE-DEPENDENT WOMEN

Half of the American women who have developed AIDS were infected through intravenous drug use, and about one fifth of these women had sexual intercourse with a male intravenous abuser (Schilling et al., 1993). Wells and Jackson (1992) have summarized the circumstances that promote the spread of HIV infection among chemically dependent women: (1) the interplay of sex and drugs, (2) the culturally reinforced female role that precludes the negotiation and adoption of safer sex behaviors,

(3) the deferential role that women generally play to maintain emotional stability in relationships, (4) the positive value of childbearing, (5) the expectation of risk, and (6) the lack of access to appropriate medical care.

Program recommendations for the HIV-positive woman in drug treatment have included AIDS education at admission, on-site HIV-related services, including counseling and medical care before and after testing, and development of comprehensive approaches that involve the women's sex partners and children (Mondanaro, 1987; Wells & Jackson, 1992). At present, little is known about the efficacy of these recommendations; predictors of sexual-risk reduction among 109 female methadone clinic patients were found to include: (1) having more than one sexual partner, (2) not being of African American descent, (3) feeling comfortable about asking partners to use condoms, (4) higher depression scores, and (5) loss of friends or family to AIDS (Schilling et al., 1993).

TREATMENT FOR OPIATE-DEPENDENT WOMEN WHO ABUSE OTHER SUBSTANCES

The problem of multiple substance use by both female and male patients in treatment for opiate dependence is well documented. Estimates of alcohol abuse in methadone patients have ranged from 20% to 53%, which is especially problematic since many studies demonstrate poorer treatment outcome when multiple substances are abused (Herd, 1993). In addition, others have demonstrated that among methadone patients who abuse alcohol, there is a tendency to abuse benzodiazepines as well (Stastny & Potter, 1991).

The problem of the pregnant addict who abuses other substances is both pervasive and particularly difficult to address. For example, 98% of 100 pregnant women treated at the multifocal Family Center Program in Philadelphia, offering medical, psychosocial, and methadone maintenance services, were found to be abusing other substances on the basis of urine toxicology screening (Leifer et al., 1983). The difficulty of affecting maternal drug use while the patient is in treatment for opiate addiction has been reported in most other subsequent studies (Edelin et al., 1988; Carroll et al., 1995). While a recent study of 92 male intravenous opiate users in methadone maintenance treatment showed that the addition of basic counseling or counseling augmented by on-site medica' psychiatric, employment, and family services reduced opiate and coc. ine use in comparison to methadone alone, the enhancements do no appear to be as effective for pregnant women (McLellan et al., 1993). The difficulty of denying treatment to the pregnant opiate addict has been raised as a possible explanation for the apparent intractability of substance abuse while in treatment.

SUMMARY

Opiate abuse and dependence in women has thus far defied facile treatment solutions. First and foremost, all available evidence indicates that most female opiate abuse and dependence is not treated and that it is more likely that the female addict pursues medical treatment for the consequences of addiction. Second, the first generation of innovations in treatment, such as utilizing female staff and limiting treatment to women, have only been partially successful. Third, more recent efforts to tailor services to pregnant addicts, such as adding prenatal care and child care, appear to improve pregnancy outcome but do not reduce maternal substance use. Thus, while some advances have been made in addressing the barriers to treatment of women opiate abusers, opportunities for improvement remain but may involve more difficult problems. These include the substance-abusing social supports frequently linked to female addicts, the greater likelihood of adverse histories of family dysfunction, sexual and other abuse, and untreated severe psychological or medical illness. Clearly, the next generation of treatment advances will need to address more deeply rooted social, medical, and psychological problems, just as what might be realistically achieved in treatment is reassessed in an era of uncertain resources.

REFERENCES

Anglin, M. D., Hser, Y. I., & McGlothlin, W. H. (1987). Sex differences in addict careers: 2. Becoming addicted. *American Journal of Drug and Alcohol Abuse, 13,* :59–79.

Carroll, K. M., Chang, G., Behr, H. M., Clinton, B., & Kosten, T. R. (1995). Improving treatment outcome in pregnant women: Results from a randomized clinical trial. *American Journal of Addictions, 4,* 56–59.

Chang, G., Carroll, K. M., Behr, H. M., & Kosten, T. R. (1992). Improving treatment outcomes in pregnant opiate dependent women. *Journal of Substance Abuse Treatment, 9,* 327–330.

Copeland, J., Hall, W., Didcott, P., & Biggs, V. (1993). A comparison of specialist women's alcohol and other drug treatment service with two traditional mixed sex services: Client characteristics and treatment outcome. *Drug and Alcohol Dependence, 32,* 81–92.

Dattel, B. J. (1990). Substance abuse in pregnancy. *Seminiars in Perinatology, 14*(2), 179–187.

Davis, S. (1994). Effects of chemical dependency in parenting women. In R. R. Watson (Ed.), *Drug and alcohol abuse reviews: Vol. 5. Addictive behaviors in women* (pp. 381–413). Totowa, NJ: Humana Press.

DeLeon, G., & Jainchill, N. (1981–1982). Male and female drug abusers: Social and psychological status two years after treatment in a therapeutic community. *American Journal of Drug and Alcohol Abuse, 8*(4), 465–497.

Edelin, K. C., Gurganious, L., Golar, K., et al. (1988). Methadone maintenance in pregnancy: Consequences to care and outcome. *Obstetrics and Gynecology, 71*(3, pt. 1), 399–404.

Ettore, E. (1992). *Women and substance use.* New Brunswick, NJ: Rutgers University Press.

Finkelstein, N. (1993). Treatment programming for alcohol and drug dependent pregnant women. *International Journal of the Addictions, 28*(13), 1275–1309.

Finnegan, L. P. (1991). Treatment issues for opioid-dependent women during the perinatal period. *Journal of Psychoactive Drugs, 23*(2), 191–201.

Gerstein, D. R., Sudd, L. L., & Rovner, S. A. (1979). Career dynamics of female heroin addicts. *American Journal of Drug and Alcohol Abuse, 6,* 1–23.

Goehl, L., Nunes, E., Quitkin, F., & Hilton, I. (1993). Social networks and methadone treatment outcome: The costs and benefits of social ties. *American Journal of Drug and Alcohol Abuse, 19*(3), 251–262.

Hagan, T. (1988). *A retrospective search for the etiology of drug abuse: A background comparison of a drug addicted population of women and a control group of non-addicted women* (NIDA Research Monograph No. 81, pp. 254–261). Rockville, MD: National Institute on Drug Abuse.

Hanke, P. J., & Faupel, C. E. (1993). Woman opiate users' perception of treatment services in New York City. *Journal of Substance Abuse Treatment, 10,* 513–522.

Hawkins, J. D., & Fraser, M. W. (1987). The social networks of drug abusers before and after treatment. *International Journal of the Addictions, 22*(4), 343–355.

Herd, D. (1993). Correlates of heavy drinking and alcohol related problems among men and women in drug treatment programs. *Drug and Alcohol Dependence, 32,* 25–35.

Johnson, E. M. (1987). Women's health: Issues in mental health, alcoholism, and substance abuse. *Public Health Reports, 102*(Suppl.), 42–48.

Katzman, M. A., Greenberg, A., & Marcus, I. D. (1991). Bulimia in opiate-addicted women: Developmental cousin and relapse factor. *Journal of Substance Abuse Treatment, 8,* 107–112.

Kosten, T. R., Rounsaville, B. J., & Kleber, H. D. (1985). Ethnic and gender differences among opiate addicts. *International Journal of the Addictions, 20,* 1143–1162.

Leifer, E. D., Goldman, J., & Finnegan, L. P. (1983). *Prevalence and implications of multi-drug abuse in a population of methadone maintained wmen* (NIDA Research Monograph No. 43, pp. 322–328). Rockville, MD: National Institute on Drug Abuse.

Marsh, K. L., & Simpson, D. D. (1986). Sex differences in opioid addiction careers. *American Journal of Drug and Alcohol Abuse, 12*(4), 309–329.

McLellan, A. T., Arndt, I. O., Metzger, D. S., Woody, G. E., & O'Brian, C. P. (1993). The effects of psychosocial services in substance abuse treatment. *Journal of the American Medical Association, 269,* 1953–1959.

Moise, R., Reed, B. G., & Conell, C. (1981). Women in drug abuse treatment programs: Factors that influence retention at very early and later stages in two treatment modalities: A summary. *International Journal of the Addictions, 16*(7), 1295–1300.

Mondanaro, J. (1987). Strategies for AIDS prevention; Motivating health behavior in drug dependent women. *Journal of Psychoactive Drugs, 19,* 143–149.

Regan, D. O., Leifer, B., & Finnegan, L. P. (1984). *The incidence of violence in the lives of pregnant and drug-dependent women* (NIDA Research Monograph No. 49, p. 330). Rockville, MD: National Institute on Drug Abuse.

Schilling, R. F., El-Bassel, N., & Gilbert, L. (1993). Predictors of changes in sexual behavior among women on methadone. *American Journal of Drug and Alcohol Abuse, 19*(4), 409–422.

Stastny, D., & Potter, M. (1991). Alcohol abuse by patients undergoing methadone treatment programmes. *British Journal of the Addictions, 86,* 307–310.

Suffet, F., & Brotman, R. (1984). A comprehensive care program for pregnant addicts: Obstetrical, neonatal, and child development outcomes. *International Journal of the Addictions, 19*(2), 199–219.

Sutker, P. B. (1981). Drug dependent women: An overview of the literature. In G. M. Breschter (Ed.), *Treatment services for drug dependent women* (NIDA Treatment Research Monograph, pp. 25–51). Rockville, MD: National Institute on Drug Abuse.

Wells, D. V. B., & Jackson, J. F. (1992). HIV and chemically dependent women: Recommendations for appropriate health care and drug treatment services. *International Journal of the Addictions, 27,* 571–585.

Zweben, J. E., & Payte, J. T. (1990). Methadone maintenance in the treatment of opioid dependence. *Western Journal of Medicine, 152,* 588–599.

Chapter 11

MEDICAL ISSUES IN THE CARE OF OPIOID-DEPENDENT PATIENTS

Patrick G. O'Connor, M.D., M.P.H.
Peter A. Selwyn, M.D., M.P.H.

Substance use disorders have long been known to be commonly accompanied by coexisting medical illness (O'Connor, 1994; Stein, 1990). The presence of medical problems are among the diagnostic criteria for psychoactive substance dependence disorders (APA, 1994). In the case of opioid dependence, the physical and medical complications can include those acute problems that are directly related to opioid use itself (e.g., intoxication and withdrawal), along with a variety of systemic or organ-specific complications that can be both acute and chronic in nature. Of particular importance when considering the medical complications seen in opioid-dependent patients is the route of administration used by an individual. Specifically, injection drug use is associated with a wide variety of medical issues that need to be considered when caring for many opioid-dependent patients (O'Connor et al., 1994; Stein, 1990).

This chapter will focus on the common medical issues seen in opioid-dependent patients, with an emphasis on medical issues that are prevalent among injection drug users. Of particular concern in this population since the 1980s has been HIV infection and AIDS (O'Connor et al., 1994a). Other important medical issues that will be reviewed will include other viral infections, important bacterial infections, and tuberculosis. In addition, we will review the general approach to providing medical care to opioid-dependent patients, including a discussion of new models of care that have been developed to provide health care services in combination with drug treatment services. Finally, we will review recent information concerning new knowledge about the impact of treatment of opioid dependence on HIV risk.

HIV INFECTION AND AIDS

The most dramatic development in the area of medical complications of drug use has been the HIV/AIDS epidemic seen in opioid-dependent patients since the early to mid-1980s. This epidemic has had major implications for the care of opioid-dependent patients, both within and outside of the drug treatment setting.

Epidemiology

A variety of studies have documented that injection drug use is a major risk factor for HIV infection (Des Jarlais et al., 1992; Centers for Disease Control and Prevention, 1993b). These data have come from multiple sites around the world, especially the Americas, Europe, and Southeast Asia (Des Jarlais et al., 1992). In the United States, injection drug use is the second most common risk factor among established AIDS cases, accounting for approximately 34% of all AIDS cases in adults (Centers for Disease Control and Prevention, 1993b). The proportion of AIDS cases attributable to injection drug use has continued to grow since it has been identified as a risk factor. Most certainly, even a higher proportion of HIV-infected persons in the United States acquired their infection through injection drug use (O'Connor et al., 1994a).

　　Within the general population there are special subpopulations whose injection drug use has contributed to even higher proportions of HIV infection. For example, among women who have AIDS, the Centers for Diseace Control and Prevention reported that 66% of documented AIDS cases in 1992 were in women who injected drugs or who reported having heterosexual contact with an injection drug user (Centers for Disease Control and Prevention, 1993b). In fact, it is likely that a significantly higher proportion of women who are HIV infected acquired their infection either directly or indirectly as a result of injection drug use (Chu & Wortley, 1995). Other studies have evaluated HIV seroprevalence among childbearing women and have documented that seroprevalence rates vary widely depending on location (Diaz et al., 1993). For example, in a study that examined seroprevalence in 1991, the rates of HIV infection in childbearing women in the District of Columbia was found to be 9 per 1,000 and in New York City was found to be 6.2 per 1,000 (Chu & Wortley, 1995). Even within cities, seroprevalence can vary. In a study completed in 1989, it was found that in some areas of New York City as many as 1 out of 22 childbearing women were HIV infected (Novick et al., 1991).

In addition, minority groups have also been shown to be at increased risk for HIV infection acquired from injection drug use (Selik et al., 1988). This is particularly true among minority women, who composed 76% of all women in the United States with AIDS in 1992 (Centers for Disease Control and Prevention, 1993c). Epidemiological data concerning the association of injection drugs and AIDS among women in minorities has had major implications for prevention strategies in these populations.

Case Definition of AIDS

In 1993 the Centers for Disease Control and Prevention revised the AIDS Case Definition (1993). These changes have had major implications for the classification of drug users and women within the category of "AIDS" cases (Table 11.1). Specifically, three common clinical conditions are prevalent in drug users: pulmonary tuberculosis, recurrent bacterial infections, and invasive cervical cancer. These conditions were added to the AIDS Case Definition, significantly increasing the proportion of injection drug users and women who would be considered under the category "AIDS Defining Illnesses" (AIDS Case Definition, 1993). The other major change in the 1993 revised AIDS Case Definition was the inclusion of all HIV-infected persons with CD4 positive T-lymphocyte counts less than 200 (AIDS Case Definition, 1993). The long-term impact of this expanded AIDS definition on how injection drug users are included in this population remains under evaluation (Chu et al., 1993). Because this definition may include more injection drug users, epidemiological surveillance of this population should become more accurate.

TABLE 11.1. 1993 Revised AIDS Case Definition

1. Clinical conditions added:
   - Pulmonary tuberculosis
   - Recurrent pneumonia
   - Invasive cervical cancer
2. CD4 T-lymphocyte criteria added:
   - Count <200
   - Percentage of total lymphocytes: <14

Note. Centers for Disease Control and Prevention (1993a) criteria.

Risk Factors Associated with HIV Infection in Injection Drug Users

The transmission of HIV infection from one individual to another among the injection-drug-using population is based on the transfer of infected blood, usually through contaminated injection equipment. However, a variety of behaviors associated with injection drug use can have a modifying impact on the risk of patients' acquiring or transmitting HIV infection (O'Connor et al., 1994a; Schoenbaum et al., 1989). For example, the risk of acquiring HIV infection through the "sharing" of injection equipment increases when the number of individuals involved in a sharing network increases (Schoenbaum et al., 1989. A particularly high-risk behavior among injection drug users is the use of "shooting galleries" (Schoenbaum et al., 1989). In these locations, individuals purchase (or "rent") injection equipment ("works") along with the drug that they are interested in injecting. The "rented equipment" used in a shooting gallery is likely to have been used by other individuals, many of whom could be HIV infected. Other injection behaviors, such as "booting" or "backloading," by which blood is drawn up into the syringe during the injection process, may further enhance the risk of HIV-infection transmission.

Along with injection behavior, other characteristics of drug use may further enhance the risk of HIV transmission. In particular, the use of cocaine that is often used with opioids has been demonstrated to enhance HIV risk (Chiasson et al., 1989; Weiss, 1989). Among the reasons that cocaine is felt to enhance one's risk of HIV infection is the fact that cocaine is often injected more frequently and is associated with increased needle-sharing behaviors (Chiasson et al., 1989; Weiss, 1989). Noninjection use of cocaine has also been shown to enhance HIV risk (Diaz & Chu, 1993). For example, crack cocaine has been demonstrated to be a risk factor for the sexual transmission of HIV infection and syphilis through the "exchange of sex for drugs" activity that has been associated with crack cocaine use (Chiasson et al., 1991; Chirgwin et al., 1991; Goldsmith, 1988). This activity is of particular concern for women (Diaz & Chu, 1993). Finally, some preliminary data has also suggested that injection drug users who use alcohol may also be at enhanced risk for HIV infection (O'Connor et al., 1992).

Medical Management of HIV Infection

In the treatment of people with HIV/AIDS over the past decade there have been many dramatic advances that have dramatically altered the natural history of HIV infection. From the treatment perspective, these advances have involved primarily the development of new antiretroviral therapies for the treatment of HIV infection and the development of strategies for the prevention and treatment of opportunistic infections and other complications associated with HIV infection. Rather than present itself as a fulminent and rapidly fatal illness, AIDS now exhibits many more characteristics of a chronic disease, albeit incurable, with exacerbations and remissions comparable to certain cancers and other life-threatening illnesses. In addition, however, the advent of the therapeutic era for AIDS has brought with it the increasing complexity of medical management decisions and the related problems of toxicity and adverse side effects from the widening range of AIDS-related medications. This section will give a brief overview of the current state of HIV-related therapeutics in 1996.

ANTIRETROVIRAL THERAPY

Concerning treatment for HIV infection itself, or antiretroviral therapy, zidovudine (ZDV), or AZT—the first drug ever used for HIV infection—was introduced in 1987, after it was shown to be effective in reducing morbidity and mortality among late-stage AIDS patients in a placebo-controlled trial (Fischl et al., 1987). Subsequent studies demonstrated a decreased progression rate from HIV infection to AIDS in asymptomatic patients who received zidovudine at less-advanced disease stages; however, these results have not been consistently reproduced, and there has been no survival benefit shown for patients who have received the drug prior to the later stages of disease (Aboulker & Swart, 1993; Cooper et al., 1993; Fischl et al., 1990; Hartigan et al., 1992; Volberding et al., 1990). In addition, although the bulk of data do suggest a benefit as far as HIV-related morbidity, if not mortality, is concerned, this benefit has been found to be transient and generally limited to the first 1–2 years after initiation of therapy (Lundgren et al., 1994; Osmond et al., 1983). This finding has prompted an intense study of other antiretroviral agents, which have been studied alone and in combination with zidovudine, including didanosine (ddi) and zalcitabine (ddc) (Collier et al., 1993; Kahn et al., 1992; Spruance et al., 1994). These agents may confer some benefit for patients who receive zidovudine and who show signs of disease progression after a period of zidovudine monotherapy, or for patients who are for other reasons unable to tolerate AZT. These medications, which are all inhibitors of the HIV reverse transcriptase enzyme, are all classified as nucleoside analogues, a class of medications that also includes stavudine (d4t), introduced commercially in 1994, and lamivudine (3TC), released in 1995. Results of clinical trials by mid-1996 had clearly demonstrated that combination therapy with two or more antiretroviral agents is superior to monotherapy, and there are therefore few indications for patients to be on monotherapy at the present time.

The evolving paradigm of HIV care underwent a dramatic change in 1996 with the emergence of new data from clinical trials of several new antiretroviral agents, including nonnucleoside reverse transcriptase inhibitors (e.g. nevirapine, delavirdine) and protease inhibitors (saquinavir, ritonavir, indinavir). In addition to the established group of nucleoside reverse transcriptase inhibitors (AZT, DDI, DDC, D4T, 3TC), these agents offered for the first time the promise of additional reverse transcriptase inhibitors, as well as inhibitors of the viral protease exzyme. This enzyme is necessary for the formation and release of progeny virions from infected cells. As with other proven strategies for antimicrobial chemotherapy (e.g., tuberculosis), the HIV protease inhibitors, when used in combination with reverse transcriptase inhibitors, allow for the possibility of interrupting replication of a pathogen at two different stages of its life cycle. Indeed, preliminiary phase I/II trials as well as clinical and virologic results of combination regimens, including both these classes of agents, have shown sustained reduction in the amount of HIV detectable in blood specimans along with sustained elevations in CD4+ T-lymphocyte counts, in some cases extending through 2 years of follow-up (Carpenter et al., 1996; Collier et al., 1996; Danner et al., 1995; D'Aquila et al., 1996; Eron et al., 1995; Markowitz et al., 1995).

The assessment of antiretroviral drug efficacy, as well as the determination of patients' prognosis and rate of disease progression, were revolutionized in 1996 with the introduction of commercial assays that quantitate the amount of HIV RNA in plasma. These blood tests, also called viral load tests, are performed by commercial laboratories, and are now routinely available. In several studies, HIV viral load measures have been shown to provide powerful new tools for estimating the risk of disease and long-term morbidity and mortality (Carpenter et al., 1996; Mellors et al., 1995, 1996; O'Brien et al., 1996). Viral load assays should be performed as part of the baseline evaluations of all HIV-infected patients and in addition should be used to assess prognosis in order to determine the appropriateness of initiating antiretroviral therapy and to evaluate responses to therapy.

The introduction of these new antiretroviral agents has raised justifiable hope of a new therapeutic era for HIV-infected patients. However, this medical advance has also introduced new complexities in patient management, particularly for injection drug users, owing in large part to potential drug toxicities and drug interations.

The principal toxicities of the nucleoside analogues consist mostly of bone marrow suppression (zidovudine); peripheral neuropathy and pancreatitis (didanosine, zalcitabine, and stavudine, to varying degrees); and, less commonly, hepatitis (zidovudine, didanosine, zalcitabine) and diarrhea (lamivudine). Some of these toxicities may be particularly important in populations of HIV-infected drug users, in whom underlying rates of peripheral nerve disease, pancreatitis (owing to coexisting alcohol abuse), and hepatitis (owing to underlying alcoholic, drug-induced, or viral hepatitis) may be very high compared to other HIV-infected populations (Cherubin & Sapira, 1993; Kreek, 1974). There is also one study suggesting that the metabolism of zidovudine may be affected by methadone—which may mean that zidovudine is not as readily metabolized in methadone-maintained patients as it is in the controls—but this possible interaction has not yet been found to result in an increased risk of zidovudine toxicity in such patients (Schwartz et al., 1992).

The principal toxicity of the nonnucleoside reverse transcriptase inhibitors (nevirapine, delavidine) is rash. The protease inhibitors, in contrast, while very potent antiretroviral agents, can have significant side effects, namely, gastrointestinal distress (saquinavir, indivanir, ritonavir) as well as liver function and lipid abnormalities (ritonavir). Of the three available by prescription in mid-1996—saquinavir, ritonavir, indinavir—saquinavir and indinavir are generally better tolerated than ritonavir, but ritonavir may be one of the more potent of the three.

In addition to drug toxicities, there are important considerations about drug interactions: all the protease inhibitors are metabolized by the hepatic cytochrome P450 microsomal enzyme system and, to varying degrees, may inhibit the metabolism of other drugs that are handled by this system. These drugs include methadone, other opioids, barbiturates, benzodiazepines, anticonvulsants, and a variety of other medications. This interaction suggests that dosing adjustments may be required and, in some cases, that certain medications may be contraindicated. Clinical and pharmaceutical studies are urgently needed to evaluate the possibly wide range of drug interactions for which HIV-infected drug users may be at risk through the use of this important new group of antiretroviral medications.

TREATMENT AND PREVENTION OF OPPORTUNISTIC INFECTIONS

Concerning the treatment and prevention of AIDS-related opportunistic infections, there has also been significant progress made over the last decade. The most dramatic advance, which has clearly altered the natural history of HIV disease, has been the widespread effective prevention of *Pneumocystis carinii* pneumonia (PCP) since the introduction of prophylactic regimens in the late 1980s. Pneumocystis, which had initially been the most common AIDS-related opportunistic infection in the United States, has decreased markedly in incidence and is now considered a virtually preventable disease (Hoover et al., 1993; Moore et al., 1992). Clinicians now have an ample number of options for the treatment and prevention of PCP (summarized in Table 11.2, together with other regimens for treatment and prevention of opportunistic infections). Notable advances in recent years include (1) the development of effective treatment for cytomegalovirus (CMV) infection, which can cause sight-threatening retinitis in AIDS patients; (2) the introduction of several systemic azole antifungal medications (e.g., fluconazole and itraconazole) for the treatment of candidiasis, cryptococcosis, histoplasmosis, and other fungal infections; (3) the development of powerful macrolide antibiotics (clarithomycin, azithromycin), which have been found to be effective in the treatment of disseminated microbacterium avium complex (MAC, or MAI) disease; and (4) the introduction of rifabutin, which may help prevent the occurrence of disseminated microbacterium avium complex (Nightingale et al., 1993).

In addition, there have been a number of effective interventions developed for treatment of HIV-related wasting, including new medications megestrol acetate (Megace) and dronabinol (Marinol), as well as testosterone, other anabolic steroids, and recombinant human growth hormone. These medications may help with anorexia and/or promote weight gain in AIDS patients, which can have a dramatic impact on quality of life and patients' self-image.

However, as noted above, one of the consequences of progress may be the occurrence of new problems or challenges, especially in drug-using populations: for example, the use of in-dwelling intravenous catheters, used for chronic suppressive medication for CMV disease (which may be used for illicit drug injection); the observation that rifabutin may result in a rifampin-like effect by accelerating methadone metabolism in certain patients, which may cause withdrawal symptoms (Sawyer et al., 1993); the possibility that dronabinol, a synthetic marijuana-like compound, may have abuse potential in patients with substance abuse problems; the likelihood that newer antiretroviral agents (especially the protease inhibitors) may have important drug interactions with opioids and other treatment-related issues that can complicate management in such patients. These issues pose a challenge to clinicians not only to remain current and up-to-date regarding the rapidly changing field of HIV therapeutics but also to appreciate and anticipate the impact of these changeson the care of opioid-abusing populations and their special needs.

TABLE 11.2. Treatment for HIV Infection and Selected Opportunistic Infections, 1996

Infection	Medication
HIV	Zidovudine (AZT)[a]
	Didanosine (ddI)[a]
	Zalcitabine (ddc)[a]
	Stavudine (d4T)[a]
	Lamivudine (3TC)[a]
	Saquinavir[a]
	Ritonavir[a]
	Indinavir[a]
	Nelfinavir[a]
	Nevirapine[a]
Pneumocystis carinii pneumonia	Trimethoprim-sulfamethoxazole
	Pentamidine
	Dapsone/Trimethoprim
	Atovaquone[a]
	Trimetrexate[a]/Leucovorin
	Clindamycin/Primaquine
Toxoplasmosis	Sulfadiazine/Pyrimethamine/ Leucovorin
	Atovaquone[a]
Mycobacterium avium complex	Clarithromycin[a]/Azithromycin[a]
	Clofazimine
	Ethambutol
	Rifabutin[a]
Mycobacterium tuberculosis	Isoniazid (INH)
	Rifampin (RIF)
	Pyrazinamide (PZA)
	Ethambutol (EMB)
	Streptomycin (STR)
Cytomegalovirus	Ganciclovir[a]
	Foscarnet[a]
	Cidofavir[a]
Candidiasis	Nystatin
	Clotrimazole
	Fluconazole[a]
Cryptococcosis	Amphotericin-B/Flucytosine
	Fluconazole[a]
Histoplasmosis	Itraconazole[a]

[a]Medication introduced after 1986.

OTHER IMPORTANT MEDICAL ISSUES
IN THE CARE OF OPIOID-DEPENDENT PATIENTS

Along with HIV infection and AIDS, a variety of medical complications have long been associated with opioid dependence in general and with injection drug use in particular (Cherubin & Sapira, 1993). Among opioid-dependent patients who are injection drug users, a variety of important viral and bacterial infections and tuberculosis are of critical importance in the care of these patients. Those who are HIV infected may have a characteristic pattern of HIV-related diseases (O'Connor et al., 1994b). In this section, we will provide an overview of the other important medical conditions seen in opioid-dependent patients (Table 11.3).

Viral Infections

Along with HIV infection, hepatitis has had a major impact on the health of opioid-dependent patients. More recently, other retroviral infections, including the human T-cell lymphotrophic virus, have been demonstrated in this population. For the most part, transmission of these viruses is primarily through needle sharing.

TABLE 11.3. Medical Conditions Commonly Seen in Opioid-Dependant Patients

1. *Viral infections*
   - HIV infection
   - Hepatitis A, B, C, and D
   - Other retroviral infections

2. *Bacterial infections*
   - Soft tissue infections
   - Pneumonia
   - Endocarditis/sepsis

3. *Tuberculosis*
   - Pulmonary
   - Extrapulmonary

4. *Sexually transmitted diseases*
   - Syphilis
   - Human papillomavirus

5. *Important noninfectious complications*
   - Cancer
   - Other substance use-related complications

Hepatitis

Each of the major forms of viral hepatitis has been associated with injection drug use, hepatitis B and C being the most important.

HEPATITIS B

Hepatitis B has long been known to be associated with drug use (Stimmel et al., 1975). A variety of studies have shown that over half of injection drug users are likely to show serological evidence of past hepatitis B infection (positive serological test for hepatitis B surface antibody and/or hepatitis B core antibody). In addition, a substantial proportion of this population will also show evidence of active hepatitis B infection (hepatitis surface antigen positive) (Chu & Wortley, 1995). These chronic carriers are at risk for transmitting hepatitis B infection and are more likely to experience chronic liver disease.

Among the major implications of hepatitis B infection in drug users is that of chronic hepatitis. In its mild form, hepatic disease in drug users manifested by abnormal liver function tests (typically elevated transaminases). In more advanced disease, patients will exhibit evidence of hepatic insufficiency, which in its most severe form includes hepatic encephalopathy and liver failure. Chronic liver disease in all its forms has major implications for medication use. For example, medications (such as isoniazid and rifampin) commonly prescribed to treat diseases like tuberculosis, that are prevalent in drug users; drugs (such as trimethopram-sulfamethoxazole) used to treat or prevent opportunistic infections; and some antiretroviral agents (such as didanosine) may have hepatotoxic implications (Kreek et al., 1976; O'Connor et al., 1994a; Sawyer et al., 1993; Schwartz et al., 1990).

HEPATITIS C

Since the development of serological testing for hepatitis C virus, this infectious agent has been demonstrated to be a very important cause of "non-A," "non-B" hepatitis. Hepatitis C is an important cause of posttransfusion hepatitis as well as hepatitis infection among injection drug users (O'Connor et al., 1994a; Cherubin & Sapira, 1993). A variety of serological studies of hepatitis C virus infection have found that, like hepatitis B, the majority (e.g., over two-thirds) of injection drug users who were examined have shown evidence of hepatitis C infection (Esteban et al., 1989; Simmonds et al., 1990). As with hepatitis B, hepatitis C is also associated with chronic liver disease, and there are similar implications concerning the use of potentially hepatotoxic drugs in such patients (O'Connor et al., 1994a; Cherubin & Sapira, 1993).

HEPATITIS A AND HEPATITIS D

While hepatitis B and C are the most prevalent forms of infectious hepatitis among drug users, those caring for that population must also be aware of the potential impact of hepatitis A and D in these patients. For example, hepatitis A which is typically transmitted through "fecal–oral" contact, was documented to occur among a population of injection drug users in Monroe County, New York (Centers for Disease Control, 1988). Presumably this transmission occurred through saliva contamination of drugs or drug injection equipment (Francis et al., 1984). Hepatitis D (or "delta") is typically seen in combination with hepatitis B infection and has been reported among injection drug users (Housset et al., 1992; Novick et al., 1988). Typically, such patients have a history of hepatitis B infection and new evidence of active hepatitis (Lettau et al., 1987).

THE IMPACT OF HIV INFECTION
ON THE CLINICAL COURSE OF HEPATITIS

Although hepatitis infection is common among all injection drug users, there has been particular concern about the impact of coinfection with hepatitis and HIV disease on the clinical course of hepatitis. Current evidence suggests that concurrent infection with HIV does not necessarily worsen the clinical course of hepatitis infections (O'Connor et al., 1994b).

However, it has been noted that the degree and duration of hepatitis B surface anginemia, as well the likelihood of coinfection with hepatitis D, may be increased among individuals who are HIV infected (Housset et al., 1992; Novick et al., 1988).

Other Retroviral Infections

Along with the HIV virus, there are other retroviral infections that have been documented to be transmitted through injection drug use (Biggar et al., 1991). Specifically, injection drug users in the United States have been shown to be the group at highest risk for infection with human T-cell lymphotrophic virus type I and/or type II (HTLV I and HTLV II) (Khabbaz et al., 1992; Williams et al., 1989). Of the two virus types, HTLV II has been documented to be the most important of these infections in prevalence (O'Connor et al., 1994b). Typically, these viruses are associated with adult T-cell leukemia/lymphoma and with tropical spastic paraparesis. On a worldwide basis, these viruses have been documented to be endemic in certain areas of Asia, Africa, and the

Caribbean. Although HTLV I and II are much less prevalent than HIV disease, there is evidence to suggest that in those patients who are coinfected with HTLV I and II and with HIV, there may be a more rapid progression of HIV disease (Page et al., 1992).

Bacterial Infections

A variety of bacterial infections have been well documented to be associated with drug use in general, and with injection drug use in particular. These infections have gained increased prominence in the area of HIV infection because individuals with advanced HIV disease are at further risk for important bacterial infections.

SKIN AND SOFT TISSUE INFECTIONS

Perhaps the most common bacterial infections seen in injection drug users are those related to the skin and soft tissue penetration of nonsterile needles (Stein, 1990; Cherubin & Sapira, 1993; Vollum, 1970; Cherubin, 1971). The typical manifestations of such infections include erythema and swelling in the area of a nonsterile injection. Cellulitis can spread from the injection site and become quite diffuse and severe. The typical bacterial organisms involved in cellulitis include staphylococcus and streptococcus species (Cherubin & Sapira, 1993; Page et al., 1992). More unusual infections can be seen in injection drug users, especially when injection equipment is contaminated by saliva or other body substances (Cherubin & Sapira, 1993). Cellulitis can be life threatening in this contamination situation and requires careful treatment and follow-up (Stein, 1990; Cherubin & Sapira, 1993; Somers & Lowe, 1986). In the most severe cases, necrotizing fasciitis can develop, a condition that frequently results in limb amputation and death. Localized cellulitic infections can be managed with local skin care and oral antibiotics such as dicloxacillin (Stein, 1990; Biderman & Hiatt, 1987). More severe infections or those that fail to show response to oral antibiotics require intravenous antibiotics.

Along with cellulitis, localized abscesses can form at injection sites. To heal properly, these infections often require incision and drainage along with antibiotic treatment.

PNEUMONIA

Bacterial pneumonias have long been known to be more prevalent among drug users than among the general population (Cherubin, 1967). In the era of HIV/AIDS, this prevalence has become even more obvious (O'Connor et al., 1994b).

Several studies have documented that HIV-infected drug users may have a risk of more than four times that of HIV-negative drug users for bacterial pneumonia (Selwyn et al., 1988). The most common organisms involved were streptococcus pneumonia and haemophilus influenzae (Selwyn et al., 1988). Other less common organisms can also be seen among drug users, especially since drug users are at higher risk for a suppressed mental status that is associated with aspiration pneumonias. Thus, the investigation of pneumonia in injection drug users requires that sputum samples be examined and that clinicians consider appropriate organisms when deciding on antibiotic therapy (Garcia-Leoni et al., 1992).

ENDOCARDITIS AND SEPSIS

Among the most common reasons that opioid-dependent injection drug users are hospitalized is for evaluation of fever and presumed endocarditis or sepsis (Fischl et al, 1987; O'Connor et al., 1994a; Stein, 1990). Bacterial endocarditis has been well documented as a prevalent condition in injection drug users (Cherubin & Sapira, 1993). Because organisms are introduced through the peripheral vascular system, the right side of the heart is commonly involved. Endocarditis skin flora such as staph aureus is also implicated, and documented cases of endocarditis require intravenous antibiotics, which for injection drug users is typically administered in the hospital setting (O'Connor et al., 1994a).

Differential Diagnosis of Fever in Injection Drug Users

Given that fever is often the reason that bacterial infections, including sepsis and endocarditis, are considered in injection drug users, a major clinical challenge is to identify which patients have important or major bacterial infection versus other causes of fever (O'Connor et al., 1994a). Two studies have examined febrile injection drug users who go to emergency departments for evaluation. Marantz et al. (1987) studied 76 febrile injection drug users in the hope of finding discriminating clinical laboratory features that might identify patients with serious bacterial infections requiring hospitalization. No such features could be found. Similarly, Samet et al. (1991), in order to identify particulars of serious illness, evaluated 296 febrile injection drug users who went to the Boston City Hospital Emergency Department. Samet's group determined that in 64% of patients the cause of the fever, which was responsible for the admission, was clinically apparent in the emergency department. Among these patients, pneumonia and cellulitis were the most common. However, the remaining 36% of cases consisted of individuals without an apparent need for hospitalization on the basis of their emergency department visit, after which some patients were found to have endocarditis on the basis of blood cultures. The etiologies of fever in patients from both studies is displayed in Table 11.4.

When taken as a whole, it is not clear how best to approach injection drug users when they come to emergency departments with fevers. Hospitalization is often recommended until the source can be identified or until major infections can be ruled out (Chu & Wortley, 1995). Alternatively, for "reliable" patients who do not have an apparent major illness, consideration could be given to obtaining blood cultures, sending the patients home, and arranging for follow-ups within 24–48 hours to review blood culture data in the patients' clinical course (O'Connor et al., 1994a).

Tuberculosis

As with bacterial infections, tuberculosis is another condition known to be prevalent in drug users prior to the AIDS epidemic (Cherubin, 1967). However, the AIDS epidemic has resulted in a major increase in the number of cases of tuberculosis, particularly among drug users (Selwyn et al., 1992). Generally, it is felt that tuberculosis in HIV-infected individuals represents reactivation of latent disease in the setting of immunosuppression. Drug users in general are thought to be at increased risk for tuberculosis infection, primarily because of environmental and "social" factors related to drug use (O'Connor et al., 1994b). For example, injection drug users are in particularly high concentration in urban areas characterized by low socioeconomic status. "Crack" cocaine use has also been associated with an increased risk of tubercu-

TABLE 11.4. Differential Diagnosis
of Fever in Injection Drug Users

Diagnosis	%
Pneumonia	26
Cellulitis	19
Endocarditis	8
Abscess	3
Other "major" illness	13
"Minor" illness	31

Note. See Marantz et al. (1987); O'Connor et al. (1994a); Samet et al. (1991).

losis, again in part because of environmental reasons (Centers for Disease Control, 1991a).

HIV-infected individuals are at particularly high risk for "extrapulmonary" manifestations of tuberculosis (Barnes et al., 1991; Braun et al., 1990), which may include infection of the gastrointestinal system or central nervous system. In addition, the emergence of multiple drug resistant tuberculosis has been described in urban areas with high concentration of drug users (Small et al., 1993; Centers for Disease Control, 1991b).

When evaluating opioid-dependent patients for tuberculosis, it is important to take a careful exposure history, as well as a history of tuberculosis-related symptoms (cough, weight loss, night sweats, fevers) and prior testing and treatment for tuberculosis. In screening for tuberculosis, skin testing with PPD should be accompanied by testing for cutaneous anergy, particularly in individuals with known or suspected HIV infection.

Although in the general population 15 mm of induration on skin testing is considered positive, drug users are considered positive with 10 mm of induration; those with HIV infection are considered positive with 5 mm of induration and thus candidates for INH (isoniazid) prophylaxis. However, because of the potential cutaneous anergy, a negative PPD does not necessarily rule out tuberculosis infection in those with HIV infection.

Sexually Transmitted Diseases

Drug users have long been known to be at increased risk for sexually transmitted diseases (Cherubin & Sapira, 1993). Syphilis in particular has been documented to be highly prevalent in this population. The diagnosis of syphilis in drug users is complicated by the fact that a significant portion of patients may have a biological false-positive screening test (VDRL or RPR) for syphilis (Sapira, 1968). "Crack" cocaine use specifically has also been shown to increase the risk of syphilis, presumably, like HIV infection, through sexual disinhibition or the exchange of sex for drugs (Chirgwin et al., 1991; Gourevitch et al., 1993). Other sexually transmitted diseases known to be highly prevalent in drug users include gonorrhea, chancroid, and herpes simplex infections.

Other Medical Complications

Along with the problems listed above, opioid-dependent individuals are at risk for a long list of potential medical problems (Cherubin & Sapira, 1993; O'Connor et al., 1994b; Stein, 1990). Two of these problems deserve special comment.

HEROIN-INDUCED NEPHROPATHY

Heroin has been associated with a form of kidney disease character-ized by focal glomerular sclerosis, which may present nephrotic syn-drome, hypertension, and renal insufficiency (Cherubin & Sapira, 1993; O'Connor et al., 1994b; Stein, 1990). In these patients, the discontinua-tion of drug use may result in decreased renal impairment. Other kid-ney diseases seen in drug users include AIDS nephropathy and glomerular nephritis secondary to bacterial endocarditis (Cherubin & Sapira, 1993; O'Connor et al., 1994b; Stein, 1990).

CANCER

Certain malignancies have been documented to be more prevalent among injection drug users, particularly those drug users with HIV in-fection (O'Connor et al., 1994a). These malignancies include cervical carcinoma, HIV-associated lymphoma, carcinoma of the lung, and car-cinoma of the oropharynx and larynx (Gachupin-Garcia et al., 1992; Monfardini et al, 1989; O'Connor et al., 1994b). Interestingly, injection drug users are less likely to develop Kaposi's carcinoma than are homosexual or bisexual men with AIDS (Beral et al., 1990). Among the reasons that drug users may be at increased risk for some of these cancers are increased sexual activity (cervical cancer) and enhanced exposure to environmental toxins such as tobacco smoke, and alcohol (oropharyngeal carcinoma and lung cancer) (O'Connor et al., 1994b).

Medical Complications Associated with Other Forms of Drug Use

Given that polysubstance use is quite prevalent among injection drug users, it is important to keep in mind that medical complications as-sociated with the use of other drugs is also important in this popula-tion. For example, clinicians need to be aware of the whole variety of alcohol-induced complications, such as central nervous system, cardi-ovascular, and gastrointestinal diseases (O'Connor, 1994). In addition, cocaine use is associated with its own complications, such as cerebral vascular disease (e.g., stroke) and cardiovascular disease (cardiac erythe-mas or ischemia/infarction) (O'Connor et al., 1992).

Models of Primary Care for Drug Users

It has long been recognized that drug users have difficulty accessing medical care. It is a population that has been generally described as "difficult" and specifically described as "hateful" (Groves, 1978). Physicians and other givers of primary care often view substance-dependent patients as unmotivated and manipulative. In their survey of primary care physicians, Gerbert et al. (1991) reported that more than half the physicians had negative attitudes about treating injection drug users. The combination of the severity of medical diseases seen in this population and their lack of access to care has resulted in the development of new models for disease prevention and management in drug-using populations.

Preventive Health Care in Drug Users

Because of the wide variety of medical illnesses seen among opioid-dependent patients, it is important to direct specific preventive health care measures toward this population. These preventive measures include screening for such complications as HIV, tuberculosis, sexually transmitted diseases, and hepatitis, as well as preventing such problems as bacterial pneumonia and hepatitis through the provision of vaccines (O'Connor et al., 1992c, 1994b). It is important that injection drug users with HIV infection receive intensive preventive health care for the important medical problems described previously (O'Connor et al., 1994b). Obviously, in this population it is important to also provide "routine" preventive services such as education about "safe sex," diet, and exercise, along with routine cancer screening such as mammography.

Models of Primary Care within Drug Treatment

Researchers in New York City, New Haven, and Boston have documented that combining medical care with drug treatment may have benefits for drug-using patients. In New York City, it was shown that HIV-infected drug users who were enrolled in methadone maintenance could effectively receive screening for tuberculosis, tuberculosis prophylaxis, and antiretroviral therapy when these services were provided "on site" within a methadone maintenance program (Selwyn et al., 1993). Similarly, researchers in New Haven demonstrated that these services can have good outcomes as far as specific HIV prevention measures are concerned when such services are offered in the context of comprehensive primary care for patients enrolled in a variety of substance abuse treatment programs (O'Connor et al., 1992c). Finally, a group at Boston University documented that a model of care that utilizes a "triage and initial intake" approach for HIV-infected drug users may be an effective way to initiate important medical services for these patients and links them to existing primary care systems (Samet et al., 1992).

RISK REDUCTION TREATMENT
FOR OPIOID DEPENDENCE AND HIV/AIDS
RISK AMONG DRUG USERS

The concept of harm reduction or risk reduction for drug injectors with or at risk for HIV infection was articulated primarily in Europe in the mid-1980s. In certain cities such as Amsterdam, where this approach was introduced even prior to the AIDS epidemic in order to prevent transmission of hepatitis B, the basis for this approach has always been that one should attempt to minimize the associated harm to drug injectors and their contacts regardless of whether society can prevent or stop the illicit injection of drugs (Engelsman, 1989). In the AIDS epidemic, the major harm reduction interventions have included education and outreach, needle disinfection and hygiene, needle and syringe exchange, and increased availability of treatment for drug use.

Concerning education and outreach, there have been numerous examples in many countries of the world to demonstrate that drug users have become aware of the risk of HIV infection and AIDS and have modified their behavior somewhat as a result of that knowledge (Becker & Joseph, 1988; Brettle, 1991; Des Jarlais et al., 1992, 1994). The most commonly reported changes in behavior have included reductions in needle sharing, reductions in the number of needle-sharing partners, and cessation of high-risk activities such as "shooting gallery" use.

However, it is also clear that relapses may occur, that sustained and consistent reductions in risk behavior may be difficult to achieve, and that, while drug-using risk behavior may have decreased, there has been little change in the sexual risk behavior of drug injectors, which has important implications for heterosexual transmission of HIV (Becker & Joseph, 1988; Watkins et al., 1994). The practice of needle disinfection and needle hygiene has most commonly involved the use of household bleach to disinfect needles that are being reused; although this practice is appealing in its simplicity, and has been proposed in areas where increased access to sterile injection equipment is not possible, several studies suggest that the use of bleach does not appear to provide protection against HIV transmission (even though undiluted bleach in a laboratory setting is effective in inactivating HIV, in the real-world practice of drug users bleach has not been found to be used consistently enough to result in a clear protective benefit) (Gleghorn et al., 1994; McCoy et al., 1994; Titus et al., 1994). The one way in which this infection might play a useful role is in that of skin cleaning prior to injection, since it has been demonstrated that skin cleaning with alcohol swabs before injection may result in a decreased incidence of skin infections and possibly od endocarditis (Vlahov et al., 1992).

A phenomenon of stabilization of HIV infection rates has been observed in recent years among selected drug-using populations, although it is not known definitively whether this stabilization has occurred as a result of the adoption of safer drug-using practices among drug injectors (Des Jarlais et al., 1994). In New York City, for example, after a rapid rise in HIV seroprevalence during the late 1970s and early 1980s, seroprevalence levels have remained close to 50%, with evidence of increased use of needle and syringe exchange and, among some users, a switch to noninjected forms of heroin use (e.g., intranasal use), parallel to the observed stabilization in HIV infection rates (Des Jarlais et al., 1992). However, it must also be noted that a stabilization in HIV seroprevalence levels does not imply the absence of new infections, since the high rates of loss from the drug-using population of HIV-infected persons (e.g., through illness, disability, or death) implies that transmission must still be occurring if the result is an apparently stable level of infection. Further, the observation that HIV infection may be acquired relatively early in drug-injecting careers (Vlahov et al., 1990), and that drug treatment programs are generally for older and more experienced injectors (McCusker et al., 1994), points out the importance of continued HIV prevention, especially in high-risk younger populations of drug users.

Needle and syringe exchange has been widely promoted as a harm reduction strategy for drug injectors, and needle exchange programs now exist in many locations in North America, Europe, and Australia (Lurie et al., 1993; Stimson, 1989; Stryker & Smith, 1993). In addition to exchanging needles and providing AIDS-condoms and related education, these programs have often served as an important link between active drug injectors and medical and social services. Studies have consistently shown that needle exchange, in addition to improving access to and engagement with needed services, is associated with decreased needle sharing and related high-risk behavior (Stimson, 1989; Stryker & Smith, 1993; Watters et al., 1994). Several studies have suggested, although none definitively, that needle exchange may be associated with a decreased risk of hepatitis B infection, and it has been suggested that a stabilization in HIV infection rates is associated with needle and syringe exchange programs (Des Jarlais et al., 1994; Stryker & Smith, 1993). Further, interesting data from an innovative needle exchange and research program in New Haven, Connecticut, suggests that the prevalence of HIV infection in used syringes in that city has steadily declined since the program was introduced, using these data, researchers have determined that the likelihood for HIV transmission via contaminated needles may have been reduced by as much as one third in this environment as a result of the increased availability of sterile needles through the needle exchange program (Kaplan et al., 1994).

Regarding the effects of drug treatment on HIV-related risk behavior and the risk of actual HIV infection, it has been clearly demonstrated that methadone treatment results in a decrease in heroin injection, overall improvement in health status and social functioning, and a reduced risk of HIV infection among opioid addicts (Ball & Ross, 1991; Hartel et al., 1995; Novick et al., 1990; Office of Technology Assessment, 1990; Schoenbaum et al., 1989). Several studies have suggested that drug injectors in long-term methadone maintenance treatment are less likely to have or acquire infection with HIV than are those out of treatment. A recent study from Philadelphia also found an HIV seroconversion rate of only 3% among drug injectors in treatment versus 22% in a comparison out-of-treatment group (Metzger et al., 1993).

SUMMARY

In summary, opioid-dependent patients represent a population with significant medical issues. A comprehensive primary care–based approach to treating this population is warranted. This approach should emphasize prevention and screening along with the care of medical complications when they occur. Clearly, joining efforts of medical care and drug treatment may be the best way to enhance the overall health of opioid-dependent patients.

REFERENCES

AIDS Case Definition. (1993). Revised classification system for HIV infection and expanded surveillance case definition for AIDS among adolescents and adults. *Morbidity and Mortality Weekly Report, 41*(RR-17), 1–19.

Aboulker, J. P., & Swart, A. M. (1993). Preliminary analysis of the Concorde trial. *Lancet, 341*, 889–890.

American Psychiatric Association. (1994). *Diagnostic and statistical manual of mental disorders* (4th ed.). Washington, DC: Author.

Ball, J. C., & Ross, A. (1991). *The effectiveness of methadone maintenance treatment.* New York: Springer-Verlag.

Barnes, P. F., Bloch, A. B., Davidson, P. T., & Snider, D. E. Jr. (1991). Tuberculosis in patients with human immunodeficiency virus infection. *New England Journal of Medicine, 324*(23), 1644–1650.

Becker, M. H., & Joseph, J. G. (1988). AIDS and behavioral change to reduce risk: a review. *American Journal of Public Health, 78*, 394–410.

Beral, V., Peterman, T. A., Berkelman, R. I., & Jaffe, H. W. (1990). Kaposi's sarcoma among persons with AIDS: A sexually transmitted infection? *Lancet, 335*, 123–128.

Biderman, P., & Hiatt, J. R. (1987). Management of soft-tissue infections of the upper extremity in parenteral drug abusers. *American Journal of Surgery, 154,* 526–528.

Biggar, R. J., Buskell-Bates, Z., Yakshe, P. N., Caussy, D., Gridley, G., & Seeff, L. (1991). Antibody to human retroviruses among drug users in three east coast American cities, 1972–1976. *Journal of Infectious Diseases, 163,* 57–63.

Braun, M. M., Byers, R. H., Heyward, W. L., Ciesielski, C. A., Bloch, A. B., Berkelman, R. L., & Snider, D. E. (1990). Acquired immunodeficiency syndrome and extrapulmonary tuberculosis in the United States. *Archives of Internal Medicine, 150,* 1913–1916.

Brettle, R. P. (1991). HIV and harm reduction for injection drug users. *AIDS, 5,* 125–136.

Carpenter, C. C. J., Fischl, M., Hammer, S. M., Hirsh, M. S., Jacobsen, D. M., Katzenstein, D. A., Montaner, J. S., Richman, D. D., Saag, M. S., Schooley, R. T., Thompson, M. A., Vella, S., Yeni, P. G., & Volberding, P. A. (1996). Antiretroviral therapy for HIV infection in 1996. *Journal of the American Medical Association, 276,* 146–154.

Centers for Disease Control. (1988). Hepatitis A among drug abusers. *Morbidity and Mortality Weekly Report, 37,* 297.

Centers for Disease Control. (1991a). Crack cocaine use among persons with tuberculosis: Contra Costa County, California, 1987–1990. *Morbidity and Mortality Weekly Report, 40,* 485–489.

Centers for Disease Control. (1991b). Nosocomial transmission of multidrug-resistant tuberculosis among HIV-infected persons: Florida and New York, 1988–1991. *Morbidity and Mortality Weekly Report, 40,* 585–602.

Centers for Disease Control and Prevention. (1993a). *HIV/AIDS Surveillance Report, 4*(February) 1–23.

Centers for Disease Control and Prevention. (1993b). *HIV/AIDS Surveillance Report, 5*(October), 1–19.

Centers for Disease Control and Prevention. (1993c). Update: Mortality attributable to HIV infection/AIDS among persons aged 25–44 years, United States, 1981–1991. *Morbidity and Mortality Weekly Report, 42,* 481–486.

Cherubin, C. E. (1967). The medical sequelae of narcotic addiction. *Annals of Internal Medicine, 67,* 23–33.

Cherubin, C. E. (1971). Infectious disease problems of narcotic addicts. *Archives of Internal Medicine, 128,* 309–313.

Cherubin, C. E., & Sapira, J. D. (1993). The medical complications of drug addiction and the medical assessment of the intravenous drug user: 25 years later. *Annals of Internal Medicine, 119,* 1017–1028.

Chiasson, R. E., Bacchetti, P., Osmond, D., Brodie, B., Sande, M. A., & Moss, A. R. (1989). Cocaine use and HIV infection in intravenous drug users in San Francisco. *Journal of the American Medical Association, 261,* 561–565.

Chiasson, R. E., Stoneburner, R. L., Hildebrandt, D. S., Ewing, W. E., Telzak, E. E., & Jaffe, H. W. (1991). Heterosexual transmission of HIV-1 associated with the use of smokable freebase cocaine (crack). *AIDS, 5,* 1121–1126.

Chirgwin, K., DeHovitz, J. A., Dillon, S., & McCormack, W. M. (1991). HIV infection, genital ulcer disease, and crack cocaine use among patients attending a clinic for sexually transmitted diseases. *American Journal of Public Health, 81,* 1576–1579.

Chu, S., Ward, J., & Fleming, P. (1993). *Impact of the expanded AIDS surveillance definition on the ascertainment of HIV morbidity in women.* American Public Health Association 121st Annual Meeting, San Francisco.

Chu, S. Y., & Wortley, P. M. (1995). Epidemiology of HIV/AIDS in women. In M. J. Minkoff & J. A. DeHovitz (Eds.), *HIV infection in women* (pp. 1–12). New York: Raven Press.

Collier, A. C., Coombs, R. W., Fischl, M. A., Skolnik, P. R., Northfelt, D., Boutin, P., Hooper, C. J., Kaplan, L. D., Volverding, P. A., Davis, L. G., et al. (1993). Combination therapy with zidovudine and didanosine compared with zidovudine alone in HIV-1 infection. *Annals of Internal Medicine, 119,* 786–793.

Collier, A. C., Coombs, R. W., Schoenfeld, D. A., Bassett, R. L., Timpone, J., Baruch, P., Jones, M., Facey, K., Whitacre, C., McAuliffe, V. J., Friedman, H. M., Merigun, J. C., Reich, R. C., Hooper, C., & Corey, L. (1996). Treatemtn of human immunodeficiency virus infection with saquinavir, zidovudine, and zalcitabine. *New England Journal of Medicine, 334,* 1011–1017.

Cooper, D. A., Gatell, J. M., Kroon, S., Clumeck, N., Millard, J., Goebel, F. D., Bruun, J. N., Stingl, G., Melville, R. L., Gonzalez-Kahoz, J., Stevens, J. W., Fiddian, A. P., & the European–Australian Collaborative Group. (1993). Zidovudine in persons with asymptomatic HIV infection and CD4+ cell counts greater than 400 per cubic millimeter. *New England Journal of Medicine, 329,* 297–303.

D'Aquila, R. T., Hughes, M. D., Johnson, V. A., Fischl, M. A., Sommadoss, J.-P., Liou, S.-H. Timpone, J., Myers, M., Basgoz, N., Niu, M., Hirsch, M. S., & the National Institute of Alergy and Infectious Diseases AIDS Clinical Trials Group Protocol 241 Investigators. (1996). Nevirapone, zidovudine, and didanosine compared with zidovudine and didanosine in patients with HIV-1 infection. *Annals of Internal Medicine, 124,* 1019–1029.

Danner, S. A., Carr, A., Leonard, J. M., Lehman, L. M., Gudiol, F., Gonzales, J., Raventos, A., Rubio, R., Bouza, E., Pintado, V., et al. (1995). A short-term study of the safety pharmacokinetics and efficacy of ritonavir, an inhibitor of HIV-1 protease. *New England Journal of Medicine, 333,* 1528–1533.

Des Jarlais, D. C., Friedman, S. R., Choopanya, K., Vanichseni, S., & Ward, T. P. (1992). International epidemiology of HIV and AIDS among injecting drug users. *AIDS, 6,* 1053–1068.

Des Jarlais, D. C., Friedman, S. R., Sotheran, J. L., Wenston, J., Maror, M., Yancovitz, S. R., Frank, B., Beatrice, S., & Mildvan, D. (1994). Continuity and change within an HIV epidemic: Injecting drug users in New York City, 1984 through 1992. *Journal of the American Medical Association, 271,* 121–127.

Diaz, T., & Chu, S. Y. (1993). Crack cocaine use and sexual behavior among people with AIDS [Letter]. *Journal of the American Medical Association, 269,* 2845–2846.

Diaz, T., Buehler, J. W., Castro, K. G., & Ward, J. W. (1993). AIDS trends among Hispanics in the United States. *American Journal of Public Health. 83,* 504–509.

Engelsman, E. L. (1989). Dutch policy on the management of drug-related problems. *British Journal of Addiction, 84,* 211–218.

Eron, J. J., Benoit, S. L., Jemsek, J., MacArthur, R. D., Santana, J., Quinn, J. B., Kuritzkes, D. R., Fallon, M. A., & Rubin, M. (1995). Treatment with lamivudine, zidovudine, or both in HIV-positive patients with 200 to 500 CD4+ cells per cubin millimeter. *New England Journal of Medicine, 333,* 1662–1669.

Esteban, J. I., Esteban, R., Viladomiu, L., Lopez-Talavera, J. C., Gonzalez, A., Hernandez, J. M., Roget, M., Vargas, V., Genesca, J., Buti, M., et al. (1989). Hepatitis C virus antibodies among risk groups in Spain. *Lancet, 2,* 294–297.

Fischl, M. A., Richman, D. D., Grieco, M. H., Gottlieb, M. S., Volberding, P. A., Laskin, O. L., Leedom, J. M., Groopman, J. E., Mildvan, D., Schooley, R. T., et al. (1987). The efficacy of 3'-azido-2', 3'-deoxythymidine (azidothymidine) in the treatment of patients with AIDS and AIDS-related complex: A double-blind placebo-controlled trial. *New England Journal of Medicine, 317,* 185–191.

Fischl, M. A., Richman, D. D., Hansen, N., Collier, A. C., Carey, J. T., Para, M. F., Hardy, W. D., Dolin, R., Powderly, W. G., ALlan, J. D., et al. (1990). The safety and efficacy of zidovudine (AZT) in the treatment of subjects with mildly symptomatic human immunodeficiency virus type 1 infection. *Annals of Internal Medicine, 112,* 727–737.

Francis, D. P., Hadler, S. C., Prendergast, T. J., Peterson, E., Ginsburg, M. M., Lookabaugh, C., Holmes, J. R. & Maynard, J. E. (1984). Occurrence of hepatitis A, B, and non-A/non-B in the United States: CDC Sentinel County Hepatitis Study I. *American Journal of Medicine, 76,* 69–74.

Gachupin-Garcia, A., Selwyn, P. A., & Budner, N. S. (1992). Population-based study of malignancies and HIV infection among injecting drug users in a New York City methadone treatment program, 1985–1991. *AIDS, 6,* 843–848.

Garcia-Leoni, M. E., Moreno, S., Rodeno, P., Cercenado, E., Vicente, T., & Bouza, E. (1992). Pneumococcal pneumonia in adult hospitalized patients infected with the human immunodeficiency virus. *Archives of Internal Medicine, 152,* 1808–1812.

Gerbert, B., Maguire, B. T., Bleecker, T., Coates, T. J., & McPhee, S. J. (1991). Primary care physicians and AIDS: Attitudinal and structural barriers to care. *Journal of the American Medical Association, 266,* 2837–2842.

Gleghorn, A. A., Doherty, M. C., Vlahov, D. D., Celentano, D. D., & Jones, T. S. (1994). Inadequate bleach contact times during syringe cleaning among injection drug users. *Journal of Acquired Immune Deficiency Syndrome, 7,* 767–772.

Goldsmith, M. F. (1988). Sex tied to drugs = STD spread. *Journal of the American Medical Association, 260,* 2009.

Gourevitch, M. N., Selwyn, P. A., Davenny, K., Buono, D., Schoenbaum, E. E., Klein, R. S., & Friedland, G. H. (1993). Effects of HIV infection on the serologic manifestations and response to treatment of syphilis in intravenous drug users. *Annals of Internal Medicine, 118,* 350–355.

Groves, J. E. (1978). Taking care of the hateful patient. *New England Journal od Medicine, 298,* 883–887.

Hartel, D. M., Schoenbaum, E. E., Selwyn, P. A., Kline, J., Davenny, K., Klein, R. S., & Friedland, G. H. (1995). Heroin use during methadone maintenance treatment: The importance of methadone dose and cocaine use. *American Journal of Public Health, 85,* 83–88.

Hartigan, P. M., Hamilton, J. D., & Simberkoff, M. S. (1992). Early zidovudine and survival in HIV infection. *New England Journal of Medicine, 327,* 814–815.

Hoover, D. R., Saah, A. J., Bacellar, H., Phair, J., Detels, R., Andersone, R., & Kaslow, R. A. (1993). Clinical manifestations of AIDS in the era of pneumocystis prophylaxis. *New England Journal of Medicine, 329,* 1922–1926.

Housset, C., Pol, S., Carnot, F., Dubois, F., Nalpas, B., Housset, B., Berthelot, P., & Brechot, C. (1992). Interactions between human immunodeficiency virus-1, hepatitis delta virus and hepatitis B virus infections in 260 chronic carriers of hepatitis B virus. *Hepatology, 15,* 578–583.

Kahn, J. O., Lagakos, S., Richman, D. D., Pettinelli, C., Liou, S. H., Brown, M., Volberding, P. A., Crumpacker, C. S., Beall, G., et al. (1992). A controlled trial comparing continued zidovudine with didanosine in human immunodeficiency virus infection. *New England Journal of Medicine, 327,* 581–587.

Kaplan, E. H., Khoshnood, K., & Heimer, R. (1994). A decline in HIV-infected needles returned to New Haven's needle exchange program: Client shift or needle exchange? *American Journal of Public Health, 84,* 1991–1994.

Khabbaz, R. F., Onorato, I. M., Cannon, R. O., Hartley, T. M., Roberts, B., Hosein, B., & Kaplan, J. E. (1992). Seroprevalence of HTLV-I and HTLV-II among intravenous drug users and persons in clinics for sexually transmitted diseases. *New England Journal of Medicine, 326,* 375–380.

Kreek, M. J. (1973). Medical safety and side effects of methadone in tolerant individuals. *Journal of the American Medical Association, 223,* 665–668.

Kreek, M. J., Garfield, J. W., Gutjahr, C. L., & Giusti, L. M. (1976). Rifampin-induced methadone withdrawal. *New England Journal of Medicine, 294,* 1104–1106.

Lettau, L. A., McCarthy, J. G., Smith, M. H., Hadler, S. C., Morse, L. J., Ukena, T., Bessette, R., Gurwitz, A., Irvine, W. G., Fields, H. A., et al. (1987). Outbreak of severe hepatitis due to delta and hepatitis B viruses in parenteral drug abusers and their contacts. *New England Journal of Medicine, 317,* 1256–1262.

Lundgren, J. D., Phillips, A. N., Pedersen, C., Clumeck, N., Gatell, J. M., Johnson, A. M., Ledergerber, B., Vella, S., & Nielsen, J. O. (1994). Comparison of long-term prognosis of patients with AIDS treated and not treated with zidovudine. *Journal of the American Medical Assocation, 271,* 1088–1092.

Lurie, P., Reingold, A. L., Bowser, B., et al. (1993). *The public health impact of needle exchange programs in the United States and abroad.* San Francisco: University of California Press.

Marantz, P. R., Linzer, M., Feiner, C. J., Feinstein, S. A., Kozin, A. M., & Friedland, G. H. (1987). Inability to predict diagnosis in febrile intrevenous drug abusers. *Annals of Internal Medicine, 106,* 823–828.

Markowitz, M., Saag, M., Powderly, W. G., Hurley, A. M., Hsu, A., Valdes, J. M., Henry, D., Sattler, F., La Marca, A., Leonard, J. M., & Ho, D. D. (1995). A preliminary study of ritonavir, an inhibitor of HIV-1 protease, to threat HIV-1 infection. *New England Journal of Medicine, 333,* 1534–1539.

McCoy, C. B., Rivers, J. E., McCoy, H. V., Shapshak, P., Weatherby, N. L., Chitwood, D. D., Page, J. B., Inciardi, J. A., & McBride, D. C. (1994). Compliance to bleach disinfection protocols among injecting drug users in Miami. *Journal of Acquired Immune Deficiency Syndromes, 7.* 773–776.

McCusker, J., Willis, G., McDonald, M., Lewis, B. F., Sereti, S. M., & Feldman, Z. T. (1994). Admissions of injection drug users to drug abuse treatment following HIV counseling and testing. *Public Health Reports, 109,* 212–218.

Mellors, J. W., Kingsley, L. A., Rinaldo, C. R., Jr., Todd, J. A., Hoo, B. S., Kokka, R. P., & Gupta, P. (1995). Quantitation of HIV-1 RNA in plasma predicts outcome after seroconversion. *Annals of Internal Medicine, 122,* 573–579.

Mellors, J. W., Rinaldo, C. R., Jr., Gupta, P., White, R. M., Todd, J. A., & Kingsley, L. A. (1996). Prognosis in HIV-1 infection predicted by the quantity of virus in plasma. *Science, 272,* 1167–1170.

Metzger, D. S., Woody, G. E., McLellan, A. T., O'Brien, C. P., Druley, P., Navaline, H., DePhilippis, D., Stolley, P., & Abrutyn, E. (1993). Human immunodeficiency virus seroconversion among intravenous drug users in- and out-of-treatment: An 18-month prospective follow-up. *Journal of Acquired Immune Deficiency Syndromes and Human Retrovirology, 6,* 1049–1056.

Monfardini, S., Vaccher, E., Pizzocaro, G., Stellini, R., Sinicco, A., Sabbatani, S., Marangolo, M., Zagni, R., Clerici, M., Foa, R., et al. (1989). Unusual malignant tumors in 49 patients with HIV infection. *AIDS, 3,* 449–452.

Moore, R. D., Keruly, J., Richman, D. D., Creagh-Kirk, T., & Chaisson, R. E. (1992). Natural history of advanced HIV disease in patients treated with zidovudine. *AIDS, 6,* 671–677.

Nightingale, S. D., Cameron, D. W., Gordin, F. M., Sullam, P. M., Cohn, D. L., Chaisson, R. E., Eron, L. J., Sparti, P. D., Bihari, B., Kaufman, D. L., et al. (1993). Two controlled trials of rifabutin prophylaxis against mycobacterium avium complex infections in AIDS. *New England Journal of Medicine, 329,* 828–833.

Novick, D. M., Farci, P., Croxson, T. S., Taylor, M. B.., Schneebaum, C. W., Lai, M. E., Bach, N., Senie, R. T., Gelb, A. M., & Kreek, M. J. (1988). Hepatitis D virus and human immunodeficiency virus antibodies in parenteral drug abusers who are hepatitis B surface antigen positive. *Journal of Infectious Diseases, 158,* 795–803.

Novick, D. M., Joseph, H., Croxson, T. S., Salsitz, E. A., Wang, G., Richman, B. L., Poretsky, L., Keefe, J. B., & Whimbey, E. (1990). Absence of antibody to human immunodeficiency virus in long-term socially rehabilitated methadone maintenance ptients. *Archives of Internal Medicine, 150,* 97–99.

O'Brien, W. A., Hartigan, P. M., Martin, D., Esinhart, J., Hill, A., Benoit, S., Rubin, M., Simberkoff, M. S., & Hamilton, J. D. (1996). Changes in plasma HIV-1 RNA and CD4++ lymphocyte counts and the risks of progression to AIDS. *New England Journal of Medicine, 334,* 426–431.

O'Connor, P. G. (1994). The general internist. *Alcohol Health and Research World, 18*(2), 110–116.

O'Connor, P. G., Chang, G., & Shi, J. (1992a). Medical complications of cocaine use. In T. R. Kosten & H. D. Kleber (Eds.), *Clinicians guide to cocaine addiction: Theory, research and treatment* (pp. 241–272). New York: Guilford Press.

O'Connor, P. G., McNelly, E. A., Kosten, T. A., Schottenfeld, R. S., Williams, A. E., & Rounsaville, B. J. (1992b). Injection drug use in HIV infection: Risk factors and current trends. *Clinical Research, 40*(2), 561A.

O'Connor, P. G., Molde, S., Henry, S., Shockcor, W. T., & Schottenfeld, R. S. (1992c). Human immunodeficiency virus infection in intravenous drug users: A model for primary care. *American Journal of Medicine, 93,* 382–386.

O'Connor, P. G., Samet, J. H., & Stein, M. D. (1994a). Management of hospitalized intravenous drug users: Role of the internist. *American Journal of Medicine, 96,* 551–558.

O'Connor, P. G., Selwyn, P. A., & Schottenfeld, R. S. (1994b). Medical care for injection-drug users with human immunodeficiency virus infection. *New England Journal of Medicine, 331*(7), 450–459.

Office of Technology Assessment. (1990). *The effectiveness of drug abuse treatment: Implications for controlling AIDS/HIV infection.* Washington, DC: U.S. Government Printing Office.

Osmond, D., Charlebois, F., Lang, W., Shiboski, S., & Moss, A. (1994). Changes in AIDS survival time in two San Francisco cohorts of homosexual men, 1983–1993. *Journal of the American Medical Association, 271,* 1083–1087.

Page, J. B., Lai, S. H., Chirwood, D. D., Klimas, N. G., Smith, P. C., & Flectcher, M. A. (1992). HTLV-I/II among intravenous drug users and person in clinics for sexually transmitted diseases. *New England Journal of Medicine, 326,* 375–380.

Samet, J. H., Gren, J., & Kalish, R. L. (1991). Initial treatment approaches for hospitalized febrile intravenous drug users without apparent major illness [Abstract]. *Clinical Research, 39,* 607A.

Samet, J. H., Libman, H., Steger, K. A., Dhawan, R. K., Chen, J., Shevitz, A. H., Dewees-Dunk, R., Levenson, S., Kufe, D. & Craven, D. E. (1992). Complications with zidovudine therapy in patients infected with human immunodeficiency virus, type 1: A cross-sectional study in a municipal hospital clinic. *American Journal of Medicine, 92,* 495–502.

Sapira, J. D. (1968). The narcotic addict as a medical patient. *American Journal of Medicine, 45,* 555–588.

Sawyer, R. C., Brown, L. S., Narong, P. K., & Li, R. (1993). Evaluation of a possible pharmacologic interaction between refabutin and methadone in HIV-seropositive injecting drug users. In *Abstracts of the Ninth International Conference on AIDS,* Berlin.

Schoenbaum, E. E., Hartel, D., Selwyn, P. A., Klein, R. S., Davenny, K., Rogers, M., Feiner, C., & Friedland, G. (1989). Risk behaviors for human immunodeficiency virus infection in intravenous drug users. *New England Journal of Medicine, 321,* 874–879.

Schwartz, E. L., Brechbuhl, A. B., Kahl, P., Miller, M. H., Selwyn, P. A., & Friedland, G. H. (1990). Altered pharmacokinetics of zidovudine in former IV drug-using patients receiving methadone. In *Abstracts of the Sixth International Conference on AIDS,* San Francisco. San Francisco: University of California Press.

Schwartz, E. L., Brechbuhl, A. B., Kahl, P., et al. (1992). Pharmocokinetics interactions of zidovudine and methadone in intravenous drug-using patients with HIV infection. *Journal of Acquired Immune Deficiency Syndrome, 5,* 619–626.

Selik, R. M., Castro, K. G., & Pappaioanou, M. (1988). Racial/ethnic differences in the risk of AIDS in the United States. *American Journal of Public Health, 78,* 1539–1545.

Selik, R. M., Castro, K. G., & Pappaioanou, M. (1988). Racial/ethnic differences in the risk of AIDS in the United States. *American Journal of Public Health, 78,* 1539–1545.

Selwyn, P. A., Budner, N. S., Wasserman, W. C., & Arno, P. S. (1993). Utilization of on-site primary care services by HIV-seropositive and -seronegative drug users in a methadone maintenance program. *Public Health Reports, 108,* 492–500.

Selwyn, P. A., Feingold, A. R., Hartel, D., Schoenbaum, E. E., Alderman, M. H., Klein, R. S., & Friedland, G. H. (1988). Increased risk of bacterial pneumonia in HIV-infected intravenous drug users without AIDS. *AIDS, 2,* 267–272.

Selwyn, P. A., Sckell, B. M., Alcabes, P., Friedland, G. H., Klein, R. S., & Schoenbaum, E. E. (1992). High risk of active tuberculosis in HIV-infected drug users with cutaneous anergy. *Journal of the American Medical Association, 268,* 504–509.

Simmonds, P., Zhang, L. Q., Watson, H. G., Rebus, S., Ferguson, E., Balfe, P., Leadbetter, G. H., Yap, P. L., Peutherer, J. F., & Ludlam, C. A. (1990). Hepatitis C quantification and sequencing in blood products, haemophiliacs, and drug users. *Lancet, 336,* 1469–1472.

Small, P. M., Shafer, R. W., Hopewell, P. C., Singh, S. P., Murphy, M. J., Desmond, E., Sierra, M. F., & Schoolink, G. K. (1993). Exogenous reinfection with multidrug-resistant mycobacterium tuberculosis in patients with advanced HIV infection. *New England Journal of Medicine, 328,* 1137–1144.

Somers, W. J., & Lowe, F. C. (1986). Localized gangrene of the scrotum and penis: A complication of heroin injection into the femoral vessels. *Journal of Urology, 136,* 111–113.

Spruance, S. L., Pavia, A. T., Peterson, D., Berry, A., Pollard, R., Patterson, T. F., Frank, I., Remick, S. C., Thompson, M., MacArthur, R. D., et al. (1994). Didanosine compared with continuation of zidovudine in HIV-infected patients with signs of clinical deterioration while receiving zidovudine: A randomized, double-blind clinical trial. *Annals of Internal Medicine, 120,* 360–368.

Stein, M. D. (1990). Medical complications of intravenous drug use. *Journal of General Internal Medicine, 5,* 249–257.

Stimmel, B., Vernac, S., & Schaffner, F. (1975). Hepatitis B surface antigen and antibody: A prospective study in asymptomatic drug abusers. *Journal of the American Medical Association, 243,* 1135.

Stimson, G. V. (1989). Syringe-exchange programmes for injecting drug users. *AIDS, 3,* 253–260.

Stryker, J., & Smith, M. D. (1993). *Dimensions of HIV prevention: Needle exchange.* Menlo Park, CA: Henry J. Kaiser Family Foundation.

Titus, S., Marmor, M., Des Jarlais, D., Kim, M., Wolfe, H., & Beatrice, S. (1994). Bleach use and HIV seroconversion among New York City injection drug users. *Journal of Acquired Immune Deficiency Syndromes, 7,* 700–704.

Vlahov, D., Munov, A., Anthony, J. C., Cohn, S., Celentano, D. D., & Nelson, K. E. (1990). Association of drug infection patterns with antibody to human immunodeficiency virus type 1 among intravenous drug users in Baltimore, Maryland. *American Journal of Epidemiology, 132,* 847–856.

Vlahov, D., Sullivan, M., Astemborski, J., Nelson, K. E. (1992). Bacterial infections and skin cleaning prior to injection among intravenous drug users. *Public Health Reports, 107,* 595–598.

Volberding, P. A., Lagakos, S. W., Koch, M. A., Pettinelli, C., Myers, M. W., Booth, D. K., Balfour, H. H., Jr., Reichman, R. C., Bartlett, J. A., Hirsch, M. S. et al. (1990). Zidovudine in asymptomatic human immunodeficiency virus infection: A controlled trial in persons with fewer than 500 CD4-positive cells per cubic millimeter. *New England Journal of Medicine, 322,* 941–949.

Vollum, D. L. (1970). Skin lesions in drug addicts. *British Medical Journal, 2,* 647–650.

Warner, E. A. (1993). Cocaine Abuse. *Annals of Internal Medicine, 119,* 226–235.

Watkins, K. E., Metzger, D., Woody, G., & McLellan, A. T. (1994). High-risk sexual behaviors of intravenous drug users in and out of treatment: Implications for the spread of HIV infection. *American Journal of Drug and Alcohol Abuse, 18,* 389–399.

Watters, J. K., Estilo, M. J., Clark, G. L., & Lorvick, J. (1994). Syringe and needle exchange as HIV/AIDS prevention for injection drug users. *Journal of the American Medical Association, 271,* 115–120.

Weiss, S. H. (1989). Links between cocaine and retroviral infection. *Journal of the American Medical Association, 261,* 607–609.

William, A. E., Fang, C. T., Slamon, D. J., et al. (1989). Seroprevalence and epidemiological correlates of HTLV-I infection in U.S. blood donors. *Science, 240,* 643–646.

Part III

THE NEW
PHARMACOTHERAPIES

Chapter 12

OPIATE MAINTENANCE THERAPY WITH LAAM

Walter Ling, M.D.
Peggy Compton, R.N., Ph.D.

The 1993 approval by the U.S Food and Drug Administration (FDA) of levo-alpha-acetylmethadol (LAAM) for the treatment of opiate addiction represents the first and only opiate substitution alternative to methadone in over 30 years of drug treatment. The pharmacological profile of LAAM is uniquely suited to the treatment of opiate addicts, and 40 years of clinical research has established its efficacy and safety in the opiate addict populations. It is a pharmacotherapeutic choice that offers untreated and undertreated opiate addicts unprecedented opportunity to more fully participate in rehabilitative and other prosocial life activities and to achieve greater autonomy from the clinic environment. The availability of LAAM to opiate addicts will reduce injection drug use and will further decrease the spread of HIV in drug-abusing populations and in the general public.

HISTORY OF DEVELOPMENT

A derivative of methadone, LAAM was first synthesized by German scientists during or soon after World War II. In preclinical studies, it

This chapter is dedicated to Pierre F. Renault, M.D., who played a significant role in the development of LAAM.

exhibited the properties of opioids and was similar in action to methadone. The first clinical studies of LAAM focused on its analgesic properties and abuse potential (Keats & Beecher, 1952).

At the Addiction Research Center in Lexington, Kentucky, Fraser
and Isbell (1952) showed LAAM's ability to relieve opiate abstinence
symptoms and to cross-substitute for morphine by several routes of administration, in single and multiple doses, in small inpatient samples
of postopiate addicts and addicts maintained on morphine. Its delayed
onset and prolonged duration of action, unique among the group of
related compounds, were recognized early and suggested the presence
of active metabolites. However, in early clinical trials, repeated dosing
resulted in severe toxicity, including coma, in several postsurgical patients, and led investigators to believe that it was too toxic an analgesic; therefore, except for minor attempts to evaluate one of its active
metabolites, N-LAAM, for use in chronic pain, further investigation was
abandoned (David et al., 1956). In the 1960s, Jaffe and colleagues (1969,
1970) piloted the use of LAAM in an outpatient opiate addiction treatment program, demonstrating its usefulness as a treatment agent for
heroin addicts within the existing methadone maintenance clinic system. These results, combined with increased recognition of the short-
comings in methadone maintenance (e.g., incomplete suppression of
abstinence owing to rapid metabolism in some patients, the need for
daily dosing, and diversion of take-home doses), motivated the Division of Narcotic Addiction and Drug Abuse (DNADA) to contract, in
1969, for a supply of LAAM to be clinically tested at several drug abuse
treatment research centers (Blachly et al., 1972; Jaffe & Senay, 1971a,
Jaffe et al., 1972; Blachly et al., 1972; Senay et al., 1974; Zaks et al., 1972).

As Director of the Special Action Office for Drug Abuse Prevention (SAODAP), Dr. Jaffe set as a top priority the approval of LAAM
as an alternative to methadone. Recognizing that LAAM's development
had been impeded by the pharmaceutical industry's lack of interest in
developing a medication for a relatively small and stigmatized market,
SAODAP took the novel strategy of using the federally funded drug
abuse research community to gather and organize the data necessary
for FDA approval.

A larger supply of LAAM was obtained in 1972, and an interagen-
cy research agenda was drafted with participation from SAODAP, the
FDA, the Veterans Administration, the National Institute of Mental
Health, and the National Academy of Sciences. Necessary toxicological and teratological preclinical data were gathered in dogs and rats,
building upon those gathered in the Phase I pharmaceutical evaluation of LAAM as an analgesic and providing further evidence of the
safety of LAAM in chronic administration. By spring of 1973, sufficient

toxicological data had accumulated to initiate the first study of the safety and efficacy of LAAM maintenance in drug-addicted veterans at three VA hospitals. This pilot was expanded into the VA Cooperative Study (Ling et al., 1976), a 40-week, controlled, clinical comparison of 80 mg of LAAM, given 3 times per week, to 100 mg daily (high dose) and 50 mg daily (low dose) methadone maintenance. Over 400 male opiate addicts participated in this 12-site VA hospitals cooperative study.

A second study, initiated in 1974 and known as the SAODAP Cooperative Study, compared open, flexible doses of LAAM to methadone maintenance. This study included 636 methadone maintenance patients, at 13 clinics, randomized to either continue on methadone or begin on LAAM.

The coordination and direction of LAAM development fell to the successor to DNADA at NIMH, namely, the National Institute on Drug Abuse (NIDA), when the agency was established in 1975. Based on the available animal and clinical data, the FDA allowed researchers to provide LAAM for up to 80 weeks and to include women of nonchildbearing potential in clinical studies (Freedman & Czertko, 1981; Judson & Goldstein, 1979; Ling et al., 1980a, 1980b; Marcovici et al., 1981; Resnick et al., 1981; Trueblood et al., 1978). As clinical research continued, NIDA sought a contractor that was willing to share the cost of continued research on LAAM in exchange for the right to submit the New Drug Application (NDA) to the FDA and to market LAAM after its approval. The pharmaceutical industry did not respond; but in 1975, Whysner Associates contracted with NIDA to collect these clinical data, which resulted in the implementation of five protocols involving over 2,000 street addicts and methadone maintenance patients. Unfortunately, the subsequent submission of an NDA, in February 1980, was insufficient for review because it did not include an adequate chemistry section. A revised submission in 1981 was also not accepted for review because the data were not tabulated in the appropriate format.

During the 1980s, addiction medication development research was halted, as drug abuse research resources were directed elsewhere. It was almost a decade later when NIDA found new support from Congress with the establishment of the Medications Development Division, which set the development of LAAM as its first priority and successfully engaged Biometric Research Institute (BRI) to bring LAAM to an NDA. BRI and NIDA compiled the already extensive existing data, highlighting results from the VA, SAODAP, Whysner, and other studies in an IND (investigational new drug) submission to the FDA in 1991. In consultation with the FDA, the LAAM Labeling Assessment Study was developed, in which the adequacy of the proposed package insert, and the safety and efficacy of LAAM were evaluated in opiate addicts of the

1990s, including polydrug abusers, HIV-positive patients, and women addicts. In addition, at the FDA's request, another pharmacokinetic study of LAAM was performed in a sample of 25 male and female opiate addicts who were maintained on methadone. Data from the labeling and pharmacokinetic studies were used to support the NDA submitted by NIDA and BRI in June 1993. The final approval came in record time, and LAAM became available to clinics in August of the same year.

As of February 1995, LAAM has been approved for the treatment of opiate addiction in 37 of the 50 states. Because each state has its own approval process for the use of opiate agonist maintenance agents, getting LAAM through the state regulatory processes, which in many cases have not been used since the introduction of methadone, has limited the rate at which LAAM has been made available to treatment-seeking opiate addicts. However, LAAM is available to patients in all VA hospitals because those hospitals are exempt from state regulations. Implementation has also been slowed by uncertainty about the funding of LAAM maintenance treatment; public assistance moneys currently fund methadone maintenance in many states, but LAAM has not yet been approved for such reimbursement. Historical, political, and social forces in the 1970s and 1980s delayed LAAM's approval time, while in the 1990s regulatory and financial concerns continue to impede its implementation.

CLINICAL PHARMACOLOGY

LAAM is a synthetic opiate agonist with action qualitatively similar to morphine, a prototype μ-agonist that affects the central nervous system and smooth muscles. The principal actions of LAAM, to which tolerance develops over time, are analgesia and sedation. An abstinence syndrome, similar to that observed with other opiates but with slower onset, less intensity, and a more protracted course, occurs on cessation after chronic dosing (Chen, 1948; Fraser & Isbell, 1952)

After subcutaneous administration, 70% of LAAM is absorbed from the injection site within the first hour. It is distributed widely throughout the body, with the highest tissue concentration in the lungs. Kidneys, spleen, liver, and fat also contain high levels of LAAM, but the levels are low in the heart, blood, and brain (Archer, 1976; Sung & Way, 1954). Despite rapid tissue uptake, the onset of opiate effect after subcutaneous administration is delayed (4–6 hours) compared to oral administration, which, while yielding lower tissue levels, results in onset of opiate effect within an hour. Less than 3% of the administered LAAM is recovered, suggesting that the bulk of the drug is metabolized. This is substantiated by the successive decrement of anal-gesic activity after administration of a metabolic inhibitor (Veach et al., 1964).

After oral administration, LAAM is well absorbed in the gastroin-testinal tract. It is metabolized by sequential n-demethylation to nor-LAAM and dinor-LAAM (Archer, 1976; McMahan et al., 1965), with a half-life of approximately 2 hours for the removal of one N-methyl group. A detectable blood level appears within 30 minutes of oral ad-ministration, peaks between 4 and 8 hours, and remains detectable for 96 hours. LAAM is excreted largely in the feces as nor-LAAM and dinor-LAAM; less than 20 percent is excreted in the urine, mostly as conjugates (Misra & Mule, 1975).

Both nor-LAAM and dinor-LAAM are potent opiate agonists, more potent in fact than the parent drug (Foldes et al., 1979; Nickander et al., 1974; Research Triangle Institute, 1984; Smits, 1974; Smits & Booher, 1973) with the former being three to six times more active than metha-done and the latter about equivalent to methadone. Moreover, both nor-LAAM and dinor-LAAM have longer half-lives than LAAM does; and, although the peak and trough blood levels for LAAM and its metabolites vary considerably after single-dose administrations, more stable steady state blood levels are achieved with repeated dosing. The combined pharmacological effects of LAAM and its active metabolites are greater after oral administration than after parenteral administra-tion. Early work by Fraser and Isbell (1952) showed that no objective opiate effects appear for 3–6 hours when 10–30 mg of LAAM is ad-ministered subcutaneously or intravenously, after which opiate effect becomes apparent over the next 12–16 hours and remains detectable for up to 72 hours. After oral administration, more-intense opiate ef-fects are observed within 90 minutes, reaching a maximum by 4 hours and, as with parenteral doses, persisting for approximately 72 hours (Fraser & Isbell, 1952). Recent work (Walsh et al., 1995) suggests that notable opiate effect can occur soon after intravenous administration. These results are consistent with self-administration studies in mon-keys that showed positive reinforcing effects occurring immediately, within minutes, but the dose level supporting self-administration was sufficiently close to toxic doses, thus detering continued self-administration in experimental animals and, by extrapolation, abuse in humans (McCarthy & Harrigan, 1975).

After multiple oral doses, the plasma concentrations of LAAM and its two principal metabolites increase from those attained after a sin-gle dose, with maximum concentration of each varying from 3- to 10-fold. The protein binding of LAAM and its metabolites in humans is weak and readily reversible and does not appear to displace the binding of the drugs. In addition, the amount of LAAM and its bound metabolites is sufficiently low so that their displacement by other drugs does not alter their pharmacological activity to a clinically significant degree (Research Triangle Institute, 1984; Toro-Goyco et al., 1980). The median terminal half-lives of nor-LAAM and dinor-LAAM are 0.7 days and 3 days, respectively, with considerable variation between individuals. The overall opiate activity after oral LAAM administration, as measured by pupillary constriction, is best represented by the time course of nor-LAAM (Misra et al., 1978). The plasma clearance of LAAM is greater in females than in males. Males evidence 42% longer terminal half-lives, primarily because of slower conversion of LAAM to nor-LAAM. Males also show a 32% longer terminal half-life for dinor-LAAM. Caucasians appear to have greater total clearance than African Americans and Hispanics. There is no trend for change in LAAM clearance as a function of dose, although naive subjects appear to be more sensitive to its agonist effects and therefore more susceptible to toxicity.

EARLY CLINICAL EXPERIENCES WITH LAAM IN OPIATE ADDICTION

Initial work by Fraser and Isbell (1952) established LAAM's ability to relieve abstinence symptoms and to cross-substitute for morphine in morphine-dependent subjects for up to 72 hours. However, interest in LAAM as an opiate substitution therapy grew only in the late 1960s and early 1970s with increasing appreciation for the success and drawbacks of methadone maintenance. Jaffe, Senay, and colleagues (Jaffe & Senay, 1971b; Jaffe et al., 1972) randomized methadone-maintained and street addicts to LAAM maintenance or methadone maintenance. In the sample of 89 LAAM-maintained patients, at an estimated dose of approximately 1.3 times the methadone dose, given three times per week, these researchers noted no significant differences from the methadone-maintained patients in opiate urine toxicology, treatment retention, clinic attendance, self-report of opiate use, and subjective complaints of anxiety. No significant adverse effects were noted in either group. In a subsequent open trial, these investigators reported slightly increased opiate toxic effects in those patients who received LAAM compared to those who received methadone. A single death occurred because of overdose.

Levine, Zaks, and colleagues (1976) also provided preliminary data on the efficacy and safety of LAAM in clinical populations. In an open comparison of methadone to LAAM, patients on 80 mg three times per week submitted the same number of opiate-positive urines as those on

100 mg of methadone daily. At doses below 80 mg three times per week, abstinence symptoms emerged before 72 hours had elapsed. LAAM side effects were rare and mild in these samples. The investigators further demonstrated that LAAM maintenance at doses above 50 mg given three times per week blocked the effects of subsequent 25-mg intravenous heroin challenges for up to 72 hours.

KEY STUDIES IN OPIATE MAINTENANCE TREATMENT

Several large-scale clinical studies have supplied the primary data that supports the approval of LAAM: the VA Cooperative Study, the SAO-DAP Cooperative Study, the Goldstein Cohort Study, the Whysner Phase III Study, and the Labeling Assessment Study. The first group of studies was performed in the early to mid-1970s, while the labeling study began in 1992.

The VA Cooperative Study, a pivotal study for FDA approval, compared LAAM to methadone (Ling et al., 1976b) in a double-blind 40-week trial at 12 VA hospitals. Four hundred thirty male patients were randomly assigned to receive either 50 mg of methadone daily, 100 mg of methadone daily, or 80 mg of LAAM three times per week (placebo was given on nondrug days). Forty-two percent of the sample completed 40 weeks of treatment. Sixty-nine percent of the LAAM group terminated early, compared to 58% in the low-dose and 48% in the high-dose methadone groups. In the last 8 weeks of the study, LAAM patients used significantly less illicit opiates than did either group of methadone patients, as evidenced by urine toxicology. Indirect measures of efficacy (retention, self-report of use, and staff global assessments) showed that LAAM and high-dose methadone were equivalent and that both were either superior to or not different from low-dose methadone. Early termination, most of which occurred in the early weeks and appeared to be related to the slow induction schedule, was higher with LAAM patients than with either of the methadone groups.

The principal supportive Phase III study for LAAM's FDA approval was the SAODAP Cooperative study that assessed the feasibility of crossing patients over from methadone to LAAM (Ling et al., 1978). The study included 636 male patients (from 16 methadone maintenance clinics) who had been stabilized on methadone for at least 3 months. Patients were randomly assigned, in an unblinded manner, (1) to cross over to LAAM on a dose equivalent to the methadone dose at which they had been stabilized or (2) to continue receiving methadone at the same dose. LAAM doses were adjusted according to individual need and physician assessment. Forty-nine percent of the sample completed the 40-week trial, with 60% of subjects dropping from the LAAM group compared to 39% of subjects from the methadone group. Rates of opiate-positive urine toxicologies did not differ between the two groups, but staff global assessments rated the LAAM patients superior on four out of eight parameters: employment/education, drug abuse, psychiatric problems, and overall adjustment. At the completion of this study, subjects were offered the option of extending the assessment period from 40 to 80 weeks; of those subjects remaining at 40 weeks, 96% of the LAAM patients opted to continue LAAM maintenance compared to 80% of the methadone patients who continued on methadone (Ling & Blaine, 1979). Thus, LAAM proved to be an acceptable pharmacotherapy. No serious adverse events were reported from either cooperative study; two deaths, unrelated to LAAM, occurred in the SAODAP study.

The Goldstein Cohort Study (Judson & Goldstein, 1979), which employed a more rapid induction schedule than the VA study did, emphasized safety outcomes as reflected by qualitative/descriptive and laboratory measurement, including quarterly electrocardiograms. One hundred sixty-nine male heroin addicts were treated for 12 months in one cohort, and 108 males were treated for 26 weeks in another. Laboratory evaluations were performed monthly and analyzed for longitudinal changes. Individual patient data were evaluated for progressive changes during treatment as far as time in treatment, dose level, and heroin use were concerned. Median retention was 10 months for the first cohort and 23 weeks for the other. There were no significant abnormal laboratory findings with chronic LAAM treatment.

Forty-seven investigators participated in the Whysner Study, which involved five separate protocols designed to establish LAAM induction, crossover from methadone, and maintenance-dosing regimens (Whysner et al., 1980). A total of 2,129 patients were enrolled, 450 street addicts and 1679 methadone maintenance patients. The first three protocols were open label; the fourth and fifth incorporated a double-blind phase prior to entering an unblinded maintenance phase. All patients received LAAM on Monday, Wednesday, and Friday. For the first two protocols, methadone maintenance patients were crossed over to LAAM at 1.2–1.3 times their daily methadone dose, and street addicts were started on 30 mg of LAAM with 5- to 10-mg increases to a target dose of 80 mg of LAAM three times per week. In the third study, crossover schedules included gradual decreases in methadone dose with concurrent gradual dose increases in LAAM. The fourth and fifth protocols inducted street addicts to LAAM by utilizing different induction schedules and a double-blind medication administration phase. In all, 0.4% of the LAAM patients in the study were eliminated because of adverse reactions, another 1.7% because of side effects, 0.9% because of feeling overmedicated during induction or crossover, and 0.2% because of other, unspecified LAAM-related reasons. Overall, 63% of LAAM patients were retained for the entire study period.

The Labeling Assessment Study was designed to address the adequacy of the proposed language for product labeling while evaluating the safety of LAAM administration in a large number of patients in the clinical environment of the 1990s (Fudala et al., 1994). Six hundred twenty-three patients, one third female, were enrolled, between June and November 1992, in 26 methadone maintenance clinics that did not have any previous experience with LAAM. Patients were either transferred to LAAM from methadone maintenance or entered LAAM treatment directly from street heroin with or without a period of methadone stabilization. No serious medical events occurred, and the response of study participants was quite positive and supportive of the value of LAAM.

In addition to the above studies, 959 patients have been treated with LAAM in eight Southern California fee-for-service methadone clinics (Tennant et al., 1986). There was no cost difference between methadone and LAAM maintenance in these settings, and many patients self-selected LAAM for the three-times-per-week dosing schedule. Patients who received LAAM decreased illicit opiate use in a magnitude comparable to those patients who received methadone. Patients who transferred from methadone performed as well as those who entered LAAM treatment from street heroin use. Two reasons given by patients for preferring LAAM over methadone were the requirement to attend the clinic less often and the perception that LAAM suppressed abstinence symptoms better. A substantial number of patients reported that if LAAM became unavailable they would rather detoxify or return to heroin use than transfer to methadone maintenance. Two patients died and two others experienced severe medical complications because of illicit drug and alcohol use early in LAAM treatment, underscoring the need for adequate patient education on the delayed onset of LAAM's opiate effect.

CLINICAL ISSUES OF LAAM TREATMENT

LAAM exerts its clinical effects in the treatment of opiate abuse by the same two mechanisms that make methadone effective (Dole & Nyswander, 1965). First, LAAM cross-substitutes for opiates of the mu-agonist type, suppressing symptoms of withdrawal in opiate-dependent individuals. Single doses of 30–60 mg of LAAM eliminate signs of abstinence for 24–48 hours in individuals maintained on high doses of morphine who are abruptly withdrawn. At higher doses (80 mg and above), suppression of withdrawal can increase to between 48 and 72 hours in most individuals. Second, repeated oral administrations of 70–100 mg of LAAM three times weekly produce cross-tolerance that blocks the subjective "high" of subsequently administered heroin for up to 72 hours.

The spectrum of safety and efficacy exhibited by LAAM is generally similar to that of methadone. In clinical trials, treatment with LAAM was found to be comparable to methadone with respect to reduction of illicit opiate use, treatment retention, employment, clinic attendance, involvement in illegal activities, and arrests. LAAM doses in the range of 60–100 mg three times per week have been shown to reduce the average frequency of urine samples positive for opiates to 15–20%, as does therapy with 50–100 mg of methadone daily. Patient acceptance and response to treatment are similar for both LAAM and methadone. LAAM appears to be most effective in patients perceived by clinicians to benefit from a reduced frequency of clinic visits and appears to be less effective in patients perceived as needing the intense support of daily clinic visits.

Potential Clinical Advantages

The clinical advantages of LAAM are related primarily to its slow onset and long duration of action. These advantages are both pharmacological and logistic. Pharmacologically, the slow onset of action makes LAAM less subject to abuse because addicts tend to seek an immediate high. With less potential for abuse, LAAM has less street value and, therefore, diminished potential for street diversion, which in turn means less loitering and drug dealing around the clinics and surrounding area, making clinics more acceptable in the community. Further, the longer duration of action provides a smoother blood level with less fluctuation between doses. Patients experience less variation of opiate effect and, because of less frequent clinic visits, have more time for pursuit of rehabilitative activities. Logistically, less frequent dosing means less paperwork, less record keeping, and less dose preparation time, enabling clinics to treat a larger number of patients. Moreover, three-times-per-week dosing diminishes the need for take-home doses, eliminating the games that patients and staff play around the issue of take-home privileges and creating a more open and honest patient–staff relationship and a more therapeutic environment at the clinic.

Clinical Management Issues

The essential requirements for LAAM maintenance are the same as for methadone maintenance. The candidate must have a documented history of opiate addiction and must be currently dependent upon opiates. LAAM is intended for use as part of a comprehensive treatment plan for opiate dependence. Supplying opiate maintenance therapy to opiate addicts for the treatment of addiction without appropriate medical evaluation, treatment planning and counseling has not been shown to be effective. Current regulations prohibit dispensing LAAM to pregnant women, nursing mothers, and persons under the age of 18, because its safety and efficacy have not been described for these groups.

Patient Selection

In general, any patient suitable for methadone maintenance can be successfully treated with LAAM. LAAM is ideally suited for patients with a moderate to severe level of dependence, for whom detoxification and other more traditional drug-free and/or opiate antagonist treatment modalities are unsuitable. In addition, there are special categories of patients who may find LAAM particularly attractive.

PERSONS WITH TRANSPORTATION OR SCHEDULING PROBLEMS

Persons reliant upon public transportation, or those who miss clinic visits because of car problems, missed rides, and so forth, can benefit from the three-times-per-week dosing schedule. Patients whose employment or education schedules conflict with daily clinic attendance often find LAAM treatment more convenient. Frequently, patients' work hours overlap dosing hours, or patients' work hours change on short notice. For parents of small children (primarily single mothers), child care arrangements can be a problem that interferes with daily clinic attendance. The 3-days-per-week LAAM schedule can significantly reduce these obstacles to treatment participation.

PERSONS WITH PAST HISTORY OF METHADONE FAILURE

Some patients rapidly metabolize on daily doses of methadone and report that it does not "hold" them for the entire 24 hours or that it causes unwanted acute sedation. The gradual onset and long duration of action associated with LAAM provide better and more complete opioid substitution than methadone does for these patients. Thus, a history of nonresponsivity to methadone may indicate more favorable response to LAAM treatment.

PERSONS WITH A FEAR OF METHADONE MAINTENANCE

Many negative myths and rumors exist about methadone. As a result, many addicts, especially those who are less involved in the drug-abusing community but who could benefit from methadone, refuse to enter methadone maintenance treatment. Others avoid methadone because of the perceived social stigma of its use. LAAM provides a fresh start as a treatment unburdened by bias and ignorance.

Induction

Patients can be inducted directly into LAAM treatment from street heroin or can be transferred to LAAM treatment after a period of methadone stabilization and maintenance. The initial dose depends upon the patient's degree of dependence. In general, the recommended starting dose for street addicts is between 20 and 40 mg with successive every-other-day dose adjustments of 5–10 mg until a pharmacokinetic and pharmacodynamic steady state is reached, usually within 1 or 2 weeks. In some cases, patients can be started on methadone to facilitate more rapid titration to an effective dose and then can be converted to LAAM maintenance after a few weeks of methadone therapy.

For patients who already are receiving methadone maintenance, most can transfer to LAAM at a three-times-per-week dose that is slightly higher than their daily methadone dose. The recommended initial dose of LAAM is 1.2 to 1.3 times the patient's daily dose of methadone, not to exceed 120 mg. Subsequent doses, administered at 48- to 72-hour intervals, can be adjusted according to clinical response. The crossover from methadone to LAAM should be accomplished in a single dose; complete transfer to LAAM is simpler and preferable to more complex regimens that involve escalating doses of LAAM and decreasing doses of methadone.

Initial dose adjustments with LAAM are somewhat more complex than with methadone because of the former's delayed onset of action. If the starting dose is too high or if the dose is escalated too rapidly for the patient's level of tolerance, excessive opioid effect may occur, namely, sedation, orthostatic hypotension, difficulty with concentration. In rare instances, opiate overdose may occur, leading to profound central nervous system and respiratory depression. Patients must be warned that the peak activity of LAAM is not immediate and that the use or abuse of other psychoactive drugs, including alcohol, may result in a fatal overdose, especially with the first few doses of LAAM, whether during initiation of treatment or after a lapse in treatment. During initiation, clonidine may be used as an adjunct to help relieve symptoms of withdrawal until the full effects of LAAM become evident. LAAM and its metabolites quickly accumulate to toxic levels if the doses intended for three-times-per-week dosing are given too frequently. It may be advisable to keep the patients in the clinic for several hours after the first LAAM dose so that its effects can be monitored and secondary drug ingestion discouraged.

Dosage Regimen

LAAM is not simply a long-acting form of methadone but is a fundamentally different medication. It is administered on a three-times-per-week dosing schedule and should never be given daily. Most patients will stabilize on LAAM doses in the range of 60–90 mg three times per week. Doses as low as 10 mg and as high as 140 mg three times per week have been used successfully in clinical trials. The maximum total amount of LAAM recommended for any patient is 140–140–140 mg or 130–130–180 mg on a thrice-weekly schedule or 140 mg every other day.

The dose of LAAM should be chosen and adjusted as needed to provide a dose high enough to suppress withdrawal, illicit drug seeking and usage, and related high-risk behaviors. As with methadone, an important explanation for continued abuse of illicit opiates relates to inadequate dosing. If opioid side effects persist once illicit drug use is controlled, the dose of LAAM may require further adjustment to minimize adverse effects. Care providers should be alert to individual differences in levels of opiate tolerance and interpatient variability in the absorption, distribution, and metabolism of both LAAM and its metabolites.

There is limited experience in detoxifying patients from LAAM in a systematic manner. The decision to discontinue LAAM maintenance depends on the patient's readiness to adopt a drug-free lifestyle. When discontinuation is considered appropriate, LAAM should be gradually reduced (5–10 mg/week) to minimize the danger of relapse.

Managing Weekends and Missed Clinic Visits

Supplemental dosing prior to the 72-hour interdose interval (i.e., the weekend for a person medicated on a Monday–Wednesday–Friday schedule) is rarely needed. If withdrawal becomes problematic during this time period, the preceding dose may be increased in 5- to 10-mg increments up to 40% over the usual dose. In some cases, an every-other-day schedule may be appropriate if clinic hours and staffing permit. Otherwise, the patient's schedule may be adjusted so that the 72-hour interval occurs during the week — which, in itself, may be sufficient, or the patient can come to the clinic to receive a small supplemental dose of LAAM or methadone. Simply changing the dosing schedule from Monday–Wednesday–Friday to Tuesday–Thursday–Saturday enables many patients to remain abstinent over the weekend.

There now are recommended protocols for planned temporary interruption of LAAM maintenance, and dose reduction following an unplanned lapse in dosing. As currently regulated, LAAM take-home doses are not permitted. Patients who would currently be eligible for take-home doses of methadone and who are unable to attend the clinic because of personal illness, crisis, or other hardship may be temporarily transferred directly to methadone. Methadone doses should be 80% of the patient's Monday and Wednesday dose, with the first dose being ingested no sooner than 48 hours after the last LAAM dose. Thus, the number of methadone take-home doses should be two less than the number of days of expected absence. Under no circumstances should the number of take-home doses exceed those allowed in methadone regulations. Upon return to the clinic, patients should resume LAAM maintenance, following the same dosing regimen prior to the temporary interruption. If more than 48 hours have elapsed since the last methadone dose, patients should be reinducted into LAAM treatment at a dose determined by clinical or toxicological evaluation by the clinic physician.

Following the lapse of one LAAM dose, if a patient returns to the clinic to be dosed on the day following the missed dose, the regular Monday and Wednesday dose should be administered and continued every other day, through the 72-hour interval, until the usual thrice-weekly schedule can be resumed. If a patient returns to the clinic on the day of the next scheduled dose, the usual dose will be well tolerated in most instances, although a reduced dose may be appropriate in cases where illicit opiate use over the missed interval is suspected. Following a lapse of more than one LAAM dose, patients should be reinducted at an initial dose of one half to three quarters of their previous LAAM dose, followed by 5- to 10-mg dose increases every dosing day (48- to 72-hour intervals) until their previous Monday and Wednesday dose is achieved. Patients who have been off LAAM for more than a week should be reinducted as previously described for the street addict.

Other Clinical Issues

Reported adverse reactions to LAAM for persons with demonstrated opiate dependence and tolerance are rare. Side effects are generally those observed with opiates and include nausea, vomiting, constipation, excessive sweating, decreased sexual interest, and delayed ejaculation. All but a few cases of LAAM overdose have involved multiple drugs and, when encountered, should be treated with naloxone once a patent airway is established. Because of the long-acting nature of LAAM, a continuous naloxone infusion to treat overdose is preferred to oral naltrexone, which may precipitate prolonged opioid withdrawal symptoms. LAAM should be used cautiously in patients with known hepatic or respiratory disease or with cardiac conduction defects. Interactions with alcohol, sedatives, tranquilizers, antidepressants, or benzodiazipines carry serious risk of overdose for persons maintained on LAAM; thus, LAAM should be administered cautiously in persons who abuse any of these drugs.

CLINICAL IMPLICATIONS OF LAAM AVAILABILITY

Impact of Treatment Philosophy

Thirty years of experience in the United States with methadone maintenance has clearly demonstrated the efficacy of opiate substitution therapy for the treatment of opiate addiction. But there remain aspects of methadone maintenance that make it less than ideal for all opiate addicts. The availability of LAAM, potentially the first of a series of alternative pharmacotherapies, affords the treatment community, as well as policy makers, an opportunity to reconsider the philosophy and treatment delivery system governing the current practice of methadone maintenance. This treatment is the most highly regulated of all medical practices and is set apart from mainstream medicine, even from the mental health system, despite wide recognition of the high prevalence of comorbidity between addictions and psychiatric disorders.

It is not always clear how the current treatment philosophy of chronic heroin addicts came about, but the fact that virtually all methadone clinics operate apart from the general medical care setting makes clear the message that society views the addict on methadone maintenance as being quite different from general medical patients. The public policy regulating methadone clinics declares to patients, clinicians, and the community at large that methadone maintenance patients are not that far removed from criminals. Unfortunately, patients often, in turn, live up to their reputations, providing policy makers further justification for their approach. A vicious cycle ensues, and over time methadone maintenance has acquired many stigmas. Few general physicians know anything about methadone maintenance treatment, and fewer still ever bother to find out. Methadone maintenance treatment is largely viewed as incompatible with general medical service. Little wonder then that only 10% of chronic heroin addicts who can benefit from methadone maintenance are in the treatment system—thousands more are turned away by the stigmatization of the treatment system. If LAAM and other new and innovative pharmacotherapies are to have a significant impact on the treatment of these patients, the entire treatment philosophy and strategy of delivery must change so that opiate substitute therapy can take its proper place among medical services. There is no compelling reason to believe that LAAM and other opiate substitute therapies, freed from the constraints of unreasonable regulation, cannot be delivered within the context of other medical and mental health services, drawing into treatment an entire population of heretofore untreated or unwilling-to-be-treated patients.

Impact of Treatment Strategy

In contrast to the required daily administration of methadone, LAAM is administered only three times per week. Hence, LAAM represents a true treatment alternative that may be optimally tailored to the needs of the patient or to the specific stage of the recovery process. During the first 2 weeks, patients need much reassurance and support to adjust to the alternate-day dosing schedule. The availability of counselors experienced with LAAM maintenance and well trained to educate and support patients during the first several weeks on LAAM is critical to the successful implementation of treatment.

LAAM benefits not only patients and clinic staff but also the larger community within which LAAM administration takes place. For a patient already receiving opiate substitution (methadone) treatment, the three-times-per-week dosing schedule provides more time for activities characteristic of a non-drug-abuse lifestyle, such as employment and educational and family activities. As noted previously, the relatively stable pharmacokinetic profile of LAAM and its metabolites provides a patient with a smoother drug response and less daily fluctuation of drug effects. Since take-home doses are often unnecessary (and unavailable, under current LAAM regulations), a patient is less tempted or pressured to abuse or sell the medication, and the danger of accidental poisoning is obviated. Because of its slow and limited onset of action, LAAM is not likely to be abused intravenously. It will have little street value, and the danger of diversion is thereby diminished. As Goldstein (1994) points out, the harm caused to society by take-home methadone diversion "could have been eliminated long ago by authorization of the use of LAAM" (p. 149).

The benefits of LAAM maintenance to clinic staff and administration are significant. Less staff and nursing hours are required to medicate the same number of patients, increasing the ability of a clinic to serve more patients. Clinics may limit their hours of service, and relatively expensive weekend medication hours can be shortened or even discontinued. Time spent evaluating which patients should receive or lose take-home dose privileges and completing the associated take-home dose preparation and documentation will be freed, further enhancing staff productivity. LAAM maintenance treatment will also benefit the local clinic community and larger society as well. Neighborhoods will welcome clinics that reduce loitering by minimizing the number of patient visits and shortening clinic hours. As drug treatment settings become increasingly integrated with health care services, three-times-per-week LAAM administration is more compatible with a general health care clinic environment. The lack of take-home opiate doses on the street will decrease street diversion and related criminal activity around the clinic. Finally, attracting currently untreated heroin addicts to treatment will help stop the spread of HIV via intravenous heroin use. In time, the greater community will better recognize the benefits of opiate substitution maintenance therapy.

Integration with Other Opiate Pharmacotherapies

LAAM may be most suitable for opiate addicts who have a significant level of dependence but who are relatively stable with respect to social, employment, legal, financial, health, and/or psychological functioning, including patients who have not yet exhausted their resources and/or are not heavily involved in the drug culture. LAAM may thus attract to treatment an entirely new subpopulation of opiate addicts.

With the availability of buprenorphine, a sequential model of opiate substitution therapy can be envisioned (see Figure 12.1). Because of its partial opiate agonist activity, daily buprenorphine can be the first substitution agent offered to treatment-seeking opiate addicts, and buprenorphine is expected to be especially effective for those with a relatively mild, short history of addiction. For these individuals, buprenorphine should effectively cross-substitute for heroin, should not significantly increase physical dependence, and should make detoxification, if desired, an easier process than withdrawal from a full agon-

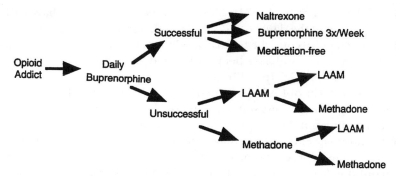

FIGURE 12.1. Sequential pharmacotherapeutic strategy for opioid dependence.

ist. Those who do well on daily buprenorphine may continue on daily doses of buprenorphine, may continue buprenorphine in one of several less-than-daily dosing schedules that are currently being evaluated, or may choose to undergo detoxification from buprenorphine with or without subsequent naltrexone therapy.

For those who do not do well on buprenorphine maintenance, LAAM and methadone should be considered next. LAAM is indicated for those patients who evidence relative stability in psychosocial, health, and economic functioning; who would benefit from the three-times-per-week dosing schedule, and/or who have found methadone maintenance to be unacceptable. Methadone is appropriate for those with more chaotic lifestyles and/or significant health and psychosocial problems (i.e., lack of housing, depression) such that daily clinic contact would help them to get off the street and to stabilize in treatment. Once illicit drug use is controlled and lifestyle stabilized, a transfer to LAAM may be considered.

Thus, if the severity of addiction and its associated lifestyle and health and social problems are conceptualized as existing on a continuum, persons with relatively mild addiction symptomatology might best respond to buprenorphine, while those severely affected may require methadone maintenance to improve. LAAM would be indicated for patients whose addiction severity falls between the two extremes, effectively widening the range of patients who can receive and benefit from opiate substitution therapy.

Remaining Research and Clinical Issues

Further research is needed to change the current LAAM dispensing regulations so that a larger population of opiate addicts can benefit from LAAM maintenance. Currently, pregnant women and adolescents are excluded from receiving LAAM therapy, although they represent subpopulations of addicts for whom LAAM may be uniquely useful. In addition, the safety and feasibility of providing take-home doses of LAAM must be empirically assessed.

LAAM IN PREGNANCY

Although it is always desirable for a woman to be drug free during pregnancy, complete abstinence is often difficult for opiate addicts to achieve. Acute opiate withdrawal can be harmful to the fetus, and relapse is frequent. Rather than run the risk of harming the pregnant woman who is using illicit opiates, it is better for the mother and the baby to be stabilized on opiate substitution therapy during pregnancy so that the mother's addiction as well as perinatal needs can be addressed. LAAM's relatively stable profile and long duration of action would seem advantageous in this context; and since LAAM is a new pharmacotherapeutic option, it may attract previously unserved pregnant opiate addicts to treatment. The preclinical data demonstrating the safety of LAAM during pregnancy and its lack of teratological effects suggest that its use in pregnancy warrants further examination.

LAAM IN ADOLESCENTS

LAAM may be a particularly helpful pharmacotherapeutic agent for adolescents who are dependent on opiates. Rather than expose adolescents daily to the methadone clinic environment and clientele, the three-times-per-week dosing schedule provides relative freedom from the treatment site and enables adolescents to participate in educational, social, and recreational activities crucial to their rehabilitation. Although opiate maintenance is never a preferred treatment modality for young addicts, a clearly effective intervention is needed for high-risk youths whose continued drug use exposes them to HIV and increased addiction severity. Future research must evaluate whether LAAM provides an acceptable treatment option for this population.

TAKE-HOME DOSES

Although the three-times-per-week dosing schedule obviates the need for take-home doses of LAAM in most clinical situations, from time to time a circumstance will arise (i.e., a personal or family hardship that entails a temporary absence from the clinic) that may require a take-home dose. Rather than transfer the patient to methadone in order to receive take-home doses, creating administrative headaches and resulting in uneven opiate substitution effects for the patient, it would be easier to simply provide patients with a dose or two of their usual medication. As noted previously, the slow onset of LAAM's opiate effects should diminish its risk of street diversion, making it a more suitable take-home medication than methadone. The current prohibition of take-home doses of LAAM is based solely on regulatory considerations. Careful clinical evaluation is needed to provide meaningful data for reconsideration of such prohibition.

CONCLUSION

The unique pharmacological properties of LAAM make it a novel alternative substitution pharmacotherapy for opiate addiction. LAAM's delayed onset and long duration of action enable dosing on a three-times-per-week schedule, making it suitable for the sizable subpopulation of opiate addicts who find methadone an ineffective or unacceptable treatment agent. Further, the introduction of LAAM into the opiate treatment arena fosters a reexamination of, and portends fundamental changes in, the current treatment delivery system of addiction pharmacotherapy. The heavily regulated and isolated methadone dispensary is quickly becoming antiquated within the rapidly changing health care delivery environment. The recent approval of LAAM provides the opportunity to explore creative integration of addiction pharmacotherapy into the comprehensive health maintenance organizations of the 1990s, minimizing the stigma and improving the quality of care associated with opiate addiction treatment.

REFERENCES

Archer, S. (1976). Preclinical studies: Pharmacology of LAAM. In J. D. Blaine & P. F. Renault (Eds), *Rx: 3×/week LAAM alternative to Methadone* (NIDA Research Monograph No. 8, pp. 10–13). Rockville, MD: National Institute on Drug Abuse.

Blachly, P. H., Aavid, N. A., & Irwin, S. (1972). Alpha-acetylmethadol (LAM): Comparison of laboratory findings, electroencephalograms, and Cornell Medical Index of patients stabilized on LAM with those on methadone. In A. Goldstein (Ed.), *Proceedings of Fourth National Conference on Methadone Treatment* (pp. 203–205). New York: National Association for Prevention of Addiction to Narcotics.

Chen, K. K. (1948). Pharmacology of methadone and related compounds. *Annals of the New York Academy of Sciences, 51*, 83–87.

David, N. A., Semler, H. J., & Burgner, P. R. (1956). Control of chronic pain by d-l-alpha-acetylmethadol. Journal of the American Medical Association, 161(7), 599–603.

Dole, U. P., & Nyswander, M. A. (1965). A medical treatment for diacetylmorphine (heroin) addiction. *Journal of the American Medical Association, 193,* 646.

Foldes, B. S., Shivaku, Y., Matsuo, S., & Morita, K. (1979). The influence of methadone derivatives on the isolated myenteric plexus-longitudinal muscle preparation of the guinea pig ileum. *Advances in Pharmacological Research and Practice: Proceedings of the 3rd Congress of the Hungarian Pharmacological Society, 5,* 165–170.

Fraser, H. F., & Isbell, H. (1952). Actions and addiction liabilities of alpha-acetylmethadols in man. *Journal of Pharmacology and Experimental Therapeutics, 105,* 458–465.F

Freedman, R. R., & Czertko, G. (1981). A comparison of thrice weekly LAAM and daily methadone in employed heroin addicts. *Drug and Alcohol Dependence, 8*(3), 215–222.

Fudala, P. J., Montgomery, A., Herbert, S., Mojsiak, J., Rosenberg, S., & Vocci, F. (1994). *A multicenter, labeling assessment study of levo-alpha-acetylmethadol (LAAM) for the maintenance treatment of opiate addicts* (NIDA Research Monograph No. 141). Rockville, MD: National Institute on Drug Abuse.

Goldstein, A. (1994). Addictive tranquility: The opiates. In A. Goldstein (Ed), *Addiction: From biology to drug policy* (pp. 137–154). New York: Freeman.

Jaffe, J. H., Schuster, C. R., Smith, B. B., et al. (1969). Comparison of DL-alpha-acetylmethadol and methadone in the treatment of narcotics addicts [Abstract]. *Pharmacologist, 11.* 256.

Jaffe, J. H., Schuster, C. R., Smith, B. B., & Blachly, P. H. (1970). Comparison of acetylmethadol and methadone in the treatment of long-term heroin users: A pilot study. *Journal of the American Medical Association, 211,* 1834–1836.

Jaffe, J. H., & Senay, E. C. (1971a). Methadone and 1-methadylacetate. Use in management of narcotics addicts. *Journal of the American Medical Association, 216,* 1303–1305.

Jaffe, J. H., & Senay, E. C. (1971b). Methadone and L-methadylacetate: Use in management of narcotic addicts. *Journal of the American Medical Association, 216,* 1834–1836.

Jaffe, J. H., Senay, E. C., Schuster, C. R., & Renault, P. R. (1972). Methadyl acetate vs. methadone: A double-blind study in heroin users. *Journal of the American Medical Association, 222,* 437–442.

Judson, B. A., & Goldstein, A. (1979). Levo-alpha-acetylmethadol (LAAM) in treatment of heroin addicts: I. Dosage schedule for induction and stabilization. *Drug and Alcohol Dependence, 4*(6), 461–466.

Keats, A. S., & Beecher, H. K. (1952). Analgesic activity and toxic effects of acetylmethadol isomers in man. *Journal of Pharmacology and Experimental Therapeutics, 105,* 210–215.

Levine, R., Zaks, A., Fink, M., & Freedman, A. M. (1976). Levomethadyl acetate: Prolonged duration of opioid effects, including cross tolerance to heroin, in man. In *Problems of drug dependence* (NIDA Research Monograph No. 8, pp. 84–85). Rockville, MD: National Institute on Drug Abuse.

Ling, W., & Blaine, J. D. (1979). The use of LAAM in treatment. In R. L. Dupont, A. Goldstein, & J. O'Donnell (Eds.), *Handbook on drug abuse* (pp. 87–96). Washington, DC: National Institute on Drug Abuse, U.S. Department of Health, Education and Welfare.

Ling, W., Blakis, E. D., Holmes, E. D., Kleet, C. J., & Carter, W. E. (1980a). Restabilization on methadone after methadyl acetate (LAAM) maintenance. *Archives of General Psychiatry, 37,* 194–196.

Ling, W., Charuvastra, V. C., Kaim, S. C., & Klett, C. J. (1976a). Methadyl acetate and mmethadone maintenance as maintenance treatments for heroin addicts. *Archives of General Psychiatry, 33,* 709–720.

Ling, W., Charuvastra, V. C., Kaim, S. C., & Klett, C. J. (1976b). ethadyl acetate and methadone maintenance treatments for heroin addicts: A Veterans Administration Cooperative Study. *Archives of General Psychiatry, 33,* 391–393.

Ling, W., Klett, C. J., & Gillis, R. D. (1978). A cooperative clinical study of methadyl acetate. *Archives of General Psychiatry, 35,* 345–353.

Ling, W., Klett, C. J., & Gillis, R. D. (1980b). A cooperative clinical study of methadyl acetate: II. Friday-only regimen. *Archives of General Psychiatry, 37,* 908–911.

Marcovici, M., O'Brien, C. P., McLellan, A. T., et al. (1981). A clinical, controlled study of acetylmethadol in the treatment of narcotic addiction. *American Journal of Psychiatry, 138*(2), 234–236.

McCarthy, D. A., & Harrigan, S. E. (1975, April 1). *Preclinical pharmacological and toxicological evaluation of compounds used in the treatment of narcotic addiction #63. Methadyl acetate self-administration by monkeys.* NIDA Contract HSM-42-72-167 (unpublished report submitted to FDA in new drug application).

McMahan, R. E., Culp, H. W., & Marshall, F. J. (1965). The metabolism of l-a-acetylmethadol in the rat: The identification of the probable active metabolite. *Journal of Pharmacology and Experimental Therapeutics, 149,* 436–445.

Misra, A. L., & Mule, S. J. (1975). L-a-Acetylmethadol (LAAM) pharmacokinetics and metabolism: Current status. *American Journal of Drug and Alcohol Abuse, 2,* 301–305.

Misra, A. L., Mule, S. J., Bloch, R., & Bates, T. R. (1978). Physiological disposition and biotransformation of l-a-[2-^{3}H] acetylmethadol (LAAM) in acutely and chronically treated monkeys. *Journal of Pharmacology and Experimental Therapeutics, 206*(2), 475–491.

Nickander, R., Booher, R., & Miles, H. (1974). L-a-Acetylmethadol and its N-demethylated metabolites have potent opiate actions in guinea pig isolated ileum. *Life Sciences, 14,* 2011–2017.

Research Triangle Institute. (1984, September). *Bioavailability and pharmacokinetics/pharmacodynamics of L-a-acetylmethadol and its metabolites: Metabolism and pharmacokinetics of drugs.* Final Report for Contract #771-80-3705, Task #2.

Resnick, R. B., Washton, A. M., Garwood, J., & Perzel, J. (1981). LAAM instead of take-home methadone. In L. S. Harris (Ed.), *Problems of drug dependence* (NIDA Research Monograph No. 41, pp. 473–475). Rockville, MD: National Institute on Drug Abuse.

Senay, E. C., Jaffe, J. H., diMenza, S., & Renault, P. F. (1974). A 48-week study of methadone, methadyl acetate, and minimal services. In S. Fisher & A. M. Freedman (Eds.), *Opiate addiction: Origins and treatment* (pp. 185–200). Washington, DC: Winston.

Smits, S. E. (1974). The analgesic activity of l-a-acetylmethadol and two of its metabolites in mice. *Research Communications in Chemical Pathology–Pharmacology, 8,* 575–578.

Smits, S. E., & Booher, R. (1973). Analgesic activity of some of the metabolites of methadone and α-acetylmethadol in mice and rats. *Federal Proceedings, 32,* 764.

Sung, C., & Way, E. L. (1954). The fate of optical isomers of a-acetylmethadol. *Journal of Pharmacology and Experimental Therapeutics, 110,* 260–270.

Tennant, F. S., Rawson, R. A., Pumphrey, E., et al. (1986). Clinical experiences with 959 opioid-dependent patients treated with levo-alpha-acetylmethadol (LAAM). *Journal of Substance Abuse Treatment, 3*(3), 195–202.

Toro-Goyco, E., Martin, B. R., & Harris, L. S. (1980). The binding of LAAM and its metabolites to blood constituents. In L. S. Harris (Ed.), *Problems of drug dependence. 1979: Proceedings of the 41st Annual Scientific Meeting of the Committee on Problems of Drug Dependence* (NIDA Research Monograph No. 27, pp. 54–60). Washington, DC, National Institute on Drug Abuse.

Trueblood, B., Judson, B. A., & Goldstein, A. (1978). Acceptability of methadyl acetate (LAAM) as compared with methadone in a treatment program for heroin addicts. *Drug and Alcohol Dependence, 3*(2), 125–132.

Veach, R. M., Adler, T. K., & Way, E. L. (1964). The importance of steric configuration in certain morphine mimetic actions of synthetic analgetics. *Journal of Pharmacology and Experimental Therapeutics, 145,* 11–19.

Walsh, S. L., Johnson, R. E., Stitzer, M. L., & Bigelow, G. E. (1995). *Acute effects of intravenous and oral LAAM in human substance abusers.* Presentation of the Committe on Problems of Drug Dependence, Scottsdale, Arizona.

Whysner, J. A., Thomas, D. B., Ling, W., & Charuvastra, C. (1980). On the relative efficacy of LAAM and methadone. In L. S. Harris (Ed.), *Problems on drug dependence: Proceedings of the 41st Annual Scientific Meeting of the Committee on Problems of Drug Dependence* (NIDA Research Monograph No. 27, pp. 429–434). Rockville, MD: National Institute on Drug Abuse.

Zaks, A., Fink, M., & Freedman, A. M. (1972). Levomethadol in maintenance treatment of opiate dependence. *Journal of the American Medical Association, 220*(6), 811–813.

Chapter 13

BUPRENORPHINE

Alison Oliveto, Ph.D.
Thomas R. Kosten, M.D.

Buprenorphine was developed as part of an intense interest in the synthesis and study of opioid compounds with mixed-action agonist–antagonist effects (Hart & McCawley, 1944; Lewis, 1982). Marketed as an injectable analgesic, buprenorphine was shown to be 25–40 times more potent than morphine (Houde, 1979; Jasinski et al., 1978; Lewis et al., 1982). Jasinski and colleagues (1978) then demonstrated that buprenorphine could relieve acute opioid withdrawal and craving and thus began more than a decade of clinical and behavioral pharmacological research on buprenorphine. This research has substantiated buprenorphine's potential as a treatment for opiate dependence, and buprenorphine is presently undergoing the U.S. Food and Drug Administration approval process.

MEDICINAL CHEMISTRY/PHARMACOKINETICS

Buprenorphine, an oripavine derivative of the opium alkaloid thebaine, is a congener of the opioid agonist etorphine and the opioid antagonist diprenorphine (Lewis, 1973). It is metabolized in the body by both N-dealkylation and conjugation and has a terminal half-life of approximately 3–5 hours (Bullingham et al., 1983), but its opioid activity can be prolonged by high doses for 3 days (Rosen et al., 1994). After sublingual administration buprenorphine has about 55% bioavailability at a 0.4- or 0.8-mg dose (Bullingham et al., 1983) and peak plasma concentrations that occur approximately 3 hours later (Jasinski et al., 1978).

PHARMACOLOGY AND SAFETY PROFILE

Opioid compounds bind to several recognition sites in the brain: μ, κ, and δ receptors. Buprenorphine binds to all three types of receptors, with an order of greatest affinity for $\mu \geq \kappa > \delta$ receptors (Richards & Sadee, 1985; Sadee et al., 1982). A unique characteristic of buprenorphine is that it dissociates very slowly from opioid receptor binding sites (Hambrook & Rance, 1976; Rance & Dickens, 1978). This binding characteristic may contribute to its very long action.

Activities at μ-opioid and κ-opioid receptors are associated with different behavioral profiles, but buprenorphine's μ activity is probably most important for treating heroin addicts. Buprenorphine has been classified as a morphine-like (μ) partial agonist (Martin et al., 1976), based on behavioral observations that buprenorphine had effects similar to morphine but produced ceiling effects on several measures. Furthermore, buprenorphine can block the analgesic effects of pure agonists such as morphine or heroin.

In nonhumans, buprenorphine's analgesic effects are complex. For instance, in some pain assays, low doses of buprenorphine produce maximal analgesic effects, whereas higher doses produce attenuated effects, producing an inverted-U-shaped function (Rance, 1979). This dose–effect configuration is highly unusual and is thought to result from some form of autoinhibition (Woods et al., 1992). When low doses of buprenorphine are administered with full opioid agonists such as morphine, buprenorphine antagonizes the analgesic effects of these compounds. The larger the dose of buprenorphine administered, the longer the duration of the antagonist effect. This characteristic is thought to result at least in part from buprenorphine's slow dissociation from opioid receptors. Overall, buprenorphine's analgesic profile is consistent with buprenorphine's partial opioid agonist activity and relatively "irreversible" binding to the μ-opioid receptor (Woods et al., 1992).

When the effects of buprenorphine and morphine on respiration were compared, morphine produced dose-related increases in arterial carbon dioxide, whereas buprenorphine produced an inverted-U-shaped dose–effect curve (Doxey et al., 1977). As buprenorphine doses rose to what might become toxic doses of a full agonist by producing respiratory suppression, this respiratory suppression began to reverse, and carbon dioxide levels in the blood dropped. Since arterial carbon dioxide levels directly reflect the risk for respiratory arrest and death from opioids, this U-shaped response suggests greater safety from overdose with buprenorphine. Furthermore, maximal increases in carbon dioxide produced by buprenorphine were much less than that produced by morphine (Doxey et al., 1977), which provides more support for the relative safety of buprenorphine.

ABUSE LIABILITY AND TREATMENT POTENTIAL

Buprenorphine's abuse liability has been examined in several animal species. Buprenorphine is readily self-administered by rhesus monkeys at doses of 0.01–0.1 mg/kg/injection (Mello et al., 1981) and by macaque monkeys at doses of 0.003–0.1 mg/kg/injection (Young et al., 1984). In contrast, the rate at which buprenorphine is self-administered in baboons is lower than that for other partial μ-opioid agonists (Lukas et al., 1983) and is similar to vehicle in postaddict rats (Khazan et al., 1984). Buprenorphine also elicits conditioned place preference with an inverted-U-shaped dose–effect function (Brown et al., 1991), suggesting that buprenorphine exhibits fewer reinforcing effects than either full agonists or other partial agonists do.

Buprenorphine has also been examined for its ability to alter the self-administration of other compounds. For instance, buprenorphine has been compared with the full opioid agonist methadone in its ability to suppress opiate self-administration by macaque monkeys (Mello et al., 1983). Buprenorphine suppressed heroin self-administration at doses equivalent to 24–48 mg/day in humans, whereas methadone did not significantly alter heroin self-administration in four of five monkeys at doses equivalent to 100–800 mg/day in humans (Mello et al., 1983). The ability of buprenorphine to suppress heroin self-administration by heroin-dependent men has also been examined (Mello & Mendelson, 1980; Mello et al., 1982). Compared to placebo, buprenorphine at 4–8 mg/day significantly suppressed the degree to which subjects self-administered heroin.

Doses of buprenorphine found to alter opiate self-administration in nonhumans also suppress cocaine self-administration in a dose-related manner (Mello et al., 1989). Interestingly, buprenorphine enhances the reinforcing effects of cocaine as measured by conditioned place preference when administered acutely (Brown et al., 1991) but attenuates cocaine-induced conditioned place preference when administered chronically (Kosten et al., 1991). The results of these studies suggest that chronic buprenorphine maintenance may be a useful treatment strategy for both opioid and cocaine abuse.

As mentioned earlier, Jasinski and colleagues were the first to examine buprenorphine's potential utility as a treatment agent for opioid dependence. In their definitive work, Jasinski and colleagues (1978) showed that buprenorphine maintenance (8 mg/day, subcutaneous) attenuated the subjective and physiological effects of high doses of morphine (60–120 mg, subcutaneous) for up to 30 hours. Upon abrupt termination of buprenorphine maintenance, a delayed withdrawal syndrome of mild severity occurred, suggesting that buprenorphine does not produce significant physical dependence in humans. These findings stimulated a host of human laboratory studies to characterize more fully buprenorphine's behavioral effects.

Several studies examined the agonist and antagonist actions of buprenorphine in both opioid-dependent and -nondependent humans. In non-dependent humans, buprenorphine at doses of 0.4 and 0.8 mg/70 kg, intramuscular, produces dose-related agonist-like effects on physiological and self-report measures, including pupillary construction, self-reported "high," and drug "liking" (Weinhold et al., 1992). When the opioid antagonist naloxone was administered concurrently with buprenorphine, buprenorphine's effects were attenuated. Another study examined the effects of larger acute doses of buprenorphine (i.e., up to 32 mg) in nondependent humans (Walsh et al., 1994). Buprenorphine produced dose-related increases in self-reported drug effects such as sedation, dysphoria, "good effects," and "high" up to doses of 4–16 mg with no further increases at higher doses. Buprenorphine produced significant long-lasting pupillary constriction but minimal respiratory depression and no effect on percentage of oxygen saturation as measured by pulse oximetry. No serious adverse effects occurred, although unpleasant side effects such as nausea, vomiting, and insomnia were reported. These findings suggest that there are ceiling effects on the self-reported and physiological effects of buprenorphine.

Buprenorphine's effects have been compared via the sublingual (1, 2, and 4 mg) and subcutaneous (1 and 2 mg) routes in nondependent opioid abusers (Jasinski et al., 1989). Regardless of route, buprenorphine produced μ-opioid agonist-like effects and miosis but no significant changes in respiration, body temperature, or cardiovascular measures. The relative potency of sublingual to subcutaneously administered buprenorphine was calculated to be approximately two thirds. These results suggest that buprenorphine's profile of effects is similar across routes of administration (Jasinski et al., 1989). Buprenorphine at doses of 0.3–1.2 mg via the intravenous route produces effects similar to that via subcutaneous and sublingual routes but with greater agonist-like effects, including miosis, decreased respiration rate, increased diastolic blood pressure, and increased ratings on "liking," "good effects," euphoria, and sedation (Pickworth et al., 1993). These results suggest that buprenorphine has higher abuse liability via the intravenous route.

The ability of buprenorphine to block the effects of the opioid agonist hydromorphone (cumulative subcutaneous doses of 0, 6, and 18 mg) was also examined in individuals who were maintained on ascending doses of buprenorphine (2, 4, 8, and 16 mg). Hydromorphone was tested after subjects were maintained on each buprenorphine dose for at least 10 days and 24 hours after the prior buprenorphine dose. Hydromorphone produced dose-related changes in physiological and self-report measures during maintenance on 2 mg of buprenorphine. As the maintenance dose of buprenorphine increased, the effects of hydromorphone were attenuated, with self-reported effects being reduced to a greater extent than physiological measures (Bickel et al., 1988a).

In humans trained to discriminate between the opioid agonist hydromorphone, the mixed-action opioid agonist/antagonist pentazocine, and saline, buprenorphine produced both hydromorphone- and pentazocine-appropriate responding (Preston et al., 1989). In contrast, the mixed-action opioid compound nalbuphine produced neither hydromorphone nor pentazocine-appropriate responding in a consistent manner. The mixed-action opioid butorphanol produced primarily pentazocine-appropriate responding. On self-reports, buprenorphine and the opioid agonist hydromorphone, but not other mixed-action opioids, produced increases in euphoria and "good effects." Similarly, in humans trained to discriminate among hydromorphone, butorphanol, and saline, buprenorphine produced hydromorphone-appropriate responding and self-reports similar to hydromorphone, whereas butorphanol did not (Bigelow & Preston, 1992). These results suggest that buprenorphine produces effects with a greater similarity to those produced by hydromorphone than to those produced by other mixed-action opioids.

Although buprenorphine's potential for abuse and dependence is much less than that of full opioid agonists, several instances of buprenorphine abuse have been reported across the globe (e.g., Pickworth et al., 1993; Strang, 1985). The abuse of buprenorphine typically occurs via the intravenous route (Sakol et al., 1989), with the user dissolving in water one or more 0.2-mg tablets intended for sublingual administration and injecting the solution intravenously (Gray et al., 1989).

TOLERANCE AND DEPENDENCE

Several studies in nonhumans have shown that tolerance develops to the behavioral effects of buprenorphine (e.g., Berthold & Moerschbaecher, 1988; Cowan et al., 1977; for exception, see Dykstra, 1983).

However, nonhuman studies that examine whether physical dependence on buprenorphine develops after chronic administration generally have negative results. For instance, both deprivation-induced withdrawal and opioid-antagonist-precipitated withdrawal are difficult to demonstrate after chronic buprenorphine administration (Woods & Gmerek, 1985). Buprenorphine has been shown to enhance dependence through an indirect procedure in which a previous chronic buprenorphine regimen facilitates the ability of morphine to produce physical dependence (Dum et al., 1981). This absence of a withdrawal syndrome after termination of chronic buprenorphine administration is thought to result from the slow dissociation of buprenorphine from the μ-opioid receptor (Rance, 1979; Woods et al., 1992).

Although buprenorphine has been shown to precipitate withdrawal in opioid-dependent nonhumans (Cowan et al., 1977; Gmerek, 1984), it has not clearly been shown to precipitate withdrawal in opioid-dependent humans. For instance, in opioid-dependent individuals maintained on methadone (25–45 mg/day, oral), buprenorphine (2 and 4 mg, sublingual) produced some withdrawal-like physiological signs, mydriasis and hypertension, but did not produce antagonist-like self-reported effects; rather, buprenorphine produced more agonist-like self-reported effects (Jasinski et al., 1983). The authors concluded that buprenorphine did not precipitate clinically significant withdrawal in opioid-dependent subjects maintained on methadone at doses up to 45 mg/day. Subsequent outpatient observations have suggested that patients who are above 35 mg of daily methadone are not likely to tolerate well a transition to buprenorphine at 2 to 4 mg, sublingual (Kosten et al., 1989).

In opioid-dependent volunteers maintained on methadone (30 mg/day), the opioid agonist hydromorphone (6 mg, subcutaneous) decreased pupil diameter and respiration and increased blood pressure and opioid-agonist-like self-report scores (Preston et al., 1988). Buprenorphine (0.2 and 0.3 mg, subcutaneous) had no significant effects, whereas the opioid antagonist naloxone (0.2 mg, subcutaneous) produced opioid-withdrawal-like effects. When buprenorphine was administered in combination with naloxone, the naloxone-induced withdrawal effects were attenuated slightly. These findings also suggest that buprenorphine does not precipitate withdrawal in this population of opioid-dependent individuals maintained at relatively low doses of methadone.

Buprenorphine at low doses (0.15–0.3 mg, sublingual) has been shown to alleviate withdrawal symptoms in methadone-maintained individuals whose methadone dose has been withheld (Callaway et al., 1991). Otherwise, the ability of buprenorphine to suppress withdrawal in opioid-dependent individuals has only been examined in the context of treatment (e.g., Bickel et al., 1988b; Jasinski et al., 1983; Johnson, et al., 1989; Kosten & Kleber, 1988; Lukas et al., 1984). For instance, Jasinski and colleagues (1983) observed that when individuals who were maintained on 25–50 mg/day of methadone were switched to buprenorphine at 2 mg, sublingual, some mild signs of withdrawal were reported; however, it was unclear whether these effects resulted from buprenorphine's failure to suppress withdrawal or from buprenorphine-precipitated withdrawal. Lukas and colleagues (1984) observed mild withdrawal signs when opioid-dependent individuals were switched from methadone (25–60 mg/day) to buprenorphine (2 mg, subcutaneous). In heroin users who were undergoing detoxification, no differences were observed between those treated with methadone and those treated with buprenorphine (Bickel et al., 1988b). Buprenophine produced agonist-like effects without signs of withdrawal for heroin users who were rapidly inducted into a maintenance dose of buprenorphine, suggesting that buprenorphine did not precipitate abstinence in these heroin-dependent individuals (Johnson et al., 1989). Heroin users and methadone-maintained patients who were abruptly switched to buprenorphine (2, 4, or 8 mg/day) reportedly experienced mild continuing withdrawal symptoms, which decreased over the 30-day test period (Kosten & Kleber, 1988). Thus, most individuals can be successfully switched from methadone or placed on buprenorphine maintenance from heroin dependence without the severity of withdrawal symptoms usually experienced after abrupt termination of opioid administration.

As mentioned previously, Jasinski and associates (1978) gave repeated administrations of buprenorphine for the purpose of examining the physical dependence potential of buprenorphine. Individuals were inducted onto a maintenance dose of buprenorphine (8 mg/day, subcutaneous). After 45–52 days of buprenorphine maintenance, the opioid antagonist naloxone (4 mg) was administered in order to determine physical dependence. Subsequently, placebo was administered instead of buprenorphine under double-blind conditions. When buprenorphine was abruptly terminated, the onset of withdrawal signs and symptoms was delayed, ranging from 1–14 days after placebo was substituted. When compared to historical data, the authors concluded that severity of withdrawal for buprenorphine when its administration is discontinued was greater than that for placebo but less than that for other opioid compounds, including morphine, nalbuphine, pentazocine, and butorphanol. These findings suggest that buprenorphine generally has a lower potential for physical dependence than other opioid compounds do.

DRUG ABUSE OUTPATIENT TREATMENT STUDIES

Buprenorphine is approved for the treatment of opiate dependence in some European countries but is not yet approved for this indication in the United States. As early as 1978, Jasinski and coworkers suggested that buprenorphine might be a promising agent for the treatment of heroin dependence. Buprenorphine may combine some of the desirable properties of both the pure opiate agonist methadone and the opiate antagonist naltrexone and may have several advantages over each of them. In addition to relative safety from overdose because of its flat dose response on respiratory suppression at high doses, buprenorphine also appears to have a relatively lower abuse potential and a milder withdrawal syndrome than do the full agonists such as methadone, as detailed earlier in this chapter.

Buprenorphine maintenance studies that have used daily doses as diverse as 1.5–16 mg daily (Kosten et al., 1991; Resnick et al., 1991, 1992) have consistently demonstrated treatment retention rates comparable to those for methadone maintenance therapy. Buprenorphine may be as efficacious as methadone in substituting for heroin, although the optimal dosage regimen has yet to be determined. Buprenorphine given sublingually at doses of 2 and 6 mg daily has been shown to be inferior to daily methadone doses of 35–65 mg in measures of retention in treatment, in opioid-free urines, and in self-reports of heroin use (Kosten et al., 1993). As far as abstinence rates from heroin are concerned, Johnson et al. (1992), using only a slightly higher dose of buprenorphine, namely, 8 mg daily sublingual, in a 17-week, randomized, double-blind, double-dummy study, showed that at this higher dose buprenorphine treatment was equivalent to methadone given at 60 mg daily (59% opiate-free urines versus 43% opiate-free urines, respectively). Dose-ranging studies (Schottenfeld et al., 1993; Bickel et al., 1988a) have suggested that further increases in buprenorphine doses to as high as 16 mg daily may further improve abstinence from opiates.

Because of its long half-life, buprenorphine may be administered by using an alternate-day or thrice-weekly schedule. Fudala et al. (1990) compared buprenorphine given at 8 mg daily with buprenorphine given on alternate days and found that only slightly greater opioid withdrawal symptoms were reported by subjects who received buprenorphine on alternate days. There was, however, increased dysphoria, a greater urge for an opioid, and measurable pupillary dilation on placebo days. Because of the substantial practical benefits of alternate-day or thrice-weekly administration, further studies to optimize alternate-day dosing are under way (O'Connor, personal communication).

Combined opioid and cocaine dependence occurs in up to 70%

of heroin addicts, and in excess of 40% of these addicts continue to use cocaine while in methadone treatment (Kosten et al., 1988, 1989). A unique characteristic of buprenorphine may be its ability to decrease use of cocaine as well as illicit opiates. Studies of nonhuman primates (Carroll et al., 1992; Mello et al., 1989, 1992; Winger et al., 1992) who have been taught to self-administer cocaine have shown robust dose-dependent decreases (up to 60–97%) in cocaine self-administration when these monkeys are treated with buprenorphine.

The effect of buprenorphine on cocaine use among human opiate addicts has been more equivocal. In an acute cocaine dosage paradigm, Mendelson et al. (1992) demonstrated that buprenorphine at doses of 4 mg daily could suppress euphoria after administration of cocaine at 30 mg intravenously. In a retrospective study, Kosten et al. (1989) showed that the percentage of patients who had at least one cocaine-positive urine was decreased in opiate-dependent patients treated with buprenorphine (3.2 mg daily) compared to a similar group treated with methadone (mean dose 46 mg daily) (23% vs. 62%). In this nonblinded study, however, groups were not controlled for severity and amount of either opiate or cocaine use. In a double-blind, placebo-controlled study (Johnson et al., 1992) that compared buprenorphine given at 8 mg sublingual daily with methadone given at 20 mg or 60 mg daily, cocaine use was comparable in all subgroups at baseline, and there was no significant difference in cocaine use in any of the treatment groups. Schottenfeld et al. (1993), on the other hand, in a buprenorphine dose-ranging study (from 4 mg to 16 mg daily), found that subjects who were dependent on both opiates and cocaine significantly decreased their cocaine use with increasing doses of buprenorphine.

In addition to its promise in treating opiate and concomitant cocaine addiction, buprenorphine has a favorable safety and diversion profile. Because of its antagonist properties at higher doses, it is possible that buprenorphine will be safer in overdose than methadone owing to less respiratory depression (see earlier in chapter). The diversion potential of buprenorphine has been theorized to be less than that of methadone because of the combined agonist–antagonist effects. It has been noted, however, that buprenorphine can be dissolved in distilled water and injected intravenously. Pickworth and co-workers (1993) have shown that even small intravenous doses of buprenorphine (i.e., 0.3–1.2 mg, intravenous) produce positive responses on rating scales for "feel drug," "liking," and euphoria; and Lavelle et al. (1991) have recently described an increase in illegal use of buprenorphine in Scotland (where the medication is approved for dispensing). To address this diversion problem, a combination of naloxone with buprenorphine is being developed.

In summary, buprenorphine shows much promise as an alternative to methadone and naltrexone maintenance. It is well accepted by patients, has a mild withdrawal syndrome that facilitates its discontinuation, it reduces opioid and possibly cocaine abuse, and it has greater safety and lower diversion potential than do full agonists such as methadone.

REFERENCES

Ball, S. A., Carroll, K. M., Babor, T. F., & Rounsaville, B. J. (1995). Subtypes of cocaine abusers: Support for a Type A–Type B distinction. *Journal of Consulting and Clinical Psychology, 63*(1), 115–124.

Berthold, C. W., & Moerschbaecher, J. M. (1988). Tolerance to the effects of buprenorphine on schedule-controlled behavior and analgesia in rats. *Pharmacology, Biochemistry and Behavior, 29,* 393–396.

Bickel, W. K., Stitzer, M. L., Bigelow, G. E., Liebson, I. A., Jasinski, D. R., & Johnson, R. E. (1988a). Buprenorphine: Dose-related blockage of opioid challenge effects in opioid dependent humans. *Journal of Pharmacology and Experimental Therapeutics, 247,* 47–53.

Bickel, W. K., Stitzer, M. L., Bigelow, G. E., Liebson, I. A., Jasinski, D. R., & Johnson, R. E. (1988b). A clinical trial of buprenorphine: Comparison with methadone in the detoxification of heroin addicts. *Clinical Pharmacology and Therapeutics, 43,* 72–78.

Bigelow, G. E., & Preston, K. L. (1992). Assessment of buprenorphine in a drug discrimination procedure in humans. In *Buprenorphine: An alternative treatment for opioid dependence* (NIDA Research Monograph No. 121, pp. 28–37). Rockville, MD: National Institute on Drug Abuse.

Brown, E. E., Finlay, J. M., Wong, J. T., Damsma, G., & Fibiger, H. C. (1991). Behavioral and neurochemical interactions between cocaine and buprenorphine: Implications for the pharmacotherapy of cocaine abuse. *Journal of Pharmocology and Experimental Therapeutics, 256,* 119–125.

Bullingham, R. E. S., McQuay. H. J., & Moore. R. A. (1983). Clinical pharmacokinetics of narcotic agonist–antagonist drugs. *Clinincal Pharmacokinetics, 8,* 332–343.

Callaway, E., Banys, P., Clark, H. W., Tusel, D., Sees, K., & Mongan, M. L. (1991, December). *Low dose buprenorphine (0.15–0.3 mg sublingual) relieves symptoms of methadone withdrawal.* Paper presented at the 30th annual meeting of the American College of Neuropsychopharmacology, San Juan, Puerto Rico.

Carroll, M. E., Carmona, G. N., May, S. A., Buzalsky, S., & Larson, C. (1992). Buprenorphine effects on self-administration of smoked cocaine base and orally delivered phencyclidine, ethanol and saccharin in rhesus monkeys. *Journal of Pharmacology and Experimental Therapeutics, 261,* 26–37.

Cowan, A., Lewis, J. W., & MacFarlane, I. R. (1977). Agonist and antagonist properties of buprenorphien, a new antinociceptive agent. *British Journal of Pharmacology, 60,* 537–545.

Doxey, J. C., Everitt, J. E., Frank, L. W., & MacKenzie, J. E. (1977). A comparison of the effects of buprenorphine and morphine on the blood gases of conscious rats. *British Journal of Pharmacology, 60,* 118P.

Dum, J., Blasig, J., & Herz, A. (1981). Buprenorphine: Demonstration of physical dependence liability. *European Journal of Pharmacology, 70,* 293–300.

Dykstra, L. A. (1983). Behavioral effects of buprenorphine and diprenorphine under multiple schedule of food presentations in squirrel monkeys. *Journal of Pharmacology and Experimental Therapeutics, 226,* 317–323.

Gmerek, D. E. (1984). The suppression of deprivation and antagonist-induced withdrawal in morphine-dependent rhesus monkeys. *Neuropeptides, 5,* 19–22.

Gray, R. F., Ferry, A., & Jauhar, P. (1989). Emergence of buprenorphine dependence. *British Journal of Addictions, 84,* 1373–1374.

Hambrook, J. M., & Rance. M. J. (1976). The interaction of buprenorphine with the opiate receptor: Lipophilicity as a determining factor in drug-receptor kinetics. In. H. Kosterlitz (Ed.), *Opiates and endogenous opioid peptides* (pp. 295–301). Amsterdam: Elsevier/North-Holland.

Hart, E. R., & McCawley, E. L. (1944). The pharmacology of N-allylnormorphine as compared with morphine. *Journal of Pharmacology and Experimental Therapeutics, 82,* 339–348.

Houde, R. W. (1979). Analgesic effectiveness of the narcotic agonist–antagonists. *British Journal of Clinical Pharmacology, 7,* 297S–308S.

Jasinski, D. R., Fudala, P. J., & Johnson, R. E. (1989). Sublingual versus subcutaneous buprenorphine on opiate abusers. *Clinincal Pharmacology and Therapeutics, 45,* 513–519.

Jasinski, D. R., Henningfield, J. E., Hickey, J. E., & Johnson, R. E. (1983). *Progress Report of the NIDA Addiction Research Center, Baltimore, Maryland* (NIDA Research Monograph No. 43). Rockville, MD: National Institute on Drug Abuse.

Jasinski, D. R., Pevnick, J. S., & Griffith, J. D. (1978). Human pharmacology and abuse potential of the analgesic buprenorphine. *Archives of General Psychiatry, 35,* 501–516.

Johnson, R. E., Cone, E. J., Henningfield, J. E., & Fudala, P. J. (1989). Use of buprenorphine in the treatment of opiate addiction: 1. Physiologic and behavioral effects during a rapid dose induction. *Clinical Pharmacology and Therapeutics, 46,* 335–343.

Johnson, R. E., Jaffe, J. H., & Fudala, P. J. (1992). A controlled trial of buprenorphine treatment for opioid dependence. *Journal of the American Medical Association, 267,* 2750–2755.

Khazan, N., Young, G. A., & Calligaro, D .(1984). Buprenorphine did not demonstrate reinforcing properties in morphine post-addict rats. *Research Communications in Substances of Abuse, 5,* 1–9.

Kosten, T. A., Marby, D. W., & Nestler, E. J. (1991). Cocaine conditioned place preference is attenuated by chronic buprenorphine treatment. *Life Sciences, 49,* 201–206.

Kosten, T. R., & Kleber, H. D. (1988). Buprenorphine detoxification from opioid dependence: A pilot study. *Life Sciences, 42,* 635–641.

Kosten, T. R., Kleber, H. D., & Morgan, C. H. (1989). Role of opioid antagonists in treating intravenous cocaine abuse. *Life Sciences, 44,* 887–892.

Kosten, T. R., Rounsaville, B. J., & Kleber, H. D. (1988). Antecedents and consequences of cocaine abuse among opioid addicts—A 2.5 year follow-up. *Journal of Nervous and Mental Disease, 176,* 176–181.

Kosten, T. R., Schottenfeld, R. Ziedoniss, D., & Falcioni, J. (1993). Buprenorphine versus methadone maintenance for opioid dependence. *Journal of Nervous Mental Disease, 181,* 358–364.

Lavelle, T. L., Hammersley, R., & Forsyth, A. (1991). The use of buprenorphine and temazepam by drug injectors. *Journal of Addictive Disease, 10,* 5–14.

Lewis, J. W., Rance, M. J., & Sanger, D. J. (1982). The pharmacology and abuse potential of buprenorphine: A new antagonist analgesic. In M. K. Mello (Ed.), *Advances in substance abuse: Behavioral and biological research* (Vol. 3., pp. 103–154). Greenwich: JAI Press.

Lewis, J. (1982). The antagonist analgesic concept. In M. M. Glatt & J. Marks (Eds.), *The dependene phenomenon* (pp. 81–102). Lancaster, England: MTP Press.

Lewis, J. W. (1973). Ring C-bridged derivatives of thebaine and oripavine. In M. C. Brause, L. S. Harris, E. L. May, J. P. Smith, & J. E. Villarreal (Eds.), *Advances in biochemical psychopharmacology: Vol. 8. Narcotic antagonists* (pp. 123–136). New York: Raven Press.

Lewis, J. W., Rance, M. J., & Sanger, D. J. (1983). The pharmacology and abuse potential of buprenorphine: A new antagonist analgesic. *Advances in Substance Abuse, 3,* 103–154.

Lukas, S. E., Griffiths, R. R., & Brady, J. V. (1983). Buprenorphine self-administration by the baboon: Comparison with other opioids. In L. S. Harris (Ed.), *Problems of drug dependence, 1982: Proceedings of the 44th Annual Scientific Meeting, The Committee on Problems of Drug Dependence* (NIDA Research Monograph No. 43, DHHS Pub. No. ADM 83-1264, pp. 178–183). Washington, DC: U.S. Government Printing Office.

Lukas, S. E., Jasinski, D. R., & Johnson, R. E. (1984). Electroencephalographic and behavioral correlates of buprenorphine administration. *Clinincal Pharmacology and Therapeutics, 36,* 127–132.

Martin, W. R., Eades, C. G., Thompson, J. A., Huppler, R. E., & Gilbert, P. E. (1976). The effects of morphine- and nalorphine-like drugs in the nondependent and morphine-dependent chronic spinal dog. *Journal of Pharmacology and Experimental Therapeutics, 197,* 517–532.

Mello, N. K., Mendelson, J. H., Bree, M. P., & Lukas, S. E. (1989). Buprenorphine suppresses cocaine self-administration by rhesus monkeys. *Science, 245,* 859–862.

Mello, N. K., Mendelson, J. H., & Kuehnle, J. C. (1982). Buprenorphine effects on human heroin self-administration: An operant analysis. *Journal of Pharmacology and Experimental Therapeutics, 223,* 30–39.

Mello, N. K., Bree, M. P., & Mendelson, J. H. (1981). Buprenorphine self-administration by rhesus monkey. *Pharmacology, Biochemistry and Behavior, 15,* 215–225.

Mello, N. K., Bree, M. P., & Mendelson, J. H. (1983). Comparison of buprenorphine and methadone effects on opiate self-administration in primates. *Journal of Pharmacology and Experimental Therapeutics, 225,* 378–386.

Mello, N. K., & Mendelson, J. H. (1990). Buprenorphine suppresses heroin use by heroin addicts. *Science, 207,* 657–659.

Mendelson, J. H., Teoh, S. K., Mello, N. K., & Ellingboe, J. (1992). Buprenorphine attenuates the effects of cocaine on adrenocorticotropin (ACTH) secretion and mood states in man. *Neuropsychopharmacology, 7,* 157–162.

Pickworth, W. B., Johnson, R. E., Holicky, B. A., & Cone, E. J. (1993). Subjective and physiologic effects of intravenous buprenorphine in humans. *Clinical Pharmocoloft and Therapeutics, 53,* 570–576.

Preston, K. L., Bigelow, G. E., Bickel, W. K., & Liebson, I. A. (1989). Drug discrimination in human post-addicts: Agonist-antagonist opioids. *Journal of Pharmacology and Experimental Therapeutics, 250,* 184–196.

Preston, K. L., Bigelow, G. E., & Liebson, I. A. (1988). Buprenorphine and naloxone alone and in combination in opioid-dependent humans. *Psychopharmacology, 94,* 484–490.

Rance, M. J. (1979). Animal and molecular pharmacology of mixed agonist–antagonist analgesic drugs. *British Journal of Pharmacology, 7,* 281S–286S.

Rance, M. J., & Dickens, J. M. (1978). The influence of drug-receptor kinetics on the pharmacological and pharmacokinetic profiles of buprenorphine. In J. M. Van Ree & L. Terenius (Eds.), *Characteristics and function of opioids* (pp. 65–68). Amsterdam: Elsevier/North-Holland.

Resnick, R. B., Galantar, M., Pycha, C., et al. (1992). Buprenorphine: An alternative to methadone for heroin dependence treatment. *Psychopharmacology, 28,* 109–113.

Resnick, R. B., Resnick, E., & Galanter, M. (1991). Buprenophine responders: A diagnostic subgroup of heroin addicts? *Progress in Neuro-Psychopharmacology and Biological Psychiatry, 15,* 531–538.

Richards, M. L., & Sadee, W. (1985). In vivo opiate receptor binding of oripavines to μ, δ and κ sites in rat brain as determined by an ex vivo labeling method. *European Journal of Pharmacology, 114,* 343–353.

Rosen, M. I., Wallace, E. A., McMahon, T. J., Pearsall, H. R., Woods, S. W., Price, L. H., & Kosten, T. R. (1994). Buprenorphine: Duration of blockage of effects of intramuscular hydromorphone. *Drug and Alcohol Dependence, 35,* 141–149.

Sadee, W., Rosenbaum, J. S., & Herz, A. (1982). Buprenorphine: Differential interaction with opiate receptor subtypes in vivo. *Journal of Pharmacology and Experimental Therapeutics, 223,* 157–162.

Sakol, M. S., Stark, C., & Sykes, R. (1989). Buprenorphine and temazepam abuse by drug takers in Galsgow: An increase. British Journal of Addictions, 84, 439–441.

Schottenfeld, R. S., Pakes, J., Ziedonis, D., & Kosten, T. R. (1993). Buprenorphine: Dose-related effects on cocaine and opioid use in cocaine-abusing opioid-dependent humans. *Biological Psychiatry, 34,* 66–74

Strang, J. (1985). Abuse of buprenorphine. *Lancet,* ii(8457), 725.

Walsh, S. L., Preston, K. L., Stitzer, M. L., Cone, E. J., & Bigelow, G. E. (1994). Clinical pharmacology of buprenorphine: Ceiling effects at high doses. *Clinical Pharmacology and Therapeutics, 55,* 569–580.

Weinhold, L. L., Preston, K., Farre, M., Liebson, I. A., & Bigelow, G. E. (1992). Buprenorphine alone and in combination with naloxone in non-dependent humans. *Drug and Alcohol Dependence, 30,* 263–274.

Winger, G., Skjoldager, P., & Woods, J. H. (1992). Effects of buprenorphine and other opioid agonists and antagonists on alfentanil- and cocaine-reinforced responding in rehesus monkeys. *Journal of Pharmacology and Experimental Therapeutics, 261,* 311–317.

Woods, J. H., France, C. P., & Winger, G. D. (1992). Behavioral pharmacology of buprenorphine: Issues relevant to its potential in treating drug abuse. In *Buprenorphine: An alternative treatment for opioid dependence* (NIDA Research Monograph No. 121, pp. 12–27). Rockville, MD: National Institute on Drug Abuse.

Woods, J. H., & Gmerek, D. E. (1985). Substitution and primary dependence studies in animals. *Drug Alcohol Dependence, 14*(3–4), 233–247.

Young, A. M., Stephens, K. R., Hein, D. W., & Woods, J. H. (1984). Reinforcing and discriminative stimulus properties of mixed agonist–antagonist opioids. *Journal of Pharmacology and Experimental Therapeutics, 229,* 118–126.

Chapter 14

CONCLUSIONS AND FUTURE DIRECTIONS IN TREATMENT MATCHING

Thomas R. Kosten, M.D.

A series of studies in the early 1980s documented the heterogeneity of opioid-dependent patients. This heterogeneity included psychiatric diagnoses such as comorbid depressive and personality disorders as well as polydrug abuse, particularly of alcohol and cocaine. Associated with this diagnostic heterogeneity has been a wide range of psychosocial and medical problems. The medical problems include severe disorders such as AIDS and its complications, as well as nondisease states such as pregnancy, which can pose difficult medical management issues in an opioid-dependent woman. The heterogeneity in psychosocial problems includes employment, legal, and family problems.

To address this heterogeneity, methadone maintenance treatment has become a multiservice modality that goes beyond dispensing methadone to a wide range of other rehabilitative and treatment services. In this book, we have covered the range of services, from an intensive day program to more limited services. These services include focused psychosocial rehabilitation for employment, family, and legal problems as well as standard psychiatric and medical evaluations.

CRITERIA FOR TREATMENT MATCHING

The simplest of matching strategies takes patients who are unemployed and who have no child care responsibilities and places them in an intensive day program. Selecting this unemployed subgroup frequently also identifies patients with multiple psychosocial and medical problems. These day treatment patients can include many who are infected with HIV. Methadone maintenance patients with AIDS frequently have special psychological issues that involve death and dying and have medical complications that distinguish them from the other methadone patients. Special medically focused programming needs to be developed for these patients. This programming focuses on the patients' primary medical care needs, including compliance with AIDS antivirals such as AZT as well as with antituberculosis medications. Another patient subgroup that benefits from specialized day treatments consists of pregnant women. During pregnancy these women are provided obstetrical services: during the postpartum period, they are given "on the job" training in appropriate childrearing and mothering behaviors.

The next level of treatment matching is dependent upon the presence of comorbid psychiatric and other substance abuse disorders. In this population, the most commonly abused drugs besides heroin are cocaine and alcohol. As many as 25% of methadone-maintained patients may also have alcohol dependence and may be in need of medical detoxification as well as ongoing alcohol relapse prevention treatment. In some cases, the management of an alcohol- and opiate-abusing patient is best done with naltrexone, as discussed below, but many other patients on methadone maintenance may benefit from a combination of disulfiram with their methadone maintenance. The aversive properties of disulfiram will markedly reduce alcohol abuse relapse, and compliance with disulfiram can be assured by its daily ingestion along with methadone.

The management of cocaine abuse and dependence among methadone-maintained patients is more complex and does not have the benefit of an established pharmacotherapy for cocaine. The management of these cocaine abusers may benefit from a comprehensive psychiatric evaluation for depressive disorders. For these depressed cocaine abusers, antidepressant medications should be considered. Other interventions under investigation for this patient subgroup include acupuncture. Acupuncture is a relatively intensive 5-days-per-week outpatient treatment that lasts about 45 minutes per day. Although the time for this treatment is less intensive than the 5 to 6 hours each day spent in a daily treatment program, it is considerably more intensive than the typical once-weekly counseling session of routine methadone maintenance treatment. Concurrent cocaine abuse also poses especially difficult management problems for patients with AIDS. Thus, within methadone maintenance, cocaine-dependent patients can receive a

range of ancillary treatment services, from the simple addition of a pharmacotherapy such as an antidepressant through a complex psychosocial
intervention such as acupuncture.

Patients can be matched to these varying levels of interventions
on the basis not only of an initial assessment but also of a sequential
escalation in intervention intensity. At the initial patient assessment,
critical factors include the severity and duration of any concurrent cocaine or alcohol dependence and the need for medical detoxification
in those patients who are alcohol dependent. Previous treatment history for concurrent substance dependence, including failures at low-
level interventions, such as the simple addition of a pharmacotherapy
to methadone maintenance, indicates the need for a higher level of
intervention. Such higher levels might include a more-than-once-weekly
intensive outpatient service or even experimental interventions such
as acupuncture. Overall, the treatment history for the patient will often
guide an escalating series of treatment interventions from lesser to
greater intensity of both the psychological and possibly pharmacological treatment.

The second area of psychiatric comorbidity for treatment matching should focus on the two most common psychiatric disorders among
opioid-dependent patients: depression and antisocial personality disorder. Because depressive disorders can be found in up to 35% of
opioid-dependent patients, a careful psychiatric evaluation of these patients is indicated. For those patients with a depressive disorder, several studies have demonstrated good efficacy both for specific
psychotherapies and for antidepressant pharmacotherapies. These treatment interventions not only reduce depressive symptoms but also
reduce illicit drug use, including the use of opiates and cocaine in those
patients with this secondary dependence. Treatment matching for these
patients involves an initial psychiatric evaluation for medications. Once
the patient becomes stabilized, at least monthly monitoring of this medication is needed. Referral to a higher-level therapist than bachelor's
level counseling staff also is typically needed for the management of
these patients. Since typical methadone maintenance counseling can
involve rather large caseloads of 40–50 patients per counselor, intensive psychotherapeutic interventions are not possible in this context.

While these large caseloads are problematic for depressed patients,
such caseloads lend themselves to group treatments and behavioral interventions that may be ideally suited to the treatment of antisocial personality disorder. These groups are also well suited to the regular urine
toxicologies and positive and negative contingencies of a well-
functioning methadone program. As described in detail elsewhere (see
Stine, Chapter 4, and Burns, Chapter 7, this volume), the therapeutic

milieu of a methadone maintenance program can be very effective in addressing some of the ego deficits of opiate-dependent patients with major personality disorders.

The treatment of other less-common psychiatric disorders, such as bipolar, panic, and psychotic disorders, also will benefit from careful psychiatric evaluation and appropriate adjunctive medications. Thus, a subgroup of methadone-maintained patients can substantially benefit from a careful psychiatric evaluation and a series of treatment interventions that address the comorbid psychopathology of methadone-maintained patients. Because psychiatric resources are generally quite limited in most methadone programs, it is important that staff be adequately trained in the use of such screening instruments as the Beck Depression Inventory for identifying depression and other treatable psychiatric disorders.

SEQUENTIAL TREATMENT MATCHING PROCESS

Multidimensional treatment matching involves a complex sequence of evaluations that are not most effectively done when the patient is applying for treatment. Indeed, treatment matching should be considered, not a static one-time process, but a dynamic one that is ongoing during the course of any methadone treatment program. Before initiating treatment, some simple aspects of treatment matching may be easily accomplished, such as the determination of employment status or the need for more-than-routine medical services for patients with AIDS or active tuberculosis. In these patients with AIDS and tuberculosis, treatment matching may include observed and monitored ingestion of an antiviral or antitubercular treatment agent as well as integration with a primary care site for coordinated management of methadone dosage with those anti-infectious agents. This coordination in dosing is essential because several of the treatment agents for tuberculosis or for AIDS interact with methadone blood levels and potentially may produce potential toxicity. For the unemployed, homeless, and heroin-dependent patient, an intensive day program may be necessary, with a provision of extensive social services that includes case management for housing and regular meals. All of these patients can be identified upon entry into treatment and can be matched with an appropriate level of service needs.

As treatment progresses and the treatment staff become more familiar with the new patients, a variety of other problems and needs or patient strengths may become evident, suggesting further stages of treatment matching. These further stages of treatment matching may include psychiatric evaluations for those patients who appear to have a major depressive or other disorder when evaluated by the counselor. Another identified area will be the persistent abuse of stimulants or alcohol that needs further pharmacologic or psychotherapeutic interventions. This may lead not only to psychiatric evaluation but also to an intensification of the treatment from once- or twice-weekly counseling to as much as a full-day program. Finally, consideration may be given to detoxification from methadone maintenance and referral to an alternative treatment modality, such as a residential treatment for those who are failing at outpatient methadone treatment. Other patients may display greater strengths than originally assessed, suggesting that a lower intensity of intervention, such as LAAM, might be used to facilitate fewer visits to the clinic. Outpatient naltrexone treatment also might be considered for the purpose of preserving an opiate-abstinent state after a successful detoxification from methadone maintenance.

MATCHING TO ALTERNATIVE PHARMACOTHERAPIES

Matching patients to alternative pharmacotherapies, such as LAAM, naltrexone, and buprenorphine therapies, is clearly in need of further study. Self-selected candidates for naltrexone therapy have frequently had relatively lower levels of dependence or have just started their addiction career (i.e., are adolescents). Other excellent candidates for naltrexone therapy include health care professionals or patients with substantial contingencies to enforce medication compliance, such as probationers in the criminal justice system. Some other patients will be appropriately matched to naltrexone therapy after they have successfully completed several years of methadone maintenance rehabilitation and have reentered the workforce. Whether matching the alcoholic opiate addict to naltrexone therapy will have success has yet to be determined, and success may be inhibited by poor naltrexone therapy compliance. Although compliance with naltrexone therapy in alcohol abusers has been excellent, the compliance with naltrexone therapy in opioid-dependent patients has been more problematic. Currently, the most effective management for the alcoholic opiate addict has involved the combined pharmacotherapy of methadone and disulfiram.

Matching appropriate patients to LAAM therapy involves an assessment of suitability for three-times-weekly dosing rather than daily methadone dosing. Because patients with multiple psychosocial impairments probably would benefit from a full-day program, LAAM may not be an appropriate therapy unless amplified with intensive psychosocial services. LAAM may, for example, be chosen over methadone if there is concern about diversion of methadone or abuse of street methadone. However, the employed opiate addict who has a variety of social supports may do extremely well if initiated on LAAM treatment. Similarly, patients who have been well stabilized on methadone and are now candidates for less-frequent clinic attendance could do well with LAAM. Other matching characteristics such as comorbid psychiatric or other substance abuse disorders have not been investigated with LAAM but may provide criteria for appropriate medication matching in the future. Overall, LAAM and methadone have many similarities in their pharmacology and might be expected to serve a similar patient population. One special group that might benefit from LAAM consists of the fast metabolizers of methadone who may have a slower metabolism of LAAM, thereby enabling better symptom stabilization. Because this group of fast metabolizers includes pregnant women, these women might benefit more from LAAM than from methadone treatment. Clinical studies will need to be completed before LAAM therapy can be recommended as a standard treatment.

The newest pharmacotherapy for opiate-dependent patients is buprenorphine. Significant research experience is accumulating in the use of this medication, although the medication is not yet available for clinical use. Preliminary studies with buprenorphine have suggested that several subgroups of patients might benefit substantially from it. First are those patients who have a fear of methadone maintenance and who would prefer to be treated with a different agent. Although some of these patients may do well on naltrexone, many others need an agent that has more reinforcing potential than naltrexone does and that does not require opiate detoxification before initiation. Buprenorphine is excellent for this patient population, and many patients who have never been treated with methadone have done well on buprenorphine. In research studies, buprenorphine patients have had equivalent outcomes compared to patients on adequate maintenance dosages of methadone. Because the withdrawal syndrome from methadone is more severe than that from buprenorphine, eventual discontinuation from buprenorphine may be easier and may facilitate transition to naltrexone with those patients for whom naltrexone is considered a subsequent optimal treatment. Thus, relatively short-term maintenance patients of a year or less might do well by being stabilized on buprenorphine and then transferred to naltrexone. Patients who abuse other drugs such as cocaine along with opiates might also be considered for buprenorphine. Some studies have suggested that buprenorphine might reduce both the opiate and cocaine abuse of those patients. Other patients who have had some response to buprenorphine are the depressed substance abusers. Several studies have indicated that patients who are refractory to other antidepressant medications may respond to buprenorphine. Other work has suggested that opioid-dependent patients with the affective instability of borderline personality disorder also may respond well to buprenorphine. Thus, matching to buprenorphine may be based on patient preference, on comorbid psychiatric disorder, and on concurrent polydrug abuse. These criteria for the future use of buprenorphine will need further examination in conjunction with other treatment alternatives, such as methadone, LAAM, and naltrexone therapies.

In summary, our most well-developed treatment intervention for chronic heroin dependence is clearly methadone maintenance, for which we have a wide range of ancillary approaches in addition to methadone itself. Optimizing methadone maintenance treatment can involve the use of other pharmacologic agents in conjunction with methadone, as well as the addition of a wide range of psychosocial interventions, from intensive day program treatment to acupuncture. Medication alternatives to methadone such as naltrexone, LAAM, and buprenorphine have been increasingly available, and their indications for matching to newly dependent patients and appropriate chronic patients are developing. Heroin-dependent patients constitute a heterogeneous group that may need a sequence of treatment interventions, beginning with high-intensity treatments and stepping down to much lower-intensity services over several years. The pharmacologic and psychosocial tools available to us have vastly increased over the 20 years since methadone was widely introduced for treatment of opioid dependence. The clinician needs to be aware of these alternatives to maintenance treatment and of advances in opiate detoxification in order to appropriately match a patient's needs to these treatment alternatives.

INDEX